The Patient-Centered Approach to Claudication

William P. Robinson III • Jessica P. Simons
Editors

The Patient-Centered Approach to Claudication

A Guide for Vascular Specialists

Springer

Editors
William P. Robinson III
Division of Vascular Surgery
Southern Illinois University School of Medicine
Springfield, IL, USA

Jessica P. Simons
Division of Vascular and Endovascular Surgery
University of Massachusetts Chan Medical School
Worcester, MA, USA

ISBN 978-3-032-02459-6 ISBN 978-3-032-02460-2 (eBook)
https://doi.org/10.1007/978-3-032-02460-2

This Springer imprint is published by the registered company Springer Nature Switzerland AG
The registered company address is: Gewerbestrasse 11, 6330 Cham, Switzerland

Dedicated to our families as well as those committed to caring for patients with vascular disease.

Contents

Contributors

Olamide Alabi Division of Vascular Surgery and Endovascular Therapy, Department of Surgery, Emory University School of Medicine, Atlanta, GA, USA

Alvaro Alonso UMass Chan Medical School, UMass Memorial Medical Center, Worcester, MA, USA

Nkiruka Arinze Division of Vascular Surgery and Endovascular Therapy, Department of Surgery, Emory University School of Medicine, Atlanta, GA, USA

Donna Bahroloomi Division of Vascular Surgery, Cedars-Sinai Medical Center, Los Angeles, CA, USA

Donald T. Baril Division of Vascular Surgery, Cedars-Sinai Medical Center, Los Angeles, CA, USA

Neal R. Barshes Division of Vascular Surgery and Endovascular Therapy, Michael E. DeBakey Department of Surgery, Baylor College of Medicine/Michael E. DeBakey Veterans Affairs Medical Center, Houston, TX, USA

Erika T. Beidelman Department of Epidemiology and Biostatistics, Indiana University School of Public Health-Bloomington, Bloomington, IN, USA

Robert N. Butler Columbia Aging Center, Columbia University Mailman School of Public Health, New York, NY, USA

Kirthi S. Bellamkonda Section of Vascular Surgery, Heart and Vascular Center, Dartmouth Hitchcock Medical Center, Lebanon, NH, USA

Laura T. Boitano Division of Vascular and Endovascular Surgery, University of Massachusetts, T.H. Chan School of Medicine, Worcester, MA, USA

Santiago Callegari Vascular Medicine Outcomes Program, Section of Cardiovascular Medicine, Department of Internal Medicine & Department of Psychiatry, Yale University, New Haven, CT, USA

Michael S. Conte Division of Vascular and Endovascular Surgery, University of California at San Francisco, San Francisco, CA, USA

Matthew A. Corriere Division of Vascular Diseases & Surgery, Department of Surgery, The Ohio State University, Columbus, OH, USA

Mark G. Davies Center for Quality, Effectiveness, and Outcomes in Cardiovascular Diseases, Houston, TX, USA

Department of Vascular and Endovascular Surgery, Ascension Health, Waco, TX, USA

Ramprakash Devadoss UMass Chan Medical School, UMass Memorial Medical Center, Worcester, MA, USA

Dominique M. Dockery Division of Vascular and Endovascular Surgery, University of Massachusetts Chan Medical School, Worcester, MA, USA

Philip P. Goodney Section of Vascular Surgery, Heart and Vascular Center, Dartmouth Hitchcock Medical Center, Lebanon, NH, USA

Joseph P. Hart Department of Surgery, Division of Vascular and Endovascular Surgery, Medical College of Wisconsin, Milwaukee, WI, USA

Center for Quality, Effectiveness, and Outcomes in Cardiovascular Diseases, Houston, TX, USA

Laura Healy, MD Division of Vascular Surgery, Southern Illinois University School of Medicine, Springfield, Illinois, USA

Caitlin W. Hicks Division of Vascular Surgery and Endovascular Therapy, Johns Hopkins University School of Medicine, Baltimore, MD, USA

Momodou L. Jammeh Department of Surgery, Medical College of Wisconsin, Milwaukee, WI, USA

Douglas W. Jones Division of Vascular and Endovascular Surgery, University of Massachusetts Chan Medical School, Worcester, MA, USA

Corey A. Kalbaugh Department of Epidemiology and Biostatistics, Indiana University School of Public Health-Bloomington, Bloomington, IN, USA

Amber B. Kernodle Department of Vascular and Endovascular Surgery, Brigham and Women's Hospital, Boston, MA, USA

Mary M. McDermott Feinberg School of Medicine, Northwestern University, Chicago, IL, USA

Carlos Mena-Hurtado Vascular Medicine Outcomes Program, Section of Cardiovascular Medicine, Department of Internal Medicine & Department of Psychiatry, Yale University, New Haven, CT, USA

Louis M. Messina Division of Vascular and Endovascular Surgery, University of Massachusetts Chan Medical School, Worcester, MA, USA

Brandi M. Mize Division of Vascular Surgery and Endovascular Therapy, Department of Surgery, Emory University School of Medicine, Atlanta, GA, USA

Reginald Nkansah Division of Vascular Surgery, University of Washington, Seattle, WA, USA

Leigh Ann O'Banion University of California San Francisco-Fresno Branch Campus, Fresno, CA, USA

Aishwarya Raja Massachusetts General Hospital, Boston, MA, USA

Interventional Cardiology and Vascular Research, Richard A. and Susan F. Smith Center for Outcomes Research, Beth Israel Deaconess Medical Center, Boston, MA, USA

William P. Robinson III Division of Vascular Surgery, Southern Illinois University School of Medicine, Springfield, IL, USA

Alejandra P. Rodriguez Division of Vascular and Endovascular Surgery, Department of Surgery, UT Southwestern Medical Center, Dallas, TX, USA

Peter Rossi Division of Vascular and Endovascular Surgery, Medical College of Wisconsin, Milwaukee, WI, USA

Eric A. Secemsky Interventional Cardiology and Vascular Research, Richard A. and Susan F. Smith Center for Outcomes Research, Beth Israel Deaconess Medical Center, Boston, MA, USA

Vascular Intervention, Interventional Cardiology and Vascular Research, Richard A. and Susan F. Smith Center for Outcomes Research, Beth Israel Deaconess Medical Center, Boston, MA, USA

Harvard Medical School, Boston, MA, USA

Jessica P. Simons Division of Vascular and Endovascular Surgery, University of Massachusetts Chan Medical School, Worcester, MA, USA

Kim G. Smolderen Vascular Medicine Outcomes Program, Section of Cardiovascular Medicine, Department of Internal Medicine & Department of Psychiatry, Yale University, New Haven, CT, USA

Department of Psychiatry, Yale School of Medicine, New Haven, CT, USA

Gale Tang Division of Vascular Surgery, Section Chief Vascular Surgery VAPSHCS, Department of Surgery, University of Washington, Seattle, WA, USA

Xiaoyi Teng Division of Vascular Diseases & Surgery, Department of Surgery, The Ohio State University, Columbus, OH, USA

Shirling Tsai Division of Vascular and Endovascular Surgery, Department of Surgery, UT Southwestern Medical Center, Dallas, TX, USA

Phong Vu University of California San Francisco-Fresno Branch Campus, Fresno, CA, USA

M. Libby Weaver Division of Vascular Surgery, University of Utah Spencer Fox Eccles School of Medicine, Salt Lake City, UT, USA

Nader Zamani Division of Vascular Surgery and Endovascular Therapy, Michael E. DeBakey Department of Surgery, Baylor College of Medicine/Michael E. DeBakey Veterans Affairs Medical Center, Houston, TX, USA

Tian Zhang Division of Vascular Surgery, Southern Illinois University School of Medicine, Springfield, IL, USA

1 A Framework for Physicians and Patients with Claudication: Toward a Patient-Centered Approach

Jessica P. Simons and William P. Robinson III

Introduction and Rationale

The evaluation and management of patients experiencing intermittent claudication (IC) secondary to peripheral artery disease (PAD) can be challenging for a host of reasons. Our objective in designing and editing this book was to facilitate care by both providing a comprehensive resource but also distilling out the key principles that can be overlooked amidst the wealth of information in clinical medicine. We sought to create a framework for a "patient-centered" approach to the treatment of patients experiencing claudication. Such an approach, centered on knowledge-sharing and shared decision-making, leads to greater patient satisfaction and improved outcomes.

We designed the book amid increasing scrutiny of claudication care in the United States that has risen to the level of exposé articles in the lay press depicting misuse and overuse of vascular procedures [1–5]. This is deeply concerning, not only that inappropriate and dangerous care may be rendered to trusting patients, but also that the media depiction of vascular specialists could have unintended consequences of deterring patients from seeking care for vascular disease. The editors sought a constructive approach that both acknowledges inappropriate use while also attempting to educate a wide audience and empower patients and providers alike to have a deeper understanding of claudication care. Well-intentioned providers may simply lack the knowledge and resources necessary to help patients understand this complicated clinical scenario, especially in a time-constrained clinic visit. Claudication is

J. P. Simons (✉)
Division of Vascular and Endovascular Surgery, University of Massachusetts Chan Medical School, Worcester, MA, USA
e-mail: Jessica.simons@umassmemorial.org

W. P. Robinson III
Division of Vascular Surgery, Southern Illinois University School of Medicine, Springfield, IL, USA
e-mail: wrobinson35@siumed.edu

W. P. Robinson III, J. P. Simons (eds.), *The Patient-Centered Approach to Claudication*, https://doi.org/10.1007/978-3-032-02460-2_1

a complex medical condition, and one surrounded by a number and variety of misconceptions from patients, primary care and other referring providers, and vascular specialists from all disciplines. For example, a cursory internet search of "intermittent claudication" yields many well-designed resources for patients and providers, from several reputable organizations, all of which lump together all forms of PAD, with very little differentiation on the important differences between asymptomatic PAD, intermittent claudication, and chronic limb threatening ischemia (CLTI). Our sincere hope is that this book highlights key differences, emphasizes why they matter, and eliminates misconceptions on goals of treatment for intermittent claudication, specifically as it differs from CLTI.

How Claudication Care Has Changed Over Time

Historically, claudication was rarely treated with revascularization. The benign natural history of IC is well established with 70–80% of patients remaining stable or improving over time without intervention [6]. The rate of lifelong progression to chronic limb-threatening ischemia is variably low (<5% to 21%), and the yearly risk of progression to amputation is less than 1% per year [7, 8]. There is no evidence to suggest that intervention on specific atherosclerotic lesions or arterial segments inhibits progression of atherosclerotic disease in the limb or improves the prognosis of the limb. In fact, failure of intervention may be associated with a natural history for the limb worse than that without intervention [9]. Guidelines from past to present have emphasized the primacy of cardiovascular risk reduction (lifestyle modification, optimal medical treatment (OMT), smoking cessation) and exercise therapy; they have stated that revascularization should be reserved for those whose IC symptoms remain disabling despite these measures [10–14]. Despite this, medical optimization is not occurring in a significant percentage of patients with IC [15–17]. Nor is smoking cessation occurring; data from the VQI demonstrates that greater than 40% of patients undergoing intervention for claudication are still active smokers [18].

In current practice, there seems to be a shift toward seeking an "immediate fix" to claudication pain using revascularization. IC is currently the most common indication for lower extremity arterial revascularization in the United States. The number of lower extremity revascularization procedures for IC increased dramatically during the early 2000s, with the annual volume of procedures for IC rising above those performed for CLTI in 2005, based upon national all-payer claims data from the Nationwide Inpatient Sample [19]. This surge of revascularization procedures was driven by a 300% increase in the number of endovascular interventions for claudication, accompanied by a 33% decrease in the number of bypass procedures performed for claudication [19]. The increase in lower extremity interventions is probably more pronounced than this data indicates. Most current administrative datasets and clinical registries fail to capture revascularization procedures performed in office-based laboratories or ambulatory surgery centers, which are the site of service for an increasing number of endovascular revascularization procedures [20, 21]. A reasonable hypothesis for the increase in endovascular revascularization for IC is that it is minimally invasive and therefore low risk. However, there is a growing body of evidence to dispute this hypothesis of a "free shot" with an endovascular-first approach. Treatment failure at any point in time may result in deterioration to CLTI and an associated risk of limb loss greater than that expected for patients with IC treated conservatively [22, 23]. Taken together, this data raises serious concerns about the consequences of overuse and premature use of lower extremity revascularization for IC.

State of the Evidence of Revascularization Strategies

In addition to concerns of overuse of intervention, there isn't clear evidence on *how* to intervene to treat IC. In the United States, practice patterns vary widely regarding the type of revascularization (surgical, endovascular, or hybrid) performed. This variability may reflect, in part, the lack of rigorous studies, which in turn leads to a lack of granular guidelines and challenges with defining quality care. The number of endovascular devices and mechanisms of action for the treatment of lower extremity occlusive disease has exploded exponentially, vastly outpacing the science to support their use or define their utility. In the limited instances in which data exists, considerable heterogeneity in study designs, patient selection, lack of conservatively managed control groups, and endpoints lacking clinical value limits our understanding of the comparative effectiveness of revascularization to non-interventional treatments and between various revascularization strategies.

In addition, practices considered unhelpful or even harmful have been increasingly utilized. For example, infra-popliteal interventions for claudication are bereft of data supporting their safety or efficacy yet appear to be increasing in frequency. In a recent analysis using Medicare claims data from 2017 to 2019, the prevalence of this practice appears to have markedly increased (28% of all index peripheral vascular interventions (PVI) for claudication) and was associated with both patient and provider-specific characteristics [24]. Despite the frequency of infrapopliteal PVI, evidence supporting tibio-peroneal artery interventions, alone or in combination with aorto-iliac and/or femoropopliteal treatment, is lacking. Decisions to treat appear to be based on local and specialty-specific practice patterns or the physician's individual treatment bias or training [24–27]. These practices are likely not without serious consequence. An analysis of the Vascular Quality Initiative data found that only 20% of combined femoropopliteal and tibial interventions were free from claudication at 2 years, which does not meet the 2015 practice guidelines set by the Society of Vascular Surgery of >50% experiencing symptom relief [27]. Of more serious concern is that infrapopliteal interventions have been associated with an increased downstream risk of major amputation [28–31]. While clear causation has not been established, the repeated signal in the data is strong enough and concerning enough to merit further study.

There are many unanswered questions pertaining to revascularization for patients experiencing claudication. Literature focused on lesion-based responses to treatment, in many ways, has been most useful in defining the potential complications, limited durability, and unfavorable natural history when revascularization fails. Broadly speaking, the goals of revascularization for IC include improved walking distance and relief of pain with presumed improvement in functional status and health-related quality of life. Improved walking ability may contribute to improved overall cardiovascular health, although data to support this hypothesis is lacking. In addition, the patient's life expectancy and the functional limitations imposed by co-existing comorbidities are critically important in considering the potential benefits of revascularization for IC. An individualized assessment and discussion of the presumed benefits of revascularization versus potential adverse events in a shared decision-making process should precede the decision to undertake revascularization.

Identifying Treatment Priorities in Patients Experiencing Claudication

While intermittent claudication due to PAD reflects the physiologic consequence of an arterial stenosis or occlusion, it is problematic to consider treatment in terms of the lesion itself. This can be an important frameshift for proceduralists given that training often focuses on the optimal technique to fix a lesion. However, in the case of IC, a lesion-based approach fails to address the more significant risks to the patient, namely, the cardiovascular morbidity and mortality that IC signifies. The findings of reduced survival and increased cardiovascular events among patients with ankle-brachial index <0.9 have been documented repeatedly; a recent meta-analysis found a 2.3-fold increased risk of the composite endpoint, myocardial infarction, stroke, and death, for these patients [32]. Of note, this analysis included patients who were asymptomatic or minimally symptomatic. For patients who present with claudication, these symptoms must be considered as a harbinger of serious cardiovascular risk. It is imperative to effectively communicate that risk to the patient.

It can be challenging to counsel a patient regarding IC for many reasons. Specifically, it is important to help patients understand the paradox of IC: the leg symptoms are not dangerous, and the risk of limb loss is very low. However, the leg symptoms are a marker of a very serious systemic disease, atherosclerosis. Clinicians need to help patients understand that IC may be the first manifestation of cardiovascular disease, and an opportunity to consider their overall health and lifestyle. It is important to both acknowledge the real negative impact that IC can have on health-related quality of life [33] and mental health [34], while also motivating patients to engage in significant risk factor modification and lifestyle changes. The importance and potential success of exercise therapy must be stressed [35, 36]. Clinicians need to help patients set realistic expectations for their physical symptoms and understand the appropriate settings for revascularization. The complexity of counseling and treating patients with IC cannot be understated. It cannot be accomplished in one office visit, nor with a lesion-focused approach. Holistic care of the patient experiencing claudication can be as rewarding as it is challenging for these reasons.

Organization of the Chapters

The editors designed this textbook with the goal of helping the practicing clinician by providing a framework for thinking of the patient with claudication from a holistic perspective, offering data and considerations for counseling and decision-making, as well as specific resources for patient education. A critical theme that carries across all chapters is the distinction between IC and the broader term, PAD. IC carries a distinctly more favorable limb prognosis than chronic limb-threatening ischemia, and it is imperative that patients and clinicians keep this at the forefront of any risk/benefit analysis. The editors believe that the obscurity of this subtle but critical differentiation may explain some of the overuse of interventions for IC.

In the early chapters of this book, the authors describe the basics of IC, starting with the pathophysiology and diagnostic considerations. The magnitude of IC as a public health problem is next considered, as well as race, ethnicity, and sex-based differences and disparities. Medical management is covered from multiple perspectives, including risk factor modification, smoking cessation, and pharmacologic therapy for limb/functional outcomes.

In the next section of the text, the authors cover topics related to the patient experience of living with intermittent claudication. The psychological impact of functional impairment and chronic pain is described. The nuances of guiding patients to achieve a successful outcome with exercise therapy are also presented.

Considerations for revascularization are next covered, according to the anatomic level of disease. This section also addresses the outcomes of revascularization, with specific attention to durability and challenges of recurrent disease. With this background, concepts of shared decision-making and patient preference science are presented.

And finally, the authors describe both the current state of IC care and future considerations. Several clinical practice guidelines are reviewed, highlighting areas of agreement and areas of controversy. Novel treatments and matters of ongoing research are described, including considerations for assessing cost-effectiveness of treatments for IC. The final section contains open-access appendices intended for use by clinicians and patients across a spectrum of settings, ranging from the primary care office to preoperative counseling by vascular specialists. This effort to re-frame the problem of IC and heighten awareness of both providers and patients regarding treatment decisions is intended to ultimately improve the quality of care provided to these patients.

References

1. Creswell J, Abelson R. Medicare payments surge for stents to unblock vessels in limbs. New York Times. Jan 29, 2015. Accessed 8 Apr 2021.
2. Waldman A. Researchers warned of possible vascular procedure abuse. *Propublica*. December 12 2023. Available from: https://www.propublica.org/article/researchers-warned-of-possible-vascular-procedure-abuse-doctors-pushed-back. Accessed 16 Mar 2024.
3. Waldman A. Steak dinners, sales reps and risky procedures. February 16, 2023. Available from: https://www.propublica.org/article/medtronic-medical-device-kickbacks-lawsuit-kansas. Accessed 16 Mar 2024.
4. Waldman A. In the "wild west" of outpatient vascular care, doctors can reap huge payments as patients risk life and limb. May 24 2023. Available from: https://www.propublica.org/article/maryland-dormu-minimally-invasive-vascular-medicare-medicaid. Accessed 2 May 2025.
5. Thomas K. They lost their legs; doctors and healthcare giants profited. New York Times. July 16, 2023. Available from: https://www.nytimes.com/2023/07/15/health/atherectomy-peripheral-artery-disease.html. Accessed 2 May 2025.
6. Hirsch AT, Haskal ZJ, Hertzer NR, et al. ACC/AHA 2005 practice guidelines for the management of patients with peripheral arterial disease (lower extremity, renal, mesenteric, and abdominal aortic): a collaborative report from the American Association for Vascular Surgery/Society for Vascular Surgery, Society for Cardiovascular Angiography and Interventions, Society for Vascular Medicine and Biology, Society of Interventional Radiology, and the ACC/AHA task force on practice guidelines (writing committee to develop guidelines for the Management of Patients with Peripheral Arterial Disease): endorsed by the American Association of Cardiovascular and Pulmonary Rehabilitation; National Heart, Lung, and Blood Institute; Society for Vascular Nursing; TransAtlantic inter-society consensus; and vascular disease foundation. Circulation. 2006;113(11):463. https://doi.org/10.1161/CIRCULATIONAHA.106.174526.
7. Norgren L, Hiatt WR, Dormandy JA, et al. Inter-society consensus for the management of peripheral arterial disease (TASC II). J Vasc Surg. 2007;45(Suppl S):5. https://doi.org/10.1016/j.jvs.2006.12.037.
8. Dormandy J, Heeck L, Vig S. The natural history of claudication: risk to life and limb. Semin Vasc Surg. 1999;12(2):123–37.
9. Kim TI, Kiwan G, Mohamedali A, et al. Multiple reinterventions for claudication are associated with progression to chronic limb-threatening ischemia. Ann Vasc Surg. 2021;72:166–74. https://doi.org/10.1016/j.avsg.2020.10.004.
10. Society for Vascular Surgery Lower Extremity Guidelines Writing Group, Conte MS, Pomposelli FB, et al. Society for Vascular Surgery practice guidelines for atherosclerotic occlusive disease of the lower extremities: management of asymptomatic disease and claudication. J Vasc Surg. 2015;61(3 Suppl):2S–41S. https://doi.org/10.1016/j.jvs.2014.12.009.
11. Gerhard-Herman MD, Gornik HL, Barrett C, et al. 2016 AHA/ACC guideline on the Management of Patients with Lower Extremity Peripheral Artery Disease: a report of the American College of Cardiology/American Heart Association task force on clinical practice guidelines. Circulation. 2017;135(12):e726–79. https://doi.org/10.1161/CIR.0000000000000471.
12. Aboyans V, Ricco J, Bartelink MEL, et al. 2017 ESC guidelines on the diagnosis and treatment of peripheral arterial diseases, in collaboration with the European Society for Vascular Surgery (ESVS): document covering atherosclerotic disease of extracranial carotid and vertebral, mesenteric, renal, upper and lower extremity arteriesEndorsed by: the European se organization (ESO)the task force for the diagnosis and treatment of peripheral arterial diseases of the European Society of Cardiology (ESC) and of the European Society for Vascular Surgery (ESVS). Eur Heart J. 2018;39(9):763–816. https://doi.org/10.1093/eurheartj/ehx095.
13. ABIM Foundation. Choosing wisely. https://www.choosingwisely.org/. Accessed 09/08, 2023.

14. Conte MS, Aulivola B, Barshes NR, et al. Society for vascular surgery clinical practice guideline on the management of intermittent claudication: focused update. J Vasc Surg. 2025;82 https://doi.org/10.1016/j.jvs.2025.04.041.
15. Subherwal S, Patel MR, Kober L, et al. Missed opportunities: despite improvement in use of cardioprotective medications among patients with lower-extremity peripheral artery disease, underuse remains. Circulation. 2012;126(11):1345–54. https://doi.org/10.1161/CIRCULATIONAHA.112.108787.
16. Pande RL, Perlstein TS, Beckman JA, Creager MA. Secondary prevention and mortality in peripheral artery disease: National Health and nutrition examination study, 1999 to 2004. Circulation. 2011;124(1):17–23. https://doi.org/10.1161/CIRCULATIONAHA.110.003954.
17. Berger JS, Ladapo JA. Underuse of prevention and lifestyle counseling in patients with peripheral artery disease. J Am Coll Cardiol. 2017;69(18):2293–300. https://doi.org/10.1016/j.jacc.2017.02.064.
18. Gabel J, Jabo B, Patel S, et al. Smoking habits of patients undergoing treatment for intermittent claudication in the vascular quality initiative. Ann Vasc Surg. 2017;44:261–8. https://doi.org/10.1016/j.avsg.2017.04.046.
19. Sachs T, Pomposelli F, Hamdan A, Wyers M, Schermerhorn M. Trends in the national outcomes and costs for claudication and limb threatening ischemia: angioplasty vs bypass graft. J Vasc Surg. 2011;54(4):1021–1031.e1. https://doi.org/10.1016/j.jvs.2011.03.281.
20. Jones WS, Mi X, Qualls LG, et al. Trends in settings for peripheral vascular intervention and the effect of changes in the outpatient prospective payment system. J Am Coll Cardiol. 2015;65(9):920–7. https://doi.org/10.1016/j.jacc.2014.12.048.
21. Giannopoulos S, Pliagas G, Armstrong EJ. Procedural and 3-year outcomes of peripheral vascular interventions performed in office-based labs: LIBERTY 360 sub-analysis. J Invasive Cardiol. 2021;33(5):E365–77. https://doi.org/10.25270/jic/20.00594.
22. Sorber R, Dun C, Kawaji Q, et al. Early peripheral vascular interventions for claudication are associated with higher rates of late interventions and progression to chronic limb threatening ischemia. J Vasc Surg. 2023;77(3):836–847.e3. https://doi.org/10.1016/j.jvs.2022.10.025.
23. Madabhushi V, Davenport D, Jones S, et al. Revascularization of intermittent claudicants leads to more chronic limb-threatening ischemia and higher amputation rates. J Vasc Surg. 2021;74(3):771–9. https://doi.org/10.1016/j.jvs.2021.02.045.
24. Bose S, Dun C, Sorber R, et al. Practice patterns surrounding the use of tibial interventions for claudication in the medicare population. J Vasc Surg. 2023;77(2):454–462.e1. https://doi.org/10.1016/j.jvs.2022.08.033.
25. Kawaji Q, Dun C, Walsh C, et al. Index atherectomy peripheral vascular interventions performed for claudication are associated with more reinterventions than nonatherectomy interventions. J Vasc Surg. 2022;76(2):489–498.e4. https://doi.org/10.1016/j.jvs.2022.02.034.
26. Weaver ML, Neal D, Columbo JA, et al. Market competition influences practice patterns in management of patients with intermittent claudication in the vascular quality initiative. J Vasc Surg. 2023;78(3):727–736.e3. https://doi.org/10.1016/j.jvs.2023.04.032.
27. Bath J, Lawrence PF, Neal D, et al. Endovascular interventions for claudication do not meet minimum standards for the society for vascular surgery efficacy guidelines. J Vasc Surg. 2021;73(5):1693–1700.e3. https://doi.org/10.1016/j.jvs.2020.10.067.
28. Bose S, McDermott KM, Dun C, et al. Infrapopliteal endovascular interventions for claudication are associated with poor long-term outcomes in Medicare-matched registry patients. Ann Surg. 2024; https://doi.org/10.1097/SLA.0000000000006368.
29. Bose S, Dun C, Solomon AJ, et al. Editor's choice – infrapopliteal peripheral vascular interventions for claudication are performed frequently in the USA and are associated with poor long term outcomes. Eur J Vasc Endovasc Surg. 2025;69(1):89–101. https://doi.org/10.1016/j.ejvs.2024.06.017.
30. Mullins CH, Novak Z, Axley JC, et al. Prevalence and outcomes of endovascular Infrapopliteal interventions for intermittent claudication. Ann Vasc Surg. 2021;70:79–86. https://doi.org/10.1016/j.avsg.2020.08.097.

31. Fashandi AZ, Mehaffey JH, Hawkins RB, Kron IL, Upchurch GRJ, Robinson WP. Major adverse limb events and major adverse cardiac events after contemporary lower extremity bypass and infrainguinal endovascular intervention in patients with claudication. J Vasc Surg. 2018;68(6):1817–23. https://doi.org/10.1016/j.jvs.2018.06.193.
32. Hajibandeh S, Hajibandeh S, Shah S, Child E, Antoniou GA, Torella F. Prognostic significance of ankle brachial pressure index: a systematic review and meta-analysis. Vascular. 2017;25(2):208–24. https://doi.org/10.1177/1708538116658392.
33. Spronk S, White JV, Bosch JL, Hunink MGM. Impact of claudication and its treatment on quality of life. Semin Vasc Surg. 2007;20(1):3–9. https://doi.org/10.1053/j.semvascsurg.2007.02.003.
34. Thomas M, Patel KK, Gosch K, et al. Mental health concerns in patients with symptomatic peripheral artery disease: insights from the PORTRAIT registry. J Psychosom Res. 2020;131:109963. https://doi.org/10.1016/j.jpsychores.2020.109963.
35. Lane R, Harwood A, Watson L, Leng GC. Exercise for intermittent claudication. Cochrane Database Syst Rev. 2017;12(12):CD000990. https://doi.org/10.1002/14651858.CD000990.pub4.
36. Treat-Jacobson D, McDermott MM, Bronas UG, et al. Optimal exercise programs for patients with peripheral artery disease: a scientific statement from the American Heart Association. Circulation. 2019;139(4):e10–33. https://doi.org/10.1161/CIR.0000000000000623.

Anatomy, Physiology, and Pathophysiology of Claudication

2

Joseph P. Hart and Mark G. Davies

Introduction

Claudication denotes painful cramping and/or muscle belly fatigue in a lower extremity muscle group during a defined amount of exercise (distance) and is relieved by rest while standing or sitting [1–4]. Exercise-induced muscle exertion-related symptoms can arise in other anatomic regions (especially the arm). However, lower extremity symptoms have the greatest clinical significance in terms of current controversy, patient volume, and variation(s) in clinical approach. The term "claudication" arises from the Latin (*claudicare*, "to limp") but has evolved to denote a painful limp induced by exercise. It is also emblematic of chronic insufficiency of arterial flow to the legs, primarily resulting from atherosclerotic occlusive disease. Claudication generally worsens in a non-linear progression over a timeline of years. Walking distance is often constant at each phase if other parameters remain the same, such as the type and gradient of the landscape and speed of walking. The severity of pain may vacillate between unchanging, improvement, or exacerbation. Critically, claudication may suddenly become acute and progress to rest pain if there is a new level of arterial obstruction, acute thrombosis of a stenotic segment, or if collateral pathways are lost.

J. P. Hart (✉)
Department of Surgery, Division of Vascular and Endovascular Surgery, Medical College of Wisconsin, Milwaukee, WI, USA

Center for Quality, Effectiveness, and Outcomes in Cardiovascular Diseases, Houston, TX, USA
e-mail: jphart@mcw.edu

M. G. Davies
Center for Quality, Effectiveness, and Outcomes in Cardiovascular Diseases, Houston, TX, USA

Department of Vascular and Endovascular Surgery, Ascension Health, Waco, TX, USA

W. P. Robinson III, J. P. Simons (eds.), *The Patient-Centered Approach to Claudication*, https://doi.org/10.1007/978-3-032-02460-2_2

The severity of symptoms in an individual patient is determined by one or more factors, such as the pattern of pain described, the degree of the obstruction, and how quickly the pain progressed. Patients with claudication typically will develop collateral arterial blood vessels (bed) around a level of stenosis with the implementation of an exercise program. How sufficient this collateral arterial bed is in delivering arterial blood supply to an exercising leg muscle determines whether claudication symptoms remain stable, worsen, or even improve if the collateral bed increases in size over time, especially if smoking cessation is accomplished.

Anatomy

Symptoms of Intermittent claudication are anatomy-dependent [5–7]. The extent of pain in the leg may reflect where the arterial occlusion is located. There are three potential levels of disease in the leg: the aorto-iliac segment, the femoro-popliteal segment, and the tibial pedal segment. The anatomy of collateral circulation is important to consider and guide understanding the management of claudication. Multiple collateral networks exist that facilitate continued perfusion in the setting of occluded named axial vessels. These include the cruciate collateral network, the genicular collateral network, and the tibioperonal-pedal network, which form around the hip-thigh, knee, and ankle respectively.

Physiology

When arterial blood supply is inadequate to maintain muscle function during exercise, ischemia ensues, which causes a muscle buildup of metabolic byproducts that stimulate the sensory nerves, leading to pain symptoms [8, 9]. At rest, when the metabolic demands of the exercising limb have reduced, the resting blood supply "catches up" and clears the imbalance of the metabolic byproducts, and pain is relieved. This cycle of pain with exercise and relief with rest repeats with the same walking distance. This pain may range from tolerable to completely disabling intensity if the patient attempts to walk beyond the distance, which elicits the pain. Patients with severe arterial insufficiency, or those who do not rest when pain develops, will have residual muscular soreness for a period thereafter because of ischemic myositis.

The physiology of vasodilation is important in compensated claudication. Vasodilation is the process whereby more distal blood vessels dilate in response to exercise-induced muscle ischemia, allowing for increased perfusion to the affected area, which mitigates pain associated with reduced blood supply due to more proximal occluded or narrowed arteries driving claudication; the arterial system attempts to compensate for the restricted inflow by dilating the more distal vessels to deliver more oxygen to the distal tissues. The physiology of coagulation relates to claudication via atherosclerosis and peripheral artery disease, which drives platelet activation and potentially additional thrombus formation due to reduced blood flow with luminal narrowing, which can further exacerbate limited blood flow to the affected muscles.

Neoangiogenesis develops as microvessels related to obstructed segments. These newly derived vessels do not have typical wall architecture and thus may not provide adequate flow distally. However, the body provides a natural system of pre-existing collateral arteries, which may bypass sites of arterial occlusion, which can grow and potentially undergo collateral regulation processes to perfuse distal ischemic tissue successfully. Figure 2.1 summarizes the mechanisms of vascular regeneration for limb perfusion as conceptualized by Cooke JP and Meng S in 2020 [10]. Muscle inactivity in claudication leads to muscle atrophy. Unused muscles involute, and protein synthesis is reduced. Muscle mass decreases (sarcopenia), leading to weakness, imbalance, and ultimately frailty.

Pathophysiology

Patients with lower extremity PAD suffer elevated cardiovascular risks due to the systemic nature of atherosclerosis; therefore, they benefit from risk factor modification. Atherosclerosis contributes to several clinical disease entities. Obstruction to arterial flow by flow-limiting atherosclerotic lesions causes ischemic limb or claudication-like symptoms as described previously. Low arterial blood perfusion with exercise, however, only partially explains the symptoms of PAD and their response to therapeutic interventions. Other potential and complex mechanisms that

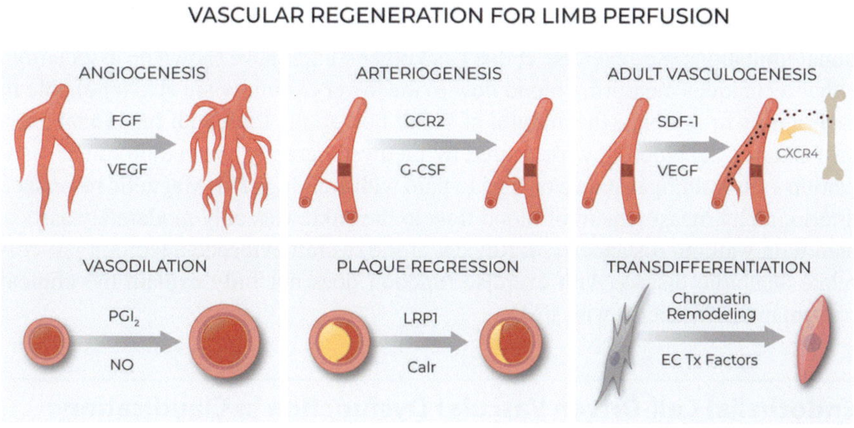

Fig. 2.1 Schematic representation of processes contributing to vascular regeneration. (CCR-2 indicates chemokine receptor 2; *EC* endothelial cell, *FGF* fibroblast growth factor, *G-CSF* granulocyte-colony stimulating factor, *LRP-1* low-density lipoprotein receptor-related protein 1, PGI_2 prostacyclin, *SDF-1* stromal-derived factor 1, *Tx* transcriptional, *VEGF* vascular endothelial growth factor). (From Cooke and Meng, with permission [10])

may drive the ischemic limb symptoms in PAD are numerous [10–20], and current evidence supporting the role of inadequate arterial blood supply, altered vascular endothelial cell function, inhibited angiogenesis, changed musculoskeletal structure, deranged mitochondrial metabolism, and inflammatory activation are discussed in this section. A broader understanding of the underlying pathophysiology of ischemic limb symptoms has the potential to better provide appropriate patient-centered care to patients with PAD.

Arterial Obstructive Lesions Reduce Limb Circulation

In a demand-ischemia model, intermittent claudication reflects the inadequate autoregulation of skeletal muscle perfusion during exercise. Obtaining an ankle brachial index (ABI) at rest and during treadmill exercise calculates the severity of lower limb atherosclerosis, reflective of reduced blood flow from the aorta to the ankle. Recently, much has been made of abnormal (exercise) ABI as a potentially additive prognostic factor for bypass/intervention and mortality compared with the resting ABI alone. Flow-limiting lesions create additive drops in both blood pressure and flow, reducing ankle pressure. With exercise, the flow to the lower extremity aggravates the pressure gradient due to the fixed lesions, increasing the sensitivity to detect PAD. Inadequate perfusion with exercise is clearly the key component underlying limb ischemia symptoms. However, multiple studies indicate that there are multiple determinants that generate limb ischemia.

Anatomic severity of obstruction imprecisely predicts clinical status and course. Prospective studies confirm that patients with an abnormal ABI will have a decline in walking ability at 2-year follow-up [19]. But the association between the magnitude of the reduction of the ABI and resulting functional abilities is less clear. Some studies have shown only a modest correlation between the ABI and extent of functional limitations (i.e., exercise ability) and other studies have shown no association. Other techniques measuring blood flow to the lower extremity are also unreliable in their ability to correlate the amount of blood flow to the limb with functional exercise status. Calf blood flow measured by plethysmography showed no direct association with walking distance or time to pain with walking [15]. Magnetic resonance arteriography measurement of blood flow to the ankle was only moderately associated with walking distance [13]. Review of the overall evidence attempting to correlate anatomic disease with exercise function does not fully explain the clinical presentation of patients with PAD.

Endothelial Cell-Driven Vascular Dysfunction in Claudication

Arterial insufficiency in PAD causes both fixed and dynamic reductions in blood flow, which can affect normal flow receptor-mediated endothelial cell functions. Multiple investigations have noted endothelial cell dysfunction in PAD. This dysfunction may limit flow-mediated dilation and increase the vasoconstrictive effects of catecholamines, thus impeding the increase of blood flow needed with exercise and exacerbating the clinical symptoms of PAD.

Nitric oxide is an important vasodilator substance that the vascular endothelial cell produces. Nitric oxide inhibits platelets, reduces smooth muscle proliferation, prevents leukocyte adhesion, and promotes angiogenesis. Reduced nitric oxide availability inhibits the increase of blood flow needed with exercise.

Other measures of endothelial cell-dependent vasodilatory functions, such as brachial artery flow-mediated vasodilation, are lower in patients with PAD. In a study comparing patients with PAD and CAD, nearly 30% patients in the PAD group had more severe vasodilator dysfunction [15]. Decreased augmentation of blood flow with exercise is associated with a decrease in functional ability. There is evidence that in patients with PAD, there is a direct association between an increase in brachial flow-mediated vasodilation and an increase in walking activity. More recent investigations have shown that reduced brachial flow-mediated dilation is correlated with a decrease in exercise capability in a 6-minute walk test [8, 15]. Of note, in patients with PAD, the severity of a flow-limiting lesion in the femoral artery was associated with a decrease in femoral artery dilation. Increased arterial stiffness, as measured by a higher pulse pressure and augmentation index, was also associated with a reduction in walking time [15, 21]. Endothelial dysfunction can predict a higher risk of adverse events after vascular surgery. However, endothelial dysfunction has not been studied in the context of whether it can be a measure of progression of exercise intolerance.

Reduced Microcirculatory Flow in the Setting of Impaired Angiogenesis

Arterial ischemia due to insufficient blood supply in patients with PAD may cause an alteration in normal vascular growth, with inhibition of angiogenesis and collateral vessel formation, thereby potentiating further impairment of exercise ability. Identified in animal models, there are multiple growth factors that regulate angiogenesis such as vascular endothelial growth factor (VEGF), fibroblast growth factor (FGF), hepatocyte growth factor, and hypoxia-inducible factor 1-alpha. MicroRNAs are also important genetic regulators of angiogenesis and appear to have lower expression in animal models of limb ischemia. When tested in animal models, therapies that enhance angiogenesis showed an increase in muscle perfusion and return of exercise function.

In humans, one study biopsied the calf muscles of patients with PAD, which showed that lower capillary vessel density was associated with decreased exercise function [12, 14, 15]. Calf blood flow measurements via MRI or contrast-enhanced ultrasound also demonstrated lower microvascular flow in patients with PAD with exercise that correlated with reduced walking time [11, 15]. These clinical studies support the hypothesis that poor microcirculation can affect exercise function in patients with PAD and therefore, pro-angiogenic therapies that enhance calf blood flow should improve functional ability. Both growth factor and cell-based therapies have been studied in human clinical trials, and none has been able to show any significant improvement in pain or ischemic wound healing. The reason that these studies in humans have not translated from animal models appears to be due to the concurrence of systemic diseases such as obesity and diabetes. Metabolic dysfunction may mediate vascular growth by upregulating anti-angiogenic growth factors and other pro-inflammatory pathways that may interfere with therapies designed to stimulate angiogenesis. For example, one study showed evidence of an upregulation of an anti-angiogenic VEGF isoform, VEGF-165b that is mediated by a pro-inflammatory pathway Wnt5a/JNK, which is activated in obesity [15]. Future pro-angiogenic therapies may need to be tested in animal models with metabolic dysfunction and target anti-angiogenic growth factors and pro-inflammatory pathways.

Mitochondrial Derangements and Skeletal Muscle Abnormalities

Persistent arterial ischemia has negative effects on the structure and metabolic properties of limb skeletal muscle, which can lead to impaired exercise function or walking ability. CT scan imaging of the limbs in patients with PAD has shown a reduced calf muscle area, lower muscle density, and higher fat content [19]. There is increased muscle cell apoptosis and reduced type I fiber content on muscle biopsy. Ischemia also damages peripheral nerves, with evidence of diminished nerve conduction in severe PAD patients.

Mitochondria are critical in skeletal muscle energy metabolism. Arterial ischemia, in PAD causes reduced mitochondrial metabolism. There is evidence of lower ATP generation, enhancement of reactive oxygen production and oxidative stress, restriction of oxygen utilization, reduced nitric oxide activity causing endothelial cell dysfunction, and impaired angiogenesis.

Coexistent systemic metabolic dysfunction in patients with PAD may also lead to impaired muscle metabolism by reduced nutrient uptake. For example, PET scan evaluation of glucose uptake in the skeletal muscle of patients with intermittent claudication shows calf muscle insulin resistance [15]. Insulin resistance is noted in patients with PAD and can predict the risk of developing the clinical manifestations of PAD. There needs to be additional studies to directly link insulin resistance to functional ability and to determine whether therapies aimed at enhancing insulin sensitivity will alleviate claudication symptoms.

There are clinical studies linking skeletal muscle abnormalities and mitochondrial dysfunction with reduced exercise functional status in patients with PAD. Patients with PAD have shown decreased calf muscle density, increased calf muscle fat, and muscle fiber damage. These are associated with decreased walking times, reduced muscle strength, and can predict functional decline in longitudinal studies. Evidence is available for mitochondrial dysfunction such as increased muscle acylcarnitine, low autophagy of mitochondria [14, 15, 21]; reduced mitochondrial respiration due to altered desmin protein levels and reduced mitochondrial biogenesis are associated with altered exercise/walking parameters and with higher overall mortality in patients with PAD [22]. Potentially, future therapies to reduce skeletal calf muscle degeneration and to support normal mitochondrial functions can improve walking parameters and decrease mortality.

Systemic and Local Inflammatory Mechanisms

Atherosclerosis is now understood to be a chronic inflammatory vascular disease. Muscle ischemia leads to systemic and local inflammation that affects the underlying cellular and molecular mechanisms of atherosclerosis and muscle metabolism. Inflammation associated with atherosclerosis can also predict clinical presentation and progression of claudication. Known biomarkers of inflammation, such as C-reactive protein (CRP), soluble intracellular adhesion molecule-1 (sICAM-1), IL-6, fibrinogen, soluble vascular cell adhesion molecule-1 (sVCAM-1), tumor necrosis factor alpha and peripheral monocyte pro-inflammatory mediator Wnt5a, are seen in higher levels in patients with PAD. These higher levels of inflammatory biomarkers are associated with progression of arterial stenosis, changes in muscle metabolism, and clinically, with decreased walking ability and walking time, and lower ABI [16, 20, 21]. Conversely, bioactivity of nitric oxide is decreased with elevated levels of vascular inflammation thereby causing a decrease in endothelium-mediated vasodilation, limiting the increase in arterial blood flow needed with exercise. Decreased calf muscle area and increased calf muscle fat are associated with an increase in systemic inflammation on imaging studies. Prospective studies investigating ambulatory function in PAD patients show that lower levels of CRP are associated with less decline of walking/exercise function. Figure 2.2 summarizes

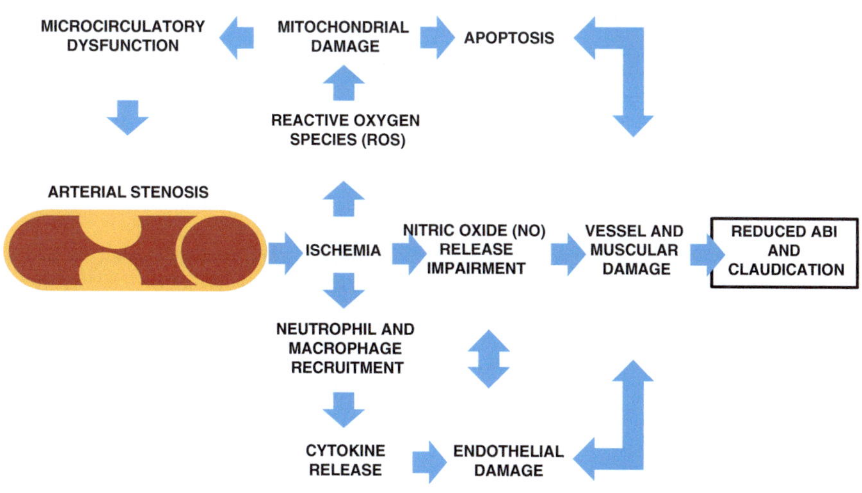

Fig. 2.2 Large/medium vessel and microcirculatory changes seen in claudication due to chronic PAD. (Adapted from Signorelli [20]. (*ABI* ankle brachial index))

the mechanisms of chronic changes in claudication due to PAD as also summarized by Signorelli SS and colleagues in 2019 [20].

This brief review of the physiology and pathophysiology of claudication outlines important implications for early and continued therapeutic intervention. Exercise (optimally in a supervised or otherwise structured format), smoking cessation, antiplatelet agent(s), statin initiation, and vasodilator therapy are all important initial therapies to consider, prior to any revascularization in nearly all, if not all, cases [21–24].

Summary

Peripheral artery disease (PAD) leads to macrovascular lesions reducing blood supply to the legs. This process reduces oxygen and metabolic substrate delivery to the legs and causes a mismatch with the metabolic requirements of skeletal muscle in the leg with exertion. However, reduced hemodynamics do not entirely account for observed exercise impairment; other mechanisms are likely to contribute to observed symptoms. The processes are due to ischemia and reperfusion at rest after exercise that are related to endothelial dysfunction, oxidant stress, inflammation, and muscle metabolic abnormalities. These phenomena provide and/or may provide opportunities for interventions aimed at the pathophysiology of exercise impairment in peripheral artery disease.

Competing Interests The authors have no competing interests.
Funding InformationThis research received no specific grant support from any funding agency in the public, commercial, or not-for-profit sectors.

References

1. Smith RB III. Claudication. In: Walker HK, Hall WD, Hurst JW, editors. Clinical methods: the history, physical, and laboratory examinations. 3rd ed. Boston: Butterworths; 1990. Chapter 13. Available from: https://www.ncbi.nlm.nih.gov/books/NBK235/.
2. Davies MG. Asymptomatic peripheral artery disease. In: UpToDate, Connor RF (Ed), Wolters Kluwer. Accessed 20 Feb 2025. https://www.uptodate.com/contents/asymptomatic-peripheral-artery-disease.
3. Meru AV, Mittra S, Thyagarajan B, Chugh A. Intermittent claudication: an overview. Atherosclerosis. 2006;187(2):221–37. https://doi.org/10.1016/j.atherosclerosis.2005.11.027.
4. Johnston AL, Vemulapalli S, Gosch KL, Aronow HD, Abbott JD, Patel MR, et al. Ankle-brachial index in patients with intermittent claudication is a poor indicator of patient-centered and clinician-based evaluations of functional status. J Vasc Surg. 2019 Mar;69(3):906–12.
5. Curci JA. Opportunities to explore the physiology of arterial insufficiency and claudication. J Vasc Surg. 2020 Mar;71(3):958.
6. Bakken AM, Palchik E, Hart JP, Rhodes JM, Saad WE, Davies MG. Impact of diabetes mellitus on outcomes of superficial femoral artery endoluminal interventions. J Vasc Surg. 2007;46(5):946–958; discussion 958. https://doi.org/10.1016/j.jvs.2007.06.047.
7. Bakken AM, Protack CD, Saad WE, Hart JP, Rhodes JM, Waldman DL, Davies MG. Impact of chronic kidney disease on outcomes of superficial femoral artery endoluminal interventions.

Ann Vasc Surg. 2009;23(5):560–8. https://doi.org/10.1016/j.avsg.2008.11.010. Epub 2009 Jan 6.
8. Brass EP, Hiatt WR, Green S. Skeletal muscle metabolic changes in peripheral arterial disease contribute to exercise intolerance: a point-counterpoint discussion. Vasc Med. 2004;9(4):293–301. https://doi.org/10.1191/1358863x04vm572ra.
9. Bapat GM, Bashir AZ, Malcolm P, Johanning JM, Pipinos II, Myers SA. A biomechanical perspective on walking in patients with peripheral artery disease. Vasc Med. 2023;28(1):77–84.
10. Cooke JP, Meng S. Vascular regeneration in peripheral artery disease. Arterioscler Thromb Vasc Biol. 2020;40(7):1627–34. 10.1161/ATVBAHA.120.312862. Epub 2020 May 21. PMID: 32434408; PMCID: PMC7357605.
11. Hiatt WR, Armstrong EJ, Larson CJ, Brass EP. Pathogenesis of the limb manifestations and exercise limitations in peripheral artery disease. Circ Res. 2015;116(9):1527–39. https://doi.org/10.1161/CIRCRESAHA.116.303566.
12. Koutakis P, Myers SA, Cluff K, Ha DM, Haynatzki G, McComb RD, et al. Abnormal myofiber morphology and limb dysfunction in claudication. J Surg Res. 2015;196(1):172–9.
13. Pipinos II, Judge AR, Selsby JT, Zhu Z, Swanson SA, Nella AA, Dodd SL. The myopathy of peripheral arterial occlusive disease: part 1. Functional and histomorphological changes and evidence for mitochondrial dysfunction. Vasc Endovasc Surg. 2007;41(6):481–9. https://doi.org/10.1177/1538574407311106.
14. Pipinos II, Judge AR, Selsby JT, Zhu Z, Swanson SA, Nella AA, Dodd SL. The myopathy of peripheral arterial occlusive disease: part 2. Oxidative stress, neuropathy, and shift in muscle fiber type. Vasc Endovasc Surg. 2008;42(2):101–12. https://doi.org/10.1177/1538574408315995. Epub 2008 Apr 7.
15. Hamburg NM, Creager MA. Pathophysiology of intermittent claudication in peripheral artery disease. Circ J. 2017;81(3):281–9. https://doi.org/10.1253/circj.CJ-16-1286. Epub 2017 Jan 26.
16. Krishna SM, Moxon JV, Golledge J. A review of the pathophysiology and potential biomarkers for peripheral artery disease. Int J Mol Sci. 2015;16(5):11294–322. https://doi.org/10.3390/ijms160511294.
17. Soto PF, Jia CX, Rabkin DG, Hart JP, Carter YM, Sardo MJ, Hsu DT, Fisher PE, Pinsky DJ, Spotnitz HM. Improvement of rejection-induced diastolic abnormalities in rat cardiac allografts with inducible nitric oxide synthase inhibition. J Thorac Cardiovasc Surg. 2000;120(1):39–46. https://doi.org/10.1067/mtc.2000.107124.
18. Hassabi M, Hassani M, Abedi-Yekta AH, Esfahani MP, Rabbani A, Salehi S, Khodabakhshian S, Aliabbar S. The calf muscle strength correlation with the severity of ischemia and outcomes in patients with chronic lower limb ischemia. J Bodyw Mov Ther. 2025;42:115–9. https://doi.org/10.1016/j.jbmt.2024.12.001. ISSN 1360-8592.
19. McDermott MM. Lower extremity manifestations of peripheral artery disease: the pathophysiologic and functional implications of leg ischemia. Circ Res. 2015;116(9):1540–50.
20. Signorelli SS, Scuto S, Marino E, Xourafa A, Gaudio A. Oxidative stress in peripheral arterial disease (PAD) mechanism and biomarkers. Antioxidants. 2019;8(9):367. https://doi.org/10.3390/antiox8090367.
21. Hamburg NM, Balady GJ. Exercise rehabilitation in peripheral artery disease: functional impact and mechanisms of benefits. Circulation. 2011;123(1):87–97. https://doi.org/10.1161/CIRCULATIONAHA.109.881888. PMID: 21200015; PMCID: PMC3061490.
22. Signorelli SS, Vanella L, Abraham NG, Scuto S, Marino E, Rocic P. Pathophysiology of chronic peripheral ischemia: new perspectives. Ther Adv Chronic Dis. 2020;11:2040622319894466. https://doi.org/10.1177/2040622319894466.
23. McDermott MM. Medical Management of Functional Impairment in peripheral artery disease: a review. Prog Cardiovasc Dis. 2018;60(6):586–92.
24. Hiatt WR. Medical treatment of peripheral arterial disease and claudication. N Engl J Med. 2001;344(21):1608–21.

3 National and International Trends in Prevalence and Incidence of Intermittent Claudication Since 1950

Erika T. Beidelman and Corey A. Kalbaugh

Vasculogenic intermittent claudication is an early-stage sequelae of peripheral artery disease (PAD) characterized by exercise-induced pain or fatigue in the lower extremities that is relieved with rest. The purpose of this chapter is to present data on the epidemiology of intermittent claudication (claudication, herein, for brevity), both nationally (United States) and internationally, with attention to trends over time. We define epidemiology as "the science that studies disease occurrence and health states in human populations" [1]. Herein, we focus on two specific measures of disease occurrence: prevalence and incidence. Prevalence is the proportion of a population with a disease at a specific time. Incidence is a measure of new events or changes in health states over time [2]. This chapter presents information only about claudication and only from studies that measured claudication specifically. Thus, studies are excluded if PAD is broadly measured or if research exclusively measured other manifestations of PAD, including chronic limb-threatening ischemia (CLTI), to the exclusion of intermittent claudication.

E. T. Beidelman
Department of Epidemiology and Biostatistics, Indiana University School of Public Health-Bloomington, Bloomington, IN, USA

Robert N. Butler Columbia Aging Center, Columbia University Mailman School of Public Health, New York, NY, USA
e-mail: ebeidelm@iu.edu

C. A. Kalbaugh (✉)
Department of Epidemiology and Biostatistics, Indiana University School of Public Health-Bloomington, Bloomington, IN, USA
e-mail: ckalbaug@iu.edu

W. P. Robinson III, J. P. Simons (eds.), *The Patient-Centered Approach to Claudication*, https://doi.org/10.1007/978-3-032-02460-2_3

A Brief History

The term claudication comes from the Latin *claudicare*, which means to limp, and is thought to have originated from Claudius, a first-century Roman Emperor who had a pronounced limp when he walked [3]. The etiology of his limp is unknown but it is likely that the cause was multi-factorial. Even fast fast-forwarding 2000 years, the cause of a limp in today's patient remains challenging to evaluate for clinicians. Similarly, epidemiologists face challenges in correctly quantifying the disease burden of claudication at a population level. First, claudication is a subtype of the more common PAD but is not always delineated as such in research studies. Instead, PAD and claudication are difficult to extract from each other in most data sources. Second, as lower extremity pain is the primary symptom, physicians face a challenge to correctly diagnose PAD-related claudication versus other causes of leg pain including sciatica, osteoarthritis, and neurogenic pain that present similarly. Third, patients may have difficulty describing their symptoms in a way that indicates a vascular cause or, because of other comorbidities like pulmonary disease, might not be able to walk far enough to produce the classic symptoms of claudication. Patients may self-limit in ways that prevent true claudication symptoms. McDermott et al. found that the majority of patients presenting with leg pain do not have classic symptoms (Fig. 3.1). To help in identifying the type of pain, they classified symptoms based on the location (calf vs. other), timing (rest and/or exercise), and the context of an individuals' activity level and ability to carry on through the pain [4]. They found that many patients with abnormal hemodynamic measurements are either asymptomatic or have leg pain symptoms that are distinctly different than classic intermittent claudication. These differences in leg pain presentation were also found to be associated with different severity of outcomes. We mention this to remind the reader that it is critically important to know if your patient has PAD, regardless of whether they have classic claudication. The ABI remains an incredibly valuable tool to diagnose broader PAD, which is vital information due to the adverse event risks of people who have PAD compared to the general population even if those with PAD are asymptomatic.

Over time, as physicians realized the difficulties in identifying true intermittent claudication, several questionnaires were created to disentangle intermittent claudication from other causes of leg pain. These questionnaires have been used as an attempt to estimate the true prevalence or incidence of claudication at a population level. Below we will detail the three claudication-specific questionnaires that have been most commonly used to estimate intermittent claudication in a defined population. Of note, we focus on studies that use both a claudication questionnaire and the ABI test to quantify both PAD and claudication (Fig. 3.2).

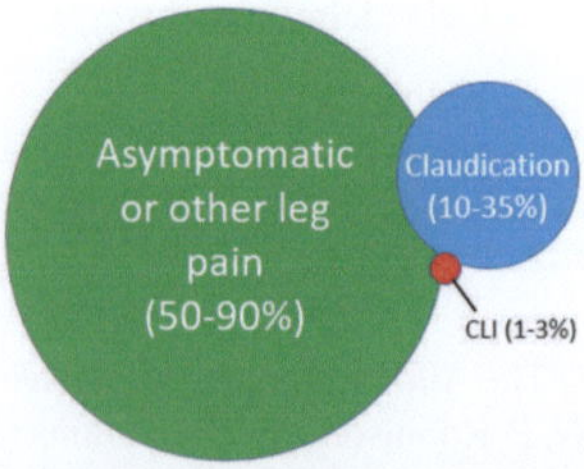

Fig. 3.1 Possible PAD manifestations

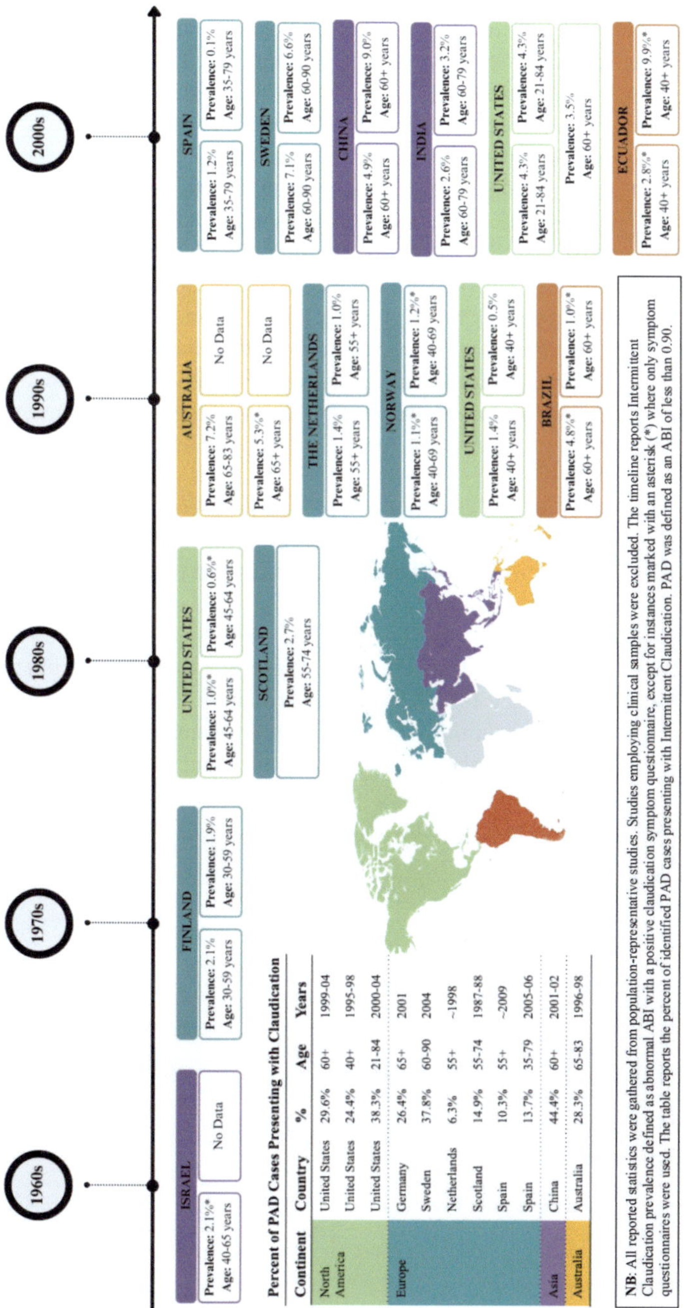

Continent	Country	%	Age	Years
North America	United States	29.6%	60+	1999-04
	United States	24.4%	40+	1995-98
	United States	38.3%	21-84	2000-04
Europe	Germany	26.4%	65+	2001
	Sweden	37.8%	60-90	2004
	Netherlands	6.3%	55+	~1998
	Scotland	14.9%	55-74	1987-88
	Spain	10.3%	55+	~2009
	Spain	13.7%	35-79	2005-06
Asia	China	44.4%	60+	2001-02
Australia	Australia	28.3%	65-83	1996-98

Fig. 3.2 Global burden of PAD over time

Measurement Tools for Intermittent Claudication

For more than 60 years, claudication has been a defined and measured disease outcome within cardiovascular studies. Within the literature, the most used objective measure to quantify the broad category of PAD is the ankle-brachial index (ABI). ABI is a non-invasive test that compares systolic blood pressure in the pedal arteries to brachial artery systolic pressure. An ABI value <0.90 or > 1.40 has been used to identify PAD and is a cut-point used to detect asymptomatic disease. The ABI test has a high sensitivity (>90%) and a high specificity (>90%) in detecting >50% occlusion of an arterial segment in contrast angiography. However, ABI is not a tool that can be used to delineate PAD from the more specific intermittent claudication, which indicates a symptomatic pathology. In clinical settings, an exercise ABI test can be used to confirm or exclude a vascular-caused claudication disorder. The use of the exercise ABI test in research studies is, however, uncommon. Most research that aims to quantify the burden of claudication relies on the use of symptom questionnaires. The various questionnaires in use are described below with a comparison provided in Table 3.1.

World Health Organization (WHO)/Rose Intermittent Claudication Questionnaire

The Rose Questionnaire (1962) was created to target the diagnosis of intermittent claudication in epidemiologic research and to facilitate international comparisons of prevalence estimates [5]. Initially, the Rose Questionnaire (RQ) was administered to 37 individuals with intermittent claudication and a control group of 18 individuals with other types of diagnosed walking-induced leg pain (control group). Thirty-four (92%) of the 37 patients with intermittent claudication met all six

Table 3.1 Claudication assessment questionnaire comparison

	Questionnaire		
Question	WHO/RQ[a]	ECQ[b]	SDCQ[c]
Do you get pain in either leg on walking?	Y	Y	Y
Do you get pain in either buttock (right or left)?			Y
Does this pain ever begin when you are standing still?	Y		Y
Does this pain ever begin when you are sitting?		Y	Y
Do you get this pain in your calf (or calves?)	Y		
Where do you get this pain or discomfort?		Y	
In what part of the leg or buttock do you feel it?			Y
Do you get it when you walk uphill or hurry?	Y	Y	Y
Do you get it when you walk at an ordinary pace on the level?	Y		Y
Does the pain ever disappear while you are still walking?	Y		Y
What do you do if you get it when you are walking?	Y		Y
What happens to it if you stand still?	Y	Y	Y
How soon?			Y

[a]World Health Organization adaptation of the Rose Questionnaire; [b]Edinburgh Claudication Questionnaire; [c]San Diego Claudication Questionnaire

criteria outlined to delineate intermittent claudication from other leg pain syndromes while none of the control group met the criteria [5].

The Rose Questionnaire was adopted by the World Health Organization (WHO/RQ, herein) in 1968 to determine PAD prevalence rates [6]. The WHO/RQ was modified in 1977 to enable self-administration [7]. Studies have found sensitivity values that range from 9% to 92% and specificity values that range from 95% to 100% [8].

Despite its ease of use and the various adaptations, there are limitations to using the WHO/RQ in population-based research. First, while false positives are exceedingly rare, false negatives are common which is consistent with the lower sensitivity reported above. Second, it is not possible to detect CLTI using this instrument. Even with the survey limitations, the WHO/RQ was commonly used to screen for claudication and was, for decades, the primary survey tool used to identify claudication in population-based research [9–12].

Edinburgh Claudication Questionnaire

While the WHO/RQ is highly specific, the moderate sensitivity results shown across several population-based studies led scientists at the London School of Tropical Medicine and Hygiene to create a new questionnaire, the Edinburgh Claudication Questionnaire (ECQ) [13]. Leng et al. (1992) found more than 50% of the false negatives generated by the WHO/RQ resulted from one question: *Does your pain disappear on walking?* [13] These investigators also found that the specificity was upheld by asking only three particular questions: 1) *Do you have pain when standing/sitting?* 2) *Do you have pain in the calf?* and 3) *Is your pain gone in 10 minutes of stopping?* [13] The investigators pre-tested new questions and piloted their new survey in 300 subjects. The ECQ had a sensitivity of 91.4% and a specificity of 99.3%, and repeatability was excellent at 6 months (kappa = 0.76) [13]. The ECQ is only moderately sensitive (~50%) in detecting PAD in high-risk patients [14, 15].

San Diego Claudication Questionnaire

Neither the WHO/RQ nor the ECQ allows for leg-specific (right versus left) assessment of claudication symptoms. While calf pain is the most typical location of pain in those with claudication, the WHO/RQ and ECQ surveys also do not allow for assessment of non-calf claudication. With these limitations in mind, the San Diego Claudication Questionnaire (SDCQ) was created and tested among 508 patients [16]. The SDCQ contains questions about anatomic location of pain and the extremity (left, right, both) affected. In the study by Criqui et al. (1996), the SDCQ identified 40% more claudication than the WHO/RQ when administered to the same participants [17].

Each of these questionnaires has benefits and drawbacks, and each has been used extensively in population-based studies of PAD and claudication. Schorr and

Treat-Jacobson reported inconsistency across studies in how these questionnaires were utilized causing biased prevalence estimates [8]. In Table 3.2, we describe the questions contained within each of these three questionnaires, highlighting the differences between the questions used to assess claudication in each questionnaire. We remind the reader that these differences make it difficult to make comparisons across studies.

Methods—Search Strategy

While we did not conduct a formal systematic review, we do intend to offer a reproducible search. After several consultations—and numerous search iterations—with our university health science librarians, we were able to refine our search to a single search term using one MeSH Major topic: "Intermittent Claudication/epidemiology" [MAJR]. MeSH Major topics are used to denote main topics of articles and their use is an effective way to narrow findings from MeSH terms, which are applied more liberally, and we found it gave us too many non-relevant studies. Our MeSH Major search yielded 157 studies to review. We then found additional studies by backward citation chasing within the bibliographies of the full texts from our search results. Our goal was to identify as many relevant populations as possible. Many of the older epidemiologic studies are not referenced in modern papers and, while laborious, the citation chasing method helped us to feel confident about our representation of the broader literature. As a specific example, there was a study based in Paris with findings written only in French, which is referenced in numerous papers that, despite our best efforts, was not identified in our PubMed search.

Incidence Estimates

The first attempts to adequately measure claudication and, to date, our best incidence data come from longitudinal cohort studies with defined populations. However, measurements of incidence remain relatively rare within the literature with no contemporary estimates available. No global-level incidence estimates for intermittent claudication currently exist. In the following section, we present detailed findings from the seminal cohort studies. We categorize studies by continent (see Table 3.1), although true incidence studies largely originate from high-income North American and European countries. Notably, the only study that considered trends over multiple decades was the Framingham Study.

Table 3.2 Hemodynamic and questionnaire-defined PAD and intermittent claudication

	ABI <0.90	ABI >0.90
Questionnaire positive	++	−+
Questionnaire negative	+−	−−

North America

The Framingham Heart Study (FHS) is a community-based cohort study from the community of Framingham, Massachusetts, an industrial and trading center of approximately 30,000 individuals [18]. A sample of 5209 participants (29 to 62 years of age at baseline), chosen based on a local census list and stratified by family size and precinct of residence, was enrolled in the study. The investigators measured the presence of intermittent claudication using criteria of cramping discomfort with exercise that was relieved with rest derived from a physician-administered questionnaire. All intermittent claudication cases were reviewed and adjudicated by a panel of investigators [19]. Over the first 14 years of follow-up in the 1950s and 1960s, 125 cases of intermittent claudication were identified with an average annual incidence of intermittent claudication of 2.6 per 1000 person-years among men and 1.2 per 1000 person-years among women. A follow-up study assessed temporal trends of intermittent claudication incidence over a fifty-year period [20]. Incident cases increased through the 1970s with a peak rate of 3.4 per 1000 from 1970 to 1979. The number of cases declined in the 1980s and 1990s and decreased to 2.2 per 1000 from 1990 to 1999 [20].

In addition to the original FHS, the Framingham Offspring Study enrolled offspring (n = 3548, ages 5 to 70) and their spouses (n = 1576) of the original cohort [21, 22]. The 12-year cumulative incidence rates for participants enrolled between 1971 and 1998, adjusted for age and sex, were 5.1 per 1000 person-years (95% CI: 2.7–7.3) among participants with a parental history of intermittent claudication, compared to 2.3 per 1000 person-years (95% CI: 1.5–3.2) among those without a parental history of intermittent claudication. This is the only study identified that examined family history of intermittent claudication as a predictor of intermittent claudication, finding that offspring that had a parent with intermittent claudication were nearly twice as likely to develop intermittent claudication than offspring whose parents did not have a history of intermittent claudication [21].

Finally, the Quebec Cardiovascular Study enrolled 4637 men aged 35–64 years old, representing approximately 2/3 of a random sample of seven Quebec City suburbs [23, 24]. The Quebec Study was designed to better understand the role of important risk factors (smoking, blood pressure, cholesterol) on the incidence of ischemic cardiovascular disease. Claudication was assessed using the WHO/RQ with diagnostic validation performed by a cardiologist. During 12 years of follow-up from 1974 to 1986, 188 participants developed intermittent claudication (4.1/1000 person-years). Investigators found important relationships of smoking history as well as increased levels of smoking (high vs low usage) with the incidence of claudication. A later study with an extended follow-up period found that 6.8% of participants developed intermittent claudication between 1974 and 1998. Additionally, this study found that participants with claudication had twice the risk of fatal and nonfatal cardiovascular events compared to those with no cardiovascular disease [25].

Europe

The Edinburgh Artery Study (EAS) examined the natural history of PAD among 1592 residents of Edinburgh, Scotland aged 55–74 years [26]. EAS investigators used ABI measurements with hyperemic drop calculation and administration of the WHO/RQ to estimate asymptomatic and symptomatic PAD, respectively [26]. Follow-up for the EAS [27] identified 116 incident intermittent claudication cases (15.5 per 1000 person-years) over 5 years of follow-up. Men had a higher incidence proportion of intermittent claudication than women (8.7% vs. 6.6%). Over 5 years of follow-up, 8.2% of those with intermittent claudication had a myocardial infarction (MI), 9.6% developed new angina, and 6.8% had a major cerebrovascular event. People with claudication had the highest mortality rate within the sample, with approximately 20% deceased at 5 years of follow-up and 13.7% deceased due to a cardiovascular-related cause [27]. They also had over two times the risk of cardiovascular death, non-cardiovascular death, and angina compared to those without claudication.

The Reykjavik Study invited men with legal residence in the city of Reykjavik and adjacent communities (Dec 1, 1966) who were 34–79 years of age [28, 29]. Claudication was defined by the WHO/RQ with physician confirmation. Over nearly 20 years of follow-up, investigators found a 66% decrease after 1970 in the incidence of claudication compared to baseline. Important risk factors included age, a history of smoking, and higher serum cholesterol. Incidence declined from 6.0 to 2.0 per 1000 person years for those aged 70+ and from 1.7 to 0.6 per 1000 person years for those aged 50–69.

Asia. The Israeli Heart Disease Project was a longitudinal study of cardiovascular disease among 10,059 Israeli male civil servants (aged ≥40 years) [30]. Intermittent claudication was assessed via the WHO-London School of Hygiene Intermittent Claudication Questionnaire. Clinician confirmation of cases was not performed. In 1963, there were 8343 participants that were free of baseline coronary heart disease and peripheral vascular disease symptoms. Over a five-year follow-up period, 360 previously healthy men were found to have intermittent claudication upon nurse-administered questionnaire. There was a crude annual incidence rate of 8.6 cases per 1000 person-years from 1963 to 1968. Five-year cumulative incidence rate was 43.1 per 1000 person-years.

Prevalence Estimates

While incidence is a measure of disease occurrence in people that were previously free of disease, prevalence is an important measure of how significant a problem is in defined populations as prevalence quantifies how many people actually have and are living with a particular disease. While contemporary global estimates for the prevalence of PAD as a whole are readily available, precise estimates for the global burden of claudication specifically remain limited. A systematic review found that 5.6% of the global population (236 million people) aged 25 years and older have some form of PAD as defined by an abnormal ABI [31]. Additionally, it is commonly reported that 10–35% of all PAD patients have classic claudication [32]. Therefore, despite a lack of global estimations, we can assume that somewhere between 23 and 75 million people worldwide currently have intermittent claudication. Importantly, an additional >50% have some form of non-classic claudication-type pain that also warrants evaluation and longitudinal outcome measurement [33].

Below we offer a summary of studies that measure the prevalence of claudication. Given the volume of studies (prevalence is reported far more frequently than incidence), we highlight representative studies from each Continent in the text. As with studies measuring incidence, we focus our prevalence studies on those that measured claudication using a claudication-specific questionnaire with ABI measurement. When available, we comment on the results by the easy-to-interpret four-category findings of (ab)normal ABI and positive/negative questionnaire (Table 3.2). Lastly, due to the readership, we also focus on studies done in clinical settings (higher risk) and on more recent studies that include information on structurally vulnerable groups where available.

North America

There are numerous cardiovascular disease-focused longitudinal studies based in the United States. A few exemplars that have measured broader PAD include the Multi-Ethnic Study of Atherosclerosis (MESA) [34], the Cardiovascular Health Study (CHS) [35], The Strong Heart Study [36], the Atherosclerosis Risk in Communities (ARIC) Study [37], and The Women's Health Initiative (WHI) [38]. Very few studies, however, have measured claudication specifically. The Jackson Heart Study is a prospective longitudinal cohort of 5306 Black adults in the American South. Of 4586 participants with ABI and SDCQ measurements, 4.2% (n = 195) had an abnormal ABI and a positive SDQC [39]. Therefore, of people with abnormal ABI (n = 509), 38% were symptomatic. In addition, 30.7% of the sample had a positive claudication questionnaire regardless of ABI status. Interestingly, the Jackson Heart Study recently reported a nearly linear trend in outcomes which they found were worst in the group with abnormal ABI (<0.90 or > 1.40) and a positive claudication survey, followed by abnormal ABI and a negative claudication survey, then normal ABI and a positive claudication survey, and the best outcomes are observed in those with normal ABI and a negative claudication survey result [39]. Additional studies from the United States have produced estimates of claudication prevalence ranging from 0.8% in adults aged 45–64 to 3.8% in adults aged 60 + [22, 40, 41]. Across the United States studies, men tended to have a slightly higher prevalence of claudication compared to women. The percentage of PAD cases exhibiting symptoms of claudication ranged from 24.4% to 38.3%.

Europe. There are numerous PAD-related prevalence studies conducted in Europe which, as in the United States, primarily use the ABI and do not include claudication-specific measurement. We recommend to the reader the Whitehall Study [42] (Smith), the Observational German Epidemiological Trial on Ankle

Brachial Index (getABI) [43], and the Limburg Peripheral Artery Occlusive Disease (PAOD) Study [44]. Within these studies, only a few examine the proportion of people with intermittent claudication. Across these European settings, findings generally showed a prevalence of claudication in older adults between 4% and 8% [10, 26, 43, 45] with the exception of the Rotterdam Study. In the Rotterdam Study [9], intermittent claudication prevalence was estimated at 1.2%. Additionally, only 6% of people with abnormal ABI reported symptoms of intermittent claudication by the WHO/RQ while ~1% of people with normal ABI reported symptoms. Across other European studies, it has been reported that approximately 10–38% of prevalent PAD cases in older adults presented with symptoms of claudication.

South America

We identified only three South American studies that measured ABI and included a claudication questionnaire. The Hearts of Brazil Project was a national, multicenter, cross-sectional study of 1170 individuals (>18 years) from 72 major Brazilian urban centers [46]. They found only 1% of individuals had abnormal ABI and a positive ECQ. Only 9% of people who had abnormal ABI values had a positive ECQ. In the Bambui Health Aging Study, a complete population study of older adults in a rural and low-income municipality of Brazil found a claudication prevalence of 4.8% among men and 1.0% among women [47]. The Atahualpa Study, a population-based study in older aged adults living in rural Ecuador, found that 26% of enrollees had an abnormal ABI [48]. However, only 3% (8/261) of enrolled participants had an abnormal ABI and a positive ECQ which accounted for only 12% (8/68) of people with an abnormal ABI.

Asia

Asian countries have significant heterogeneity in terms of health status. While higher income countries like Japan, South Korea, and Singapore have among the highest life expectancies in the world, countries in Western Asia (e.g., Yemen, Afghanistan) tend to have among the lowest life expectancies. As with overall health, estimates of PAD and claudication vary widely across Asian countries. A population-based study in Wanshoulu Community of Haidian District in Beijing, China, found that 11.3% of people 60 years of age or older had abnormal ABI and a positive WHO/RQ and that 44.4% of participants with PAD defined by abnormal ABI had evidence of claudication [11]. A study in Kerala, South India, found 7% of participants had a positive WHO/RQ but only 11% of the abnormal ABI group also had the positive WHO/RQ. Overall, only 3% of people had both abnormal ABI and a positive WHO/RQ [49].

Africa

We know that African countries have among the highest prevalences of PAD in the world [50]. A systematic review of sub-Saharan African countries found PAD prevalence ranging from 3.1% in healthy adults to 52% among people with diabetes. The Health and Aging in Africa: Longitudinal Studies in South Africa (HAALSA) [51] cohort is one of few well-designed prospective studies that measured PAD. Still, there are few studies of intermittent claudication on the African continent and population-representative studies of burden are especially lacking. One study enrolled patients with pre-existing diabetes from the Korle-Bu Teaching Hospital in Accra, Ghana (2009–2010) and an age- and gender-matched healthy cohort recruited from communities surrounding the Hospital (Yeboah) [52]. Using ABI and the ECQ, investigators found that 3.5% of all study participants had both low ABI and classic claudication, including 2.6% of the diabetes group and 0.9% of the healthy controls. Okella et al [53] found that 10.5% of patients with diabetes from a clinic in Southwestern Uganda had abnormal ABI and positive Edinburgh questionnaire.

Australia

Australia was an important participant in The Reduction of Atherothrombosis for Continued Health (REACH) registry, a large multi-national study of patients at high risk of developing a cardiovascular disease. Australia was the only country that recruited patients from primary care settings and subsequently performed ABI and a claudication survey on all 2489 eligible participants [54]. Investigators found 4.7% of people (117/2489) had an abnormal ABI and a positive ECQ. An additional 6.2% (154/2489) had a positive ECQ but normal ABI and another 23.1% (576/2489) of participants had an abnormal ABI but negative ECQ. This high-risk population was then followed for 1 year and an additional 6% were found to have developed intermittent claudication. In a second study, which measured claudication among a sample of men from the Western Australia State Electoral role, investigators found that 2.5% (167/6582) of participants had an abnormal ABI and a positive Edinburgh questionnaire [55]. They also found that only 28% of people with abnormal ABI had a positive Edinburgh, concluding that 70% of people with PAD were either asymptomatic or had non-classic claudication.

Summary

Current research on the burden of intermittent claudication, though limited, suggests that a significant proportion of older adults globally are affected by the condition. Across population-representative studies measuring claudication as both an abnormal ABI and positive symptom questionnaire, we estimated a pooled prevalence of approximately 4.4%. The highest claudication prevalences were observed in China, Germany, and Sweden. However, the majority of prevalence estimates fell between approximately 3% and 7%. As expected, studies performed in older populations showed higher claudication burdens. This was true across all geographic locations except for the Jackson Heart Study set in Mississippi. Despite a population including adults as young as 21 years old, claudication prevalence was estimated to be 4.2%. In comparison, other studies including younger adults most commonly estimated prevalence at <1%. This difference may be due to the primary low-income and minority population, suggesting a higher risk among vulnerable groups.

The WHO/RQ was commonly used as the diagnostic tool for claudication in available studies. However, this tool is no longer used in practice and researchers generally agree that studies that used the WHO/RQ likely underestimated the burden of claudication. Indeed, in our review of the literature, studies employing the WHO/RQ produced some of the lowest estimates of claudication prevalence. The Edinburgh Claudication Questionnaire is most frequently used in studies outside of the United States, and the San Diego Claudication Questionnaire is mostly used in US-based settings. This illustrates the significant heterogeneity in the diagnostic assessment of claudication across studies, making cross-study comparisons difficult. Additionally, age inclusion criteria are largely varied across the literature. The age structure of the sample should be taken into account when interpreting burden estimations.

The majority of longitudinal studies on intermittent claudication have focused on men in the dominant race and ethnicity group where the study was completed (e.g., White Americans in the United States). Despite the focus on men, from available studies including women we can see that they generally have a lower prevalence of claudication compared to men. However, this focus has created the obvious issue of having limited data on how claudication impacts structurally vulnerable groups [56], such as women and racial and ethnic minority groups. Here we want to remind clinicians that diseases where pain is a presenting symptom tend to be underestimated in structurally vulnerable populations. In the United States, there has been a tendency to blame the patient. It is not uncommon to hear that Black patients have a genetic predisposition to more severe disease or are late care seekers. We suggest that anyone treating patients who have leg pain have an opportunity to not further propagate disparities.

Even after a successful diagnosis, all people with claudication who have a revascularization are at a higher risk of subsequent amputation and other poor vascular outcomes [57]. Most troubling, however, is that research has shown that structurally vulnerable groups [56] are more likely to undergo early and potentially harmful surgical management for claudication, contributing to well-documented disparities in treatment outcomes. Black patients are more likely to undergo early peripheral revascularizations for claudication (within the first 6 months of diagnosis) compared to their White peers [58, 59] and are also more likely to undergo surgical interventions on below the knee arteries, which for claudication, are considered risk greater than benefit and are not supported by current professional guidelines [60–62]. Additionally, Black patients are >2 times as likely to experience an adverse event following a procedure as their White peers, including a 2–4 times increased risk of major limb amputation. Women, and particularly women from minoritized groups, and people with limited education and lower income are also more likely to undergo premature surgical management and have poor post-operative outcomes.

What Are the Trends and Why Do They Matter?

At the time of this writing, new data is continuing to emerge in high-income countries that the trends in coronary heart disease-related mortality, which had precipitously declined since the 1950s, are slowing, if not beginning to increase. Will these same trends hold true for the incidence of other conditions associated with high mortality, like intermittent claudication? The answer remains unclear as no population-representative studies on the burden of claudication post the early 2000s were available. Still, from available data, we can see that the percentage of PAD cases presenting with claudication may be increasing over time with the most recent studies showing the highest proportions (26–44% of cases). This skews higher than the commonly reported figure that 10–30% of PAD cases have claudication. Clinicians should remain vigilant to the risk of claudication within their patients given this trend.

Currently, 9 out of 10 people with clinically defined claudication die from a cardiovascular cause [63]. Within 1 year of diagnosis, 34% of patients with PAD-related claudication have one or more major adverse vascular events, such as myocardial infarction (4%), stroke (8%), or death (12%) [64–66]. Patients who experience a major adverse vascular event are particularly expensive to manage with costs ranging from $58 K per patient year following an ischemic stroke to $108 K per patient year among patients who required a limb amputation [67]. These expenses are not sustainable and are overburdening our health systems.

The good news here is that these poor outcomes remain largely preventable. The Global Burden 2019 Study found that nearly 70% of PAD is preventable with aggressive risk factor modification. Patients with PAD across all subtypes should be prescribed and should complete guideline directed medical therapy (GDMT), which is clearly defined and consists of antiplatelet therapy, cholesterol management with a high-intensity statin, blood pressure management with antihypertensives, diabetes management via diet and medication, and smoking cessation counseling [60, 68]. However, only <1 in 5 patients with PAD ever complete GDMT [69] and not completing GDMT definitely increases the risk of major adverse vascular events. We reported that compared to patients who receive 6 months of GDMT, patients undergoing surgical revascularization for claudication prematurely have a two-fold risk of conversion to CLTI, a 2.6-fold risk of major lower extremity amputation, and a nearly seven-fold risk of repeat invasive peripheral vascular intervention [70].

All studies we reviewed found increasing prevalence and incidence of claudication with age. Given the definitive correlation between age and disease burden, countries with aging populations will likely see increases in claudication. While people may be smoking less now, at least in high-income countries, the proportion of the population with diabetes is dramatically increasing. As such, the etiology of claudication may be changing and becoming more challenging to identify and manage. Demonstrated by the association with severe adverse outcomes including mortality, it remains critical to prevent and diagnose claudication within this changing landscape. Notably in regard to prevention, diabetes is thought to be the most relevant modifiable risk factor in people with younger populations and smoking is the leading modifiable risk factor in older aged populations [71]. Trends in the prevalence of these and other critical risk factors will need to be closely monitored.

Remaining Gaps and Future Directions

Despite the relatively high proportion of PAD cases presenting with claudication in the most recent studies, health professional and public awareness of all PAD-related disorders remain low in comparison with awareness of other cardiovascular diseases. Up to 50% of those with PAD are unaware they have the disease and physicians often fail to evaluate for the presence of PAD [72]. Generally, PAD and all its sequelae have been understudied for decades. The majority of studies with longitudinal follow-up began—and ended for most—in the twentieth century. More recently, claudication has been the subject of fewer studies than CLTI, despite at least a tenfold higher burden. Due to this, clinicians should remain aware that the current burden of claudication is largely unknown with evidence pointing to increasing burdens.

Nearly 70% of all people with a PAD sequela live in low- and middle-income countries (LMICs) yet there is very little data on the burden of claudication in LMICs. The limited data we found suggested that people living in low-income contexts are more likely to develop PAD and claudication at an earlier age than their peers in high-income countries. PAD and claudication can be challenging to identify in lower resourced settings as many lack the tools required to perform the test. Claudication questionnaires have not been translated into many languages and the ABI requires both tools and training. The ABI is also unreliable in patients with diabetes due to calcification of arteries or the presence of skin wounds, necessitating an additional modality such as the toe-brachial index. While the toe-brachial index (TBI) is useful, there are major issues regarding the usage of different detection systems and experimental conditions such as skin temperature. The relationship of TBI to the diagnosis of PAD requires further study. Increasing awareness—and providing resources—to LMIC settings is paramount in places where people may be at earlier risk.

We continue to need better data for the myriad of vascular diseases, and it is the opinion of these authors that PAD and all its sequelae (including intermittent claudication) are vastly underestimated—in measures of disease occurrence and all the attributable outcomes that are missed as a result of underestimating disease occurrence. This is evident from the large proportion of available studies employing the WHO/RQ for claudication diagnosis. From a data standpoint, we need to unify definitions across our study populations and agree upon criteria for these definitions. As is the purpose of this book, we need to further define what matters to the patient with intermittent claudication as it may differ based on symptomatology. Related, while intermittent claudication is clinically defined by either Fontaine's classification [73] or Rutherford's categories [74], we were unable to find any data indicating what proportion of symptoms fall within each disease stage. And we currently do not know why ABI is an effective measure of asymptomatic disease but is not directly correlated with symptoms or functional limitations. Lastly, we remain unsure as to how the vascular community might overcome a disease with serious branding issues. In naming a disease "peripheral" with a subtype that is called "intermittent," we should not wonder why others outside our vascular community see these problems as unimportant (*peripheral* artery disease) or only occasionally problematic (*intermittent* claudication). We must put some of our energy into this problem so that people understand the significance of PAD and its sequelae.

References

1. Rothman KJ, Lash TL, Haneuse S, VanderWeele TJ. The scope of epidemiology. In: Modern epidemiology; 2021. p. 3–15.
2. Lash TL, Rothman KJ, Lash T, VanderWeele T, Haneuse S, Rothman K. Measures of occurrence. In: Modern epidemiology. Wolters Kluwer; 2021. p. 53–77.
3. Meru AV, Mittra S, Thyagarajan B, Chugh A. Intermittent claudication: an overview. Atherosclerosis. 2006;187:221–37. https://doi.org/10.1016/j.atherosclerosis.2005.11.027.
4. McDermott MM, Greenland P, Liu K, Guralnik JM, Criqui MH, Dolan NC, Chan C, Celic L, Pearce WH, Schneider JR, et al. Leg symptoms in peripheral arterial disease: associated clinical characteristics and functional impairment. JAMA. 2001;286:1599–606. https://doi.org/10.1001/jama.286.13.1599.
5. Rose GA. The diagnosis of ischaemic heart pain and intermittent claudication in field surveys. Bull WHO. 1962;27:645–58.
6. Rose GA, Blackburn H. Cardiovascular survey methods. Monogr Ser. 1968;56:1–188.
7. Rose G, McCartney P, Reid DD. Self-administration of a questionnaire on chest pain and intermittent claudication. Br J Prev Soc Med. 1977;31:42–8.
8. Schorr EN, Treat-Jacobson D. Methods of symptom evaluation and their impact on peripheral artery disease (PAD) symptom prevalence: a review. Vasc Med. 2013;18:95–111. https://doi.org/10.1177/1358863X13480001.
9. Meijer WT, Hoes AW, Rutgers D, Bots ML, Hofman A, Grobbee DE. Peripheral arterial disease in the elderly : the Rotterdam study. Arterioscler Thromb Vasc Biol. 1998;18:185–92. https://doi.org/10.1161/01.atv.18.2.185.
10. Sigvant B, Wiberg-Hedman K, Bergqvist D, Rolandsson O, Andersson B, Persson E, Wahlberg E. A population-based study of peripheral arterial disease prevalence with special focus on critical limb ischemia and sex differences. J Vasc Surg. 2007;45:1185–91. https://doi.org/10.1016/j.jvs.2007.02.004.
11. He Y, Jiang Y, Wang J, Fan L, Li X, Hu FB. Prevalence of peripheral arterial disease and its association with smoking in a population-based study in Beijing, China. J Vasc Surg. 2006;44:333–8. https://doi.org/10.1016/j.jvs.2006.03.032.
12. Criqui MH, Fronek A, Barrett-Connor E, Klauber MR, Gabriel S, Goodman D. The prevalence of peripheral arterial disease in a defined population. Circulation. 1985;71:510–5.
13. Leng GC, Fowkes FGR. The Edinburgh claudication questionnaire: an improved version of the WHO/Rose questionnaire for use in epidemiological surveys. J Clin Epidemiol. 1992;45:1101–9.

14. Sprynger M, Fassotte C, Verhaeghe R. The ankle-brachial pressure index and a standardized questionnaire are easy and useful tools to detect peripheral arterial disease in non-claudicating patients at high risk. Int Angiol. 2007;26:239–44.
15. Missault L, Krygier C, Lukito G, Mary-Rabine L. Occurrence of peripheral arterial disease in a Belgian cohort of patients with cardiovascular history of atherothrombosis. Acta Chir Belg. 2007;107:508–14.
16. Criqui MH, Denenberg JO, Bird CE, Fronek A, Klauber MR, Langer RD. The correlation between symptoms and non-invasive test results in patients referred for peripheral arterial disease testing. Vasc Med. 1996;1:65–71.
17. Criqui MH, Denenberg JO, Bird CE, Fronek A, Klauber MR, Langer A. The correlation between symptoms and non-invasive test results in patients referred for peripheral arterial disease testing. Vasc Med. 1996;1:65–71.
18. Dawber TR, Meadors GF, Moore FE. Epidemiological approaches to heart disease: the Framingham study. Am J Public Health. 1951;41:279–86.
19. Kannel WB, Skinner JJ, Schwartz MJ, Shurtleff D. Intermittent claudication: incidence in the Framingham study. Circulation. 1970;41:875–83. https://doi.org/10.1161/01.cir.41.5.875.
20. Murabito JM, Evans JC, D'Agostino RB, Wilson PWF, Kannel WB. Temporal trends in the incidence of intermittent claudication from 1950 to 1999. Am J Epidemiol. 2005;162:430–7.
21. Prushik SG, Farber A, Gona P, Shrader P, Pencina MJ, D'Agostino RB Sr, Murabito JM. Parental intermittent claudication as risk factor for claudication in adults. Am J Cardiol. 2012;109:736–41. https://doi.org/10.1016/j.amjcard.2011.10.032.
22. Murabito JM, Evans JC, Nieto K, Larson MG, Levy D, Wilson PWF. Prevalence and clinical correlates of peripheral arterial disease in the Framingham offspring study. Am Heart J. 2002;143:961–5. https://doi.org/10.1067/mhj.2002.122871.
23. Dagenais GR, Robitaille NM, Lupien PJ, Christen A, Gingras S, Moorjani S, Meyer F, Rochon J. First coronary heart disease event rates in relation to major risk factors: Quebec cardiovascular study. Can J Cardiol. 1990;6:274–80.
24. Dagenais GR, Maurice S, Robitaille NM, Gingras S, Lupien PJ. Intermittent claudication in Quebec men from 1974-1986: the Quebec cardiovascular study. Clin Invest Med. 1991;14:93–100.
25. St-Pierre A, Cantin B, Lamarche B, Auger D, Després J, Dagenais GR. Intermittent claudication: from its risk factors to its long-term prognosis in men. The Quebec cardiovascular study. Can J Cardiol. 2010;26:17–21. https://doi.org/10.1016/s0828-282x(10)70328-7.
26. Fowkes FGR, Housley E, Cawood EH, Macintyre CC, Ruckley CV, Prescott RJ. Edinburgh artery study: prevalence of asymptomatic peripheral arterial disease in the general population. Int J Epidemiol. 1991;20:384–92.
27. Leng GC, Lee AJ, Fowkes FG, Whiteman M, Dunbar J, Housley E, Ruckley CV. Incidence, natural history and cardiovascular events in symptomatic and asymptomatic peripheral arterial disease in the general population. Int J Epidemiol. 1996;25:1172–81.
28. Sigurdsson E, Thorgeirsson G, Sigvaldason H, Sigfusson N. Prevalence of coronary heart disease in Icelandic men 1968-1986. The Reykjavik Study. Eur Heart J. 1993;14:584–91. https://doi.org/10.1093/eurheartj/14.5.584.
29. Björnsson O, Davidsson D, Olafsson H, Olafsson O, Sigfusson N. Thorsteinsson Th. Health survey in the Reykjavík area Men Stages I-III. 1967;1968:1970–1.
30. Bowlin SJ, Medalie JH, Flocke SA, Zyzanski SJ, Goldbourt U. Epidemiology of intermittent claudication in middle-aged men. Am J Epidemiol. 1994;140:418–30. https://doi.org/10.1093/oxfordjournals.aje.a117264.
31. Song P, Rudan D, Zhu Y, Fowkes FJI, Rahimi K, Fowkes FGR, Rudan I. Global, regional, and national prevalence and risk factors for peripheral artery disease in 2015: an updated systematic review and analysis. Lancet Glob Health. 2019;7:e1020–30. https://doi.org/10.1016/S2214-109X(19)30255-4.
32. Fowkes FG, Aboyans V, Fowkes FJ, McDermott MM, Sampson UK, Criqui MH. Peripheral artery disease: epidemiology and global perspectives. Nat Rev Cardiol. 2017;14:156–70. https://doi.org/10.1038/nrcardio.2016.179.

33. Wang JC, Criqui MH, Denenberg JO, McDermott MM, Golomb BA, Fronek A. Exertional leg pain in patients with and without peripheral arterial disease. Circulation. 2005;112:3501–8. https://doi.org/10.1161/CIRCULATIONAHA.105.548099.
34. Allison MA, Criqui MH, McClelland RL, Scott JM, McDermott MM, Liu K, Folsom AR, Bertoni AG, Sharrett AR, Homma S, et al. The effect of novel cardiovascular risk factors on the ethnic-specific odds for peripheral arterial disease in the multi-ethnic study of atherosclerosis (MESA). J Am Coll Cardiol. 2006;48:1190–7. https://doi.org/10.1016/j.jacc.2006.05.049.
35. Newman AB, Shemanski L, Manolio TA, Cushman M, Mittelmark M, Polak JF, Powe NR, Siscovick D. Ankle-arm index as a predictor of cardiovascular disease and mortality in the cardiovascular health study. Arterioscler Thromb Vasc Biol. 1999;19:538–45.
36. Fabsitz RR, Sidaway AN, Go O, Lee ET, Welty TK, Devereux RB, Howard BV. Prevalence of peripheral arterial disease and associated risk factors in American Indians: the strong heart study. Am J Epidemiol. 1999;149:330–8.
37. Zheng ZJ, Rosamond WD, Chambless LE, Nieto FJ, Barnes RW, Hutchinson RG, Tyroler HA, Heiss G. Lower extremity arterial disease assessed by ankle-brachial index in a middle-aged population of African Americans and whites: the atherosclerosis risk in communities (ARIC) study. Am J Prev Med. 2005;29:42–9.
38. Hsia J, Criqui MH, Rodabough RJ, Langer RD, Resnick HE, Phillips LS, Allison M, Bonds DE, Masaki K, Caralis P, et al. Estrogen plus progestin and the risk of peripheral arterial disease: the Women's Health Initiative. Circulation. 2004;109:620–6. https://doi.org/10.1161/01.CIR.0000115309.63979.92.
39. Lee M, Smolderen KG, Ionescu C, Hillegass WB, Romain G, Mena-Hurtado C. Lower extremity symptoms and ankle-brachial index screening as predictors of cardiovascular outcomes in Black adults. Vasc Med. 2023;28:197–204. https://doi.org/10.1177/1358863x231151729.
40. Zheng ZJ, Sharrett AR, Chambless LE, Rosamond WD, Nieto FJ, Sheps DS, Dobs A, Evans GW, Heiss G. Associations of ankle-brachial index with clinical coronary heart disease, stroke and preclinical carotid and popliteal atherosclerosis: the atherosclerosis risk in communities (ARIC) study. Atherosclerosis. 1997;131:115–25.
41. Ostchega Y, Paulose-Ram R, Dillon CF, Gu Q, Hughes JP. Prevalence of peripheral arterial disease and risk factors in persons aged 60 and older: data from the National Health and nutrition examination survey 1999-2004. J Am Geriatr Soc. 2007;55:583–9. https://doi.org/10.1111/j.1532-5415.2007.01123.x.
42. Smith GD, Shipley MJ, Rose G. Intermittent claudication, heart disease risk factors, and mortality. The Whitehall Study. Circulation. 1990;82:1925–31. https://doi.org/10.1161/01.cir.82.6.1925.
43. Diehm C, Schuster A, Allenberg JR, Darius H, Haberl R, Lange S, Pittrow D, von Stritzky B, Tepohl G, Trampisch H-J. High prevalence of peripheral arterial disease and co-morbidity in 6880 primary care patients: cross-sectional study. Atherosclerosis. 2004;172:95–105. https://doi.org/10.1016/s0021-9150(03)00204-1.
44. Hooi JD, Kester ADM, Stoffers EJHH, Overdijk MM, van Ree JW, Knottnerus JA. Incidence of and risk factors for asymptomatic peripheral arterial occlusive disease: a longitudinal study. Am J Epidemiol. 2001;153:666–72.
45. Blanes JI, Cairols MA, Marrugat J. Prevalence of peripheral artery disease and its associated risk factors in Spain: the ESTIME study. Int Angiol. 2009;28:20–5.
46. Makdisse M, Pereira Ada C, Brasil Dde P, Borges JL, Machado-Coelho GL, Krieger JE, Nascimento Neto RM, Chagas AC. Prevalence and risk factors associated with peripheral arterial disease in the hearts of Brazil project. Arq Bras Cardiol. 2008;91:370–82. https://doi.org/10.1590/s0066-782x2008001800008.
47. Passos VM, Barreto SM, Guerra HL, Firmo JO, Vidigal PG, Lima-Costa MF. The Bambuí health and aging study (BHAS). Prevalence of intermittent claudication in the aged population of the community of Bambuí and its associated factors. Arq Bras Cardiol. 2001;77:453–62. https://doi.org/10.1590/s0066-782x2001001100006.
48. Del Brutto OH, Sedler MJ, Zambrano M, Mera RM, Phelan KJ, Gruen JA, Cusick EH, Moral CF, Del Brutto VJ, Castillo PR, et al. Comparison of field questionnaires with the ankle-brachial

index for the detection of peripheral artery disease. A population-based study in rural Ecuador. Int J Cardiol. 2014;177:703–4. https://doi.org/10.1016/j.ijcard.2014.09.188.
49. Krishnan MN, Geevar Z, Mohanan PP, Venugopal K, Devika S. Prevalence of peripheral artery disease and risk factors in the elderly: a community based cross-sectional study from northern Kerala, India. Indian Heart J. 2018;70:808–15. https://doi.org/10.1016/j.ihj.2017.11.001.
50. Johnston LE, Stewart BT, Yangni-Angate H, Veller M, Upchurch GR Jr, Gyedu A, Kushner AL. Peripheral arterial disease in sub-Saharan Africa: a review. JAMA Surg. 2016;151:564–72. https://doi.org/10.1001/jamasurg.2016.0446.
51. Beidelman ET, Rosenberg M, Wade AN, Crowther NJ, Kalbaugh CA. Prevalence of and risk factors for peripheral artery disease in rural South Africa: a cross-sectional analysis of the HAALSI cohort. J Am Heart Assoc. 2024;13:e031780. https://doi.org/10.1161/jaha.123.031780.
52. Yeboah K, Puplampu P, Ainuson J, Akpalu J, Gyan B, Amoah AG. Peripheral artery disease and exertional leg symptoms in diabetes patients in Ghana. BMC Cardiovasc Disord. 2016;16:68. https://doi.org/10.1186/s12872-016-0247-x.
53. Okello S, Millard A, Owori R, Asiimwe SB, Siedner MJ, Rwebembera J, Wilson LA, Moore CC, Annex BH. Prevalence of lower extremity peripheral artery disease among adult diabetes patients in southwestern Uganda. BMC Cardiovasc Disord. 2014;14:75. https://doi.org/10.1186/1471-2261-14-75.
54. Si S, Golledge J, Norman P, Nelson M, Chew D, Ademi Z, Bhatt DL, Steg GP, Reid CM. Prevalence and outcomes of undiagnosed peripheral arterial disease among high risk patients in Australia: an Australian REACH sub-study. Heart Lung Circ. 2019;28:939–45. https://doi.org/10.1016/j.hlc.2018.04.292.
55. Fowler B, Jamrozik K, Norman P, Allen Y. Prevalence of peripheral arterial disease: persistence of excess risk in former smokers. Aust N Z J Public Health. 2002;26:219–24.
56. Bourgois P, Holmes SM, Sue K, Quesada J. Structural vulnerability: operationalizing the concept to address health disparities in clinical care. Acad Med. 2017;92:299–307. https://doi.org/10.1097/acm.0000000000001294.
57. Hicks CW, Holscher CM, Wang P, Black JH 3rd, Abularrage CJ, Makary MA. Overuse of early peripheral vascular interventions for claudication. J Vasc Surg. 2020;71(121–130):e121. https://doi.org/10.1016/j.jvs.2019.05.005.
58. Hicks CW, Wang P, Bruhn WE, Abularrage CJ, Lum YW, Perler BA, Black JH 3rd, Makary MA. Race and socioeconomic differences associated with endovascular peripheral vascular interventions for newly diagnosed claudication. J Vasc Surg. 2020;72:611–621 e615. https://doi.org/10.1016/j.jvs.2019.10.075.
59. Kalbaugh CA, Witrick B, Howard KA, McGinigle KL, Lesko CR. Abstract P105: bypasses to below-knee arteries may expedite amputation in patients with claudication. Circulation. 2022;145:AP105.
60. Conte M, Pomposelli F, Clair D, Geraghty P, McKinsey J, Mills J, Moneta G, Murad M, Powell R, Reed A, et al. Society for vascular surgery practice guidelines for atherosclerotic occlusive disease of the lower extremities: management of asymptomatic disease and claudication. J Vasc Surg. 2015;61:2s–41s.
61. Woo K, Siracuse JJ, Klingbeil K, Kraiss LW, Osborne NH, Singh N, Tan TW, Arya S, Banerjee S, Bonaca MP, et al. Society for Vascular Surgery appropriate use criteria for management of intermittent claudication. J Vasc Surg. 2022;76:3–22 e21. https://doi.org/10.1016/j.jvs.2022.04.012.
62. Bose S, Dun C, Keegan A, McDermott KM, Stonko DP, Black JH, Columbo JA, Conte MS, Deery SA, Goodney PP, et al. Infrapopliteal peripheral vascular interventions for claudication are associated with poor long-term outcomes regardless of anatomic and disease severity. 2023 vascular annual meeting. National Harbor, MD; 2023.
63. Steg P, Bhatt D, Wilson P, D'Agostino R, Ohman E, Röther J, Liau C, Hirsch A, Mas J, Ikeda Y, et al. One-year cardiovascular event rates in outpatients with atherothrombosis. JAMA. 2007;297:1197–206.

64. Bloor K. Natural history of arteriosclerosis of the lower extremities. Ann R Coll Surg Engl. 1961;28:36–51.
65. Breslau PJ, Jorning PJG, Dassen P. The natural history of intermittent claudication, a prospective study. Presented at 2nd International Vascular Symposium. 1986.
66. Aquino R, Johnnides C, Makaroun M, Whittle JC, Muluk VS, Kelley ME, Muluk SC. Natural history of claudication: long-term serial follow-up study of 1244 claudicants. J Vasc Surg. 2001;34:962–70. https://doi.org/10.1067/mva.2001.119749.
67. Desai U, Kharat A, Hess CN, Milentijevic D, Laliberte F, Zuckerman P, Benson J, Lefebvre P, Hiatt WR, Bonaca MP. Healthcare resource utilization and costs of major atherothrombotic vascular events among patients with peripheral artery disease after revascularization. J Med Econ. 2021;24:402–9. https://doi.org/10.1080/13696998.2021.1891089.
68. Gerhard-Herman M, Gornik H, Barrett C, Barshes N, Corriere M, Drachman D, Fleisher L, Fowkes F, Hamburg N, Kinlay S, et al. 2016 AHA/ACC guideline on the management of patients with lower extremity peripheral artery disease: executive summary: a report of the American College of Cardiology/American Heart Association task force on clinical practice guidelines. J Am Coll Cardiol. 2017;69:1465–508.
69. Saxon JT, Safley DM, Mena-Hurtado C, Heyligers J, Fitridge R, Shishehbor M, Spertus JA, Gosch K, Patel MR, Smolderen KG. Adherence to guideline-recommended therapy-including supervised exercise therapy referral-across peripheral artery disease specialty clinics: insights from the international PORTRAIT registry. J Am Heart Assoc. 2020;9:e012541. https://doi.org/10.1161/JAHA.119.012541.
70. Sorber R, Dun C, Kawaji Q, Abularrage CJ, Black JH 3rd, Makary MA, Hicks CW. Reprint of: early peripheral vascular interventions for claudication are associated with higher rates of late interventions and progression to chronic limb threatening ischemia. J Vasc Surg. 2023;77:1720–1731.e1723. https://doi.org/10.1016/j.jvs.2023.04.023.
71. Eid MAMK, Barnes JA, Wanken Z, Columbo JA, Stone DH, Goodney P, Mayo SM. The global burden of peripheral artery disease. J Vasc Surg. 2022;77:5214. https://doi.org/10.1016/j.jvs.2022.12.015. Epub ahead of print.
72. Hirsch AT, Criqui MH, Treat-Jacobson D, Regensteiner JC, Creager MA, Olin JW, Krook SH, Hunninghake DB, Comerota AJ, Walsh ME, et al. Peripheral arterial disease detection, awareness, and treatment in primary care. JAMA J Am Med Assoc. 2001;286:1317–24.
73. Fontaine R, Kim M, Kieny R. Surgical treatment of peripheral circulation disorders. Helv Chir Acta. 1954;21:499–533.
74. Rutherford RB, Baker JD, Ernst C, Johnston KW, Porter JM, Ahn S, Jones DN. Recommended standards for reports dealing with lower extremity ischemia: revised version. J Vasc Surg. 1997;26:517–38.

Making the Diagnosis of Vasculogenic Claudication

4

Laura Healy

Vasculogenic claudication refers to the symptoms a patient experiences when there is inadequate blood supply to the muscles of the legs because of stenoses or occlusions of the arteries of the lower extremities. This stenosis or occlusion, in turn, leads to a reduced oxygen supply to the muscles of the lower extremity, causing pain, cramping, and discomfort in the affected muscle groups, particularly during physical activity such as walking or climbing stairs. The pain typically resolves with rest, as the demand for oxygen decreases.

Differentiating vasculogenic claudication from other sources of lower extremity pain or discomfort is crucial to identifying patients who can benefit from medical or surgical intervention under the direction of a vascular surgeon. The first step in whittling down the diagnosis is to take a thorough history to determine the nature of the patient's leg pain and their medical conditions that may contribute to atherosclerotic disease. The diagnosis can be made through this detailed history combined with a physical examination and diagnostic testing. Understanding the nuances of diagnosis is crucial for instituting appropriate management.

History of Present Illness

The patient's chief complaint should always be the focus of the history. While many consults may be accompanied by pre-visit testing, it is important that this does not cloud the initial conversation or allow it to veer away from the main concerns and chief complaint according to the patient.

The onset, location, duration, character, aggravating and alleviating factors, timing, and severity of the pain should all be reviewed. Vasculogenic pain tends to

L. Healy (✉)
Division of Vascular Surgery, Southern Illinois University School of Medicine, Springfield, Illinois, USA

W. P. Robinson III, J. P. Simons (eds.), *The Patient-Centered Approach to Claudication*, https://doi.org/10.1007/978-3-032-02460-2_4

progress over time with patients gradually walking shorter and shorter distances before they feel pain. This progression from mild discomfort after walking long distances to being unable to tolerate walking one block may have been gradual over months or even years. The symptoms are often associated with climbing stairs or walking on an incline and can vary in location depending on the location of disease. Patients often describe these as "cramps" or "Charlie horses" that come on with exercise. Some patients may not describe it strictly as "pain;" instead they may describe a sensation of leg fatigue or heaviness. Some will say their leg "gives out" when they walk. Regardless of the specific descriptor, the correspondence of the symptoms to exertion should be present. The symptoms are relieved with rest, as the lactic acid is cleared. If the patient resumes walking, the symptoms recur at approximately the same distance.

Relief with rest is a crucial characteristic of claudication pain as it is a demand ischemia of the muscles of the lower extremities. This key fact can help isolate vasculogenic claudication from musculoskeletal or neurogenic claudication.

Patients may minimize or ignore this pain, attributing it to being "out of shape" or "getting old" or simply reflective of arthritis. It is therefore crucial to thoroughly discuss their symptoms, how they are affecting their life, and to elucidate any concurrent medical problems that may interfere with a diagnosis, such as musculoskeletal injuries, joint replacements, or a history of low back pain.

The location of pain is the muscle group downstream from any areas of hemodynamic stenosis secondary to atherosclerosis. Most commonly, pain from intermittent claudication is in the calf muscles due to disease in the common femoral, superficial femoral, or popliteal artery. Buttock or thigh pain implicates the iliac arteries as the area of stenosis.

Central to the history of claudication are the implications for the patient's health-related quality of life. This will vary greatly depending on the patient's baseline functional status, degree of physical activity, and amount of daily ambulation. It is important to ask about the patient's livelihood and if/how these symptoms are affecting it. Do they use any illicit drugs? Cocaine in particular is a potent vasoconstrictor and can worsen symptoms of claudication or PAD. In the event that the patient is unable to maintain their job or activities of daily living secondary to their pain, intervention is more strongly considered after medical optimization. Asking pointed questions about the distance the patient can walk before having symptoms is a key feature of the diagnosis and can help determine how greatly the pain is affecting the patient's life.

Past Medical History

Atherosclerosis causing hemodynamically significant arterial narrowing is at the root of the pain in claudication. A demand ischemia in the muscles leads to a buildup of lactic acid and resulting cramping. Because of this, a thorough past medical history should be taken with a particular focus on the patient's risk factors for atherosclerosis and peripheral artery disease (PAD). These medical issues should be optimized with medications and lifestyle changes and include hypertension, hyperlipidemia, diabetes, and smoking. Age is also a contributing factor but is non-modifiable.

Management of atherosclerosis should include a statin and aspirin. Smoking is the most significant modifiable risk factor and should therefore be addressed in a patient's initial consultation. Efforts to quit should be encouraged and reinforced with adjuncts such as medications, patches, and gum, depending on the patient's preferences for method of cessation.

A thorough family history should also be taken, with care to address any family history of connective tissue disorders, aneurysms, or early PAD. While the role genetics plays in the progression of atherosclerosis is largely unknown and not often implicated, early onset of severe PAD in first-degree relatives is certainly worthy of note.

Review of Systems

While the musculoskeletal positives for calf, thigh, or buttock pain would be central to the diagnosis of intermittent claudication, other pertinent positives should also be investigated. These include cardiovascular; chest pain with exertion or at rest, dyspnea on exertion, and orthopnea can be symptoms of coronary atherosclerosis. If the coronary arteries have been found to have atherosclerosis, the likelihood that this disease is similar in another vascular bed, such as the lower extremities, is highly likely. Neurologic symptoms of numbness or tingling are more typical of peripheral neuropathy or neurogenic claudication but can also be present in vasculogenic claudication. Cold feet, hair loss, or delayed capillary refill are dermatologic signs of peripheral vascular disease. In men, impotence can be a urologic manifestation of aortoiliac occlusive disease.

Physical Exam

The physical examination of a patient with suspected claudication is often grossly normal, with only subtle findings. By definition, they have no wounds on their feet or rest pain which would instead be the hallmarks of chronic limb-threatening ischemia. On initial inspection, patients with claudication should be observed as they walk into the office and examination room. Are they stopping after walking down the hall? Do they favor one leg over another? Are they limping? Or do they have a smooth and symmetric gait?

Vital signs should be obtained with particular attention paid toward in-office hypertension. Inspection of the patient's legs may reveal skin or hair changes. The shins and calves in particular should be closely examined for loss of hair as reduced blood flow inhibits hair follicle function and can therefore be a sign of PAD before non-healing wounds develop.

Following inspection, the pulse examination may be the most revealing. The femoral artery, popliteal artery, dorsalis pedis (dp) artery, and posterior tibial (pt) artery should all be examined and, in a patient with normal anatomy, should be palpable. If pulses are challenging to palpate or appear diminished, this is also valuable information. In the absence of palpable distal pulses, a Doppler should be employed to detect signals in the dp and pt. arteries bilaterally. Their audible signals should be described as monophasic or multiphasic and are revealing about the location and severity of disease.

One test that can supplement a physical exam for intermittent claudication or any form of PAD is the Buerger's test or the Elevational Pallor Test. For this test, the patient lies flat on their back while the physician elevates the patient's leg to a 45-degree angle. The legs are then observed to determine if there is a color change after 2–3 minutes. The legs are then rapidly lowered to horizontal and the feet are once more observed. If the feet become pale, poor arterial inflow is implicated. Arterial insufficiency is also diagnosed if there is a reactive hyperemia when the feet are returned to horizontal. This is dependent rubor and is also a sign of severe PAD.

Differential Diagnosis

After one's clinical suspicions have been raised that a patient is having leg pain due to claudication which is vascular in origin, it is important to rule out other causes before proceeding with counseling and treatment.

Neurogenic claudication is a common condition that can present with symptoms similar to vasculogenic claudication, particularly in older patients. It is typically caused by lumbar spinal stenosis, where narrowing of the spinal canal leads to compression and irritation of the nerves, most commonly the lumbar nerve roots but also possibly in the spinal cord from spinal stenosis. This presents as leg pain, cramping, or weakness during walking, but the pain tends to be relieved by flexing the spine (such as bending forward or sitting down), unlike vasculogenic claudication, which is relieved by rest rather than position changes but worsens with activity. Neurogenic claudication is often in the lower back and legs and can be accompanied by numbness, tingling, or feelings of weakness in the legs. Patients may describe neurogenic claudication as "burning" or "tingling" pain rather than the cramping or aching found in vascular claudication. Physical examination may reveal lower extremity weakness or sensory changes (such as diminished sensation in the feet), and diagnostic tests like an MRI of the lumbar spine can confirm the presence of spinal stenosis.

Leg pain can also be secondary to musculoskeletal causes. An overuse injury or muscle strain may present similarly to claudication in the early stages but is largely localized to the injured muscle. A thorough history is important to determine if there was a distinct event which led to the pain and if it is localized to one particular area of the lower extremity. Musculoskeletal pain is also aggravated by physical activity but does not have the characteristic relief with rest that is quintessential in vasculogenic claudication. Patients will be tender to palpation over the injured muscle, which can also help distinguish it from having a vascular origin. While the entire lower extremity is subject to injury or strain, gastrocnemius muscle strains or shin splints are the most likely diagnoses to mimic intermittent claudication in their location and presentation.

Chronic venous insufficiency must also be ruled out as a potential cause of leg pain. The patient's history will likely involve worsening symptoms with standing for prolonged periods of time. The pain is usually aching in nature and worse at the end of the day. Impaired venous drainage of the lower extremities due to valve incompetence leads to swelling, aching, and heaviness in the legs. This is usually absent in the mornings and improves with elevation. Visible signs will likely be present on physical exam as well including hyperpigmentation, varicosities, edema, hyperkeratosis, or even ulcerations. Gaiter distribution of hyperpigmentation or wounds can help easily distinguish chronic venous insufficiency from peripheral arterial disease.

While swelling from chronic venous insufficiency can present with leg pain, so too can acute venous hypertension caused by an acute deep vein thrombosis (DVT). Swelling, tenderness, and leg pain can be the result of a DVT depending on its location. A thorough history is often revealing in this instance as DVTs are more common in immobile or sedentary patients. It can also be secondary to a hypercoagulable condition such as malignancy or oral contraceptive use. Patients with DVTs experience continuous pain from the thrombus, associated with edema and warmth in the affected site. The diagnosis of an acute thrombus can be made with ultrasound which can easily assess the arterial and venous flow simultaneously.

Osteoarthritis or other joint disorders are common in elderly patients and can present with lower extremity pain that increases with walking or physical activity. While pain may increase with movement, the pain is usually isolated to the joints themselves, namely the hip or knee joint. It can be accompanied by stiffness, swelling, or reduced range of motion. Physical examination findings can be revealing as the joints are often tender to palpation and exhibit decreased mobility. X-rays can be used to help make the diagnosis of degenerative joint disease.

A rare cause of lower extremity pain is popliteal artery entrapment syndrome (PAES). The popliteal artery is compressed by surrounding muscle or tendon which creates claudication-like symptoms. The main distinguishing factor in this disease process is that patients tend to be young, healthy, athletes rather than older patients with vascular risk factors including tobacco use, as in vasculogenic claudication. The patients experience very similar physical findings of intermittent claudication with symptoms resolving with rest in both populations. However, the artery has a narrowed lumen secondary to external compression rather than internal atherosclerosis. In severe cases, patients can develop chronic ischemia. Provocative maneuvers such as forced plantar flexion on physical exam can help to reproduce symptoms. Crucial to a final diagnosis in PAES is imaging. MRA can provide images of the popliteal artery as it is surrounded by muscle or tendon. If the diagnosis cannot be confirmed by MRI but suspicion is still high, angiography with provocative maneuvers (flexing/extending the leg) can be employed.

Testing

Once the physician's suspicions have been raised that peripheral arterial disease is responsible for the patient's symptoms of cramping pain with exercise, testing is necessary to confirm the diagnosis. The workhorse test in claudication is an Ankle-Brachial Index (ABI). The ankle brachial index is aptly named, as it compares the systolic occlusion pressure of the ankle (DP and PT) to the systolic occlusion pressure of the arm (brachial artery) using a Doppler device. A lower ABI is suggestive of peripheral arterial disease, specifically an ABI less than 0.9 and is consistent with a diagnosis of claudication. Normal ABIs are between 1.0 and 1.4. The degree of arterial disease is proportional to the decrement in ABI.

In the event that a patient has a strong story for intermittent claudication but his/her ABIs are normal, an exercise ABI can be ordered. This test has the patient have their ABI tested before and after exercise on a treadmill. The increase in demand for arterial blood flow in the lower extremity muscles with exercise can help unveil arterial disease that may be mild and therefore will appear to be normal at rest. In normal arteries, exercise induces dilation to meet the increasing demand for oxygenated blood. However, in patients with peripheral artery disease, the stenosed, calcified, or occluded arteries are unable to meet this increased demand. A drop in ABI after exercise reveals a functional arterial obstruction or insufficiency.

This is a dynamic and functional assessment of the arterial flow during physical activity. A key diagnostic indicator in exercise ABI testing is the degree of ABI drop after exercise. A reduction of more than 20% from the baseline ABI is generally considered indicative of significant PAD. In some cases, a post-exercise ABI that falls below 0.9 or does not recover to baseline levels within 5–10 minutes of rest may indicate severe arterial obstruction.

ABIs are non-invasive, fast, inexpensive, and immensely helpful in guiding treatment for patients with claudication. However, it does have several pitfalls including the inability to compress calcified arteries as is often seen in patients with diabetes mellitus and end-stage renal disease. These calcified arteries will result in falsely elevated ABIs and inaccurate readings. In addition, the technique in measuring blood pressure in the upper extremities is crucial to the resultant ABI. An inappropriately sized cuff or inappropriate placement can lead to altered results. ABIs can also be inaccurate when it is difficult to obtain a reliable arterial signal as is the case in obesity or lower extremity edema. The index uses the brachial pressure as the baseline and standard. This can also be problematic if there is subclavian stenosis bilaterally as the denominator of the ABI will be reduced, leading to potentially falsely elevated ABIs.

Another diagnostic test available that is non-invasive is an arterial Duplex, using Doppler ultrasound. This is a useful tool to assess the velocity of blood flow through the lower extremity arteries. Through an analysis of their speed and waveforms, one can determine if there is a more proximal stenosis or occlusion. Color Doppler can also be employed during imaging and will allow the physician to visualize blood flow patterns in real time and to evaluate collateral circulation as well.

Increasing in invasiveness but also in resolution of images and adding anatomic landmarks to the picture, a CT angiography (CTA) is another viable option. CTA provides high-resolution images of the vascular tree. It allows the physician to localize the area of peripheral arterial disease more accurately and also gives information about the extent and severity of these areas of arterial stenosis. CTA uses contrast dye which is administered intravenously and then timed to obtain a maximum opacity during the arterial phase. This can be particularly helpful when evaluating the iliac, femoral, and popliteal arteries, as are commonly affected in vasculogenic claudication.

Similarly invasive but significantly more costly in terms of time, labor, and money is an MR angiography (MRA) which uses magnetic fields and radio waves rather than ionizing radiation as in CTA. MRA is often sometimes preferred in patients with kidney disease, as it does not involve the use of iodinated contrast, which can strain kidney function. However, gadolinium has also been found to negatively affect renal function.

Both CTA and MRA provide clear, high-resolution images of the arteries, making them invaluable for pre-surgical planning.

The most invasive test and considered the gold standard for assessing the arterial system is contrast angiography. A catheter is placed into an artery, most commonly the contralateral common femoral artery, and contrast dye is injected in order to visualize arterial flow in conjunction with X-ray. Contrast angiography is helpful in patients where you suspect you will be able to intervene endovascularly as it provides a diagnosis and the potential for intervention simultaneously. While this test has many benefits including accuracy and detail of information useful for surgical planning, if necessary, it does carry the risk of bleeding from the access site and contrast-induced nephropathy.

Summary

Vasculogenic claudication is demand ischemia of the muscles of the buttock and/or lower extremity during physical activity. It differs from other leg pain such as musculoskeletal or neurogenic claudication, in terms of its underlying cause, pain characteristics, and the timing of its occurrence. Vasculogenic claudication is caused by PAD resulting in a hemodynamic stenosis or occlusion and presents as cramping leg pain or fatigue that worsens with exertion and improves with rest in the absence of distal wounds. Accurate diagnosis is essential for appropriate treatment which includes lifestyle changes and medications and may be escalated to include additional medications or even surgical intervention.

The Natural History of the Limb in Patients with Intermittent Claudication

5

Phong Vu and Leigh Ann O'Banion

Epidemiology of Peripheral Artery Disease

Incidence and Prevalence

Lower extremity peripheral artery disease (PAD) encompasses a wide range of clinical symptoms resulting from the gradual narrowing of the arteries, ranging from asymptomatic disease, intermittent claudication (IC), and in its most severe form, chronic limb-threatening ischemia (CLTI). Over the last decade, the worldwide incidence of PAD has steadily increased, primarily due to population expansion and aging, as well as the increasing prevalence of modifiable risk factors, including smoking, diabetes mellitus (DM), hypertension, and dyslipidemia [1, 2].

Recent epidemiologic studies have estimated that approximately 113 million individuals were affected by PAD in 2019 worldwide. Of note, over 40% occurred in nations with low to middle socio-demographic indices, with females having an increased prevalence in this demographic. In addition, PAD was more common among older individuals, with a prevalence of 14.91% in those aged 80–84 years [2]. In the United States (US), few estimates of PAD prevalence have been published. The most quoted estimate is 8–12 million, based on studies conducted in the late 1990s or early 2000s [3]. However, in the past decades, the US population has aged with increasing rates of DM, two major risk factors for PAD. A more recent study estimated that at least 21 million Americans have PAD, and this number could exceed 26 million [4]. Studies have also demonstrated a higher prevalence of PAD in Black individuals relative to non-Hispanic White individuals in the US. An analysis from 6 different community-based cohorts indicated that almost 30% of Black individuals are projected to develop PAD throughout their lifetime, in contrast to an estimated 20% for White and Hispanic individuals [5]. The rise in prevalence

P. Vu · L. A. O'Banion (✉)
University of California San Francisco-Fresno Branch Campus, Fresno, CA, USA
e-mail: Phuong.Vu2@ucsf.edu; LeighAnn.O'banion@ucsf.edu

W. P. Robinson III, J. P. Simons (eds.), *The Patient-Centered Approach to Claudication*, https://doi.org/10.1007/978-3-032-02460-2_5

highlights the importance of improved understanding of the natural history of PAD as not only does the disease negatively impact patient's health outcomes and social life but also our healthcare system. PAD is associated with increased risk of cardiovascular and cerebrovascular events, disability, depression, and limb amputation [6]. The need for revascularization procedures, wound care, hospitalization, and in extreme cases, limb loss imposes a significant social burden on patients and their families, as well as a substantial financial strain on the healthcare system [7].

Clinical Syndromes of Peripheral Arterial Disease

Patients with PAD can be classified according to their symptoms or clinical presentation, with most individuals being clinically asymptomatic. The 2024 ACC/AHA/Multisociety PAD Guidelines classify PAD into 4 clinical categories: asymptomatic PAD, chronic symptomatic PAD (which encompasses IC and other ischemia-related exertional leg symptoms), CLTI, and acute limb ischemia (ALI) [6]. Individuals with PAD may experience advancing symptoms as their condition progresses, transitioning between various categories depending on interventions. For instance, chronic symptomatic PAD can worsen into CLTI or ALI, while patients may improve following treatment into an asymptomatic PAD category.

Despite advancements in the management of PAD over the past decades, many widely used interventions globally (medical and surgical) are not based on high-level evidence. Significant geographical variations and discrepancies exist in the application of revascularization strategies. In addition, PAD is often underdiagnosed, and medical therapy is underutilized and frequently not maximized. Therefore, clinicians need to have a clear understanding of the manifestations of PAD and its disease progression, particularly in those patients in early stages, presenting with intermittent claudication.

Asymptomatic Peripheral Artery Disease

The majority of individuals with PAD are asymptomatic and unaware of their condition, with only a minority exhibiting typical symptoms. Depending on the specific population studied and the method of assessment, between 20% and 59% of individuals with verified PAD report having no symptoms [8–11]. Asymptomatic PAD results when the imbalance between oxygen supply and demand that triggers claudication symptoms is not present either from lack of hemodynamically significant atherosclerotic burden, or physical inactivity [12]. Some patients with PAD experience muscle discomfort during ambulation but fail to report these symptoms, as they consider them a normal aspect of aging, highlighting the health illiteracy that predominates across the US, specifically in socioeconomically disadvantaged regions.

Diagnosis

The diagnosis of asymptomatic PAD is determined by the presence of relevant risk factors and an abnormal resting ankle-brachial index (ABI), defined as ≤0.9 [13]. The ABI, which is the ratio of systolic occlusion pressure at the ankle to that of the brachial artery, is the most frequently used test for screening and diagnosing PAD. A systematic review of studies assessing ABI as a screening tool for PAD in asymptomatic individuals found an overall detection rate of 17%, with a range from 1% to 42%. The detection rate of ABI testing in younger, asymptomatic individuals without atherosclerosis risk factors is low (1–4%), and routine testing for PAD in this population is not recommended [6, 14, 15]. For individuals at moderate-to-high risk for cardiovascular disease, the ESVS 2024 Clinical Practice Guidelines on the Management of PAD and IC recommends performing ABI testing to detect lower extremity PAD. Individuals at risk encompass adults aged 65 years and older, and those aged 50–64 years with additional atherosclerotic risk factors (DM, smoking history, dyslipidemia, hypertension, chronic kidney disease, or those with family history of PAD). Additionally, individuals under 50 years of age with diabetes and at least one other atherosclerotic risk factor are also considered at risk [13]. ABI testing should also be considered for individuals with known atherosclerotic disease in another vascular bed. In patients exhibiting symptoms of PAD, the resting ABI demonstrates a sensitivity ranging from 69% to 79% and a specificity between 83% and 99% when compared to imaging studies that reveal significant arterial stenoses [16, 17].

ABI testing, while straightforward and informative for diagnostic purposes, does possess certain limitations. The sensitivity is limited in individuals with significant arterial calcification, notably in populations with diabetes, end-stage renal disease, and the elderly. ABI testing in these individuals may yield results within the normal range (1–1.3) or the supernormal range (above 1.3), indicating the presence of non-compressible vessels [16, 17]. In these cases, a toe-brachial index (TBI), which is the ratio of toe systolic occlusion pressure to brachial systolic occlusion pressure, can be used to diagnose PAD. Digital arteries are typically unaffected by arterial calcification, resulting in lower susceptibility to measurement errors in TBI compared to ABI, a factor of particular significance in patients with DM and renal disease. A TBI of ≤0.70 is deemed abnormal and is consistent with the diagnosis of PAD in patients with an ABI >1.4 who present with a relevant history or physical examination findings indicative of PAD [6].

When PAD is suspected but the resting ABI is normal, post-exercise ABI measurements can be useful [18]. Exercise reduces vascular resistance and increases blood flow to the active extremities. An arterial stenosis of less than 70% is unlikely to substantially reduce blood flow at rest or generate a systolic pressure gradient. Exercise in these patients can enhance blood flow and amplify the pressure gradient across stenoses, improving the sensitivity for detecting PAD. A post-exercise ABI reduction of at least 20% or an absolute ABI pressure decrease of 30 mmHg or greater confirms the presence of PAD [16].

Management

Evidence highlights the association between asymptomatic PAD and a higher risk of myocardial infarction, stroke, and overall mortality. The elevated mortality risk is attributed to cardiovascular factors, as well as nonvascular causes, predominantly neoplasms associated with smoking [19, 20]. The management of asymptomatic PAD includes risk factor modification to mitigate disease progression and complications, maintain functional status, and lower the risk of future adverse cardiovascular events.

Lifestyle modifications, such as smoking cessation, exercise, and a healthy diet, are essential initial steps and are recommended for all patients diagnosed with PAD. Exercise programs have demonstrated efficacy in reducing functional impairment in individuals with asymptomatic PAD. A prospective cohort study of 417 individuals with PAD found that asymptomatic patients who exercised by walking three or more times per week experienced a smaller annual decline in six-minute walking performance compared to those who walked less frequently [21–23].

Due to the systemic nature of atherosclerotic disease, the 2024 ACC/AHA/Multisociety PAD Guidelines recommend antiplatelet therapy as reasonable, given that patients are at an increased risk of major adverse cardiovascular events (MACE), including mortality [6]. In terms of lipid-lowering therapy, statin medications have demonstrated efficacy in enhancing lower extremity outcomes and reducing MACE in various studies, and are recommended for all patients with PAD [6, 23]. A meta-analysis of 39 studies involving 275,670 patients found that statin use was linked to a 42% reduction in all-cause mortality, a 43% decrease in cardiovascular death, and a 35% lower risk of MACE [24]. Despite substantial evidence of its benefits, statin therapy is under prescribed in patients with PAD relative to those with other atherosclerotic cardiovascular conditions, particularly coronary artery disease (CAD). Statin therapy should be aimed at reducing the initial low-density lipoprotein (LDL) level by ≥50% or achieving an LDL target of <70 mg/dL in high-risk individuals. Other conditions associated with cardiovascular disease should also be optimized, including hypertension and DM [25].

Guideline-directed medical therapy for PAD, specifically in those with DM, emphasizes preventive foot care as a key aspect of management, to prevent ulceration and the associated risk of CLTI. Patients should have their feet regularly examined by clinicians during office visits. When possible, referring them to a foot care specialist for ongoing foot evaluations and monitoring is advisable [26].

Symptomatic Peripheral Artery Disease

Intermittent Claudication

The most commonly appreciated symptom associated with PAD is IC, which results from impaired blood flow to the lower extremity muscles during exertion. Patients may describe their pain as aching, burning, cramping, discomfort, or heaviness in the muscles one level below the anatomical level of obstruction. For example, walking may cause discomfort in the buttocks and thighs in patients with aortoiliac disease, or calf pain in those with femoropopliteal disease, which subsides after a brief period of rest. Depending on the extent of arterial stenosis or occlusion, the effectiveness of collateral vascular channels, and the intensity of exercise, patients may experience a range of symptom severity. Patients' perceptions of claudication can vary from minor discomfort to disabling pain that significantly affects quality of life and adversely impacts work capability.

In 2001, Hirsch et al. reported that <10% of patients with PAD exhibit the characteristic signs of intermittent claudication based on the Rose questionnaire, with a majority having atypical leg symptoms [9]. These patients may be able to continue walking despite pain, while others may require a period of rest or are unable to continue walking. PAD patients with asymptomatic or atypical leg symptoms have been shown to have functional impairment comparable to patients with typical IC [8]. This highlights the importance of a meticulous history and patient-centric focus during any encounter with a patient with risk factors for PAD.

The severity of IC is typically assessed by the initial claudication distance or claudication onset time, measured during daily activities or a treadmill test. Patients with severe intermittent claudication typically cannot complete a standard 5-minute treadmill protocol set at 2 mph with a 12% incline. They frequently report the onset of symptoms within minutes of walking, necessitating cessation of activity, which results in considerable disability and diminished quality of life. Functional testing of patients with intermittent claudication reveals a wide spectrum of deficits in lower limb strength, balance, and related mobility limitations. Furthermore, the progression of functional decline in individuals with IC is substantial and correlates with the severity of PAD [27].

Fortunately, the ACC/AHA/Multisociety PAD Guideline and the Society for Vascular Surgery (SVS) guidelines for the management of PAD suggest that the incidence of IC that progresses to CLTI is 1–3% per 5 years [6, 23]. This low rate of progression to limb threat is important to bear in mind when counseling patients regarding the risks and benefits of procedural intervention for claudication. The indication for intervention is *not* prevention of progression to CLTI or limb loss. Through lifestyle modifications and advancement of medical management of risk factors (including an emphasis on exercise therapy), this statistic, however, may decrease further.

The ACC/AHA/Multisociety PAD Guideline as well as the SVS guidelines strongly advocate for exercise therapy as the first line of therapy in patients with IC [6, 23]. A recent meta-analysis of exercise therapy trials, including 1816 participants with stable leg pain, found a mean increase of 82.11 meters in pain-free walking distance, along with improvements in quality-of-life measures [28]. An additional review of 21 studies involving a total of 1400 participants also demonstrated that supervised exercise therapy programs are more effective than home-based therapy while achieving comparable adherence rates [29]. The benefits of exercise therapy were also found to extend significantly beyond the conclusion of prescribed programs lasting up to 7 years after a 28-week supervised intervention [30].

The SVS Appropriate Use Criteria (AUC) for IC included a systematic review and gap analysis of all critical publications on IC from 2000 to 2022. The resulting publications from these efforts strongly support the initial recommendation of supervised exercise therapy for patients with IC and no evidence of CLTI [31, 32]. Also highlighted was the existing gaps in the literature on patient-reported outcomes and comparative effectiveness of exercise therapy vs revascularization as initial therapy.

In the subset of patients who ultimately receive revascularization therapies, supervised exercise therapy has been shown to effectively improve walking performance, functional status, and quality of life when administered concomitantly. The Revascularization and Supervised Exercise (ERASE) trial randomized 212 PAD patients with aortoiliac or femoropopliteal artery stenoses, or both, to either supervised exercise training with stenting or supervised exercise training alone. The study found that the combination of endovascular revascularization and supervised exercise training, compared to exercise training alone, resulted in increased walking distance and improved quality of life at 3, 6, and 12 months [33]. This supports the continuous provision of supervised exercise therapy to individuals with claudication, whether as a monotherapy or paired with revascularization. Despite evidence supporting the effectiveness of supervised exercise therapy, access is limited and unavailable to many patients. Additionally, even when it is accessible, uptake and adherence rates remain low [34]. Advocating for the development of supervised exercise therapy programs is essential to improving outcomes for patients with claudication due to PAD.

Patients with claudication who have responded well to guideline-directed medical therapy, including structured exercise, and no longer experience significant impairment in functional status, walking performance, or quality of life should continue their prescribed therapies to minimize progression of disease. Patients with lifestyle-limiting claudication who have not shown significant improvement after optimal medical and exercise therapy may be considered for revascularization. Revascularization is a highly personalized treatment approach, focused on patient-centered goals derived from clinical assessment, and should include consideration of the limited durability of results of revascularization. The primary aim is functional improvement, considering the potential benefits for quality of life and exercise rehabilitation, rather than prevention of limb loss. It is crucial to assess the severity of the patient's disability (such as pain-free walking distance and maximum walking distance) and how these limitations affect their daily activities.

Several studies have indicated that revascularization in patients with intermittent claudication is linked to an increased risk of disease progression and amputation [35, 36]. A retrospective review of 1051 patients with intermittent claudication who underwent revascularization found that revascularization was associated with a higher risk of progression to CLTI (hazard ratio [HR] 2.9, 95% CI 2.0–4.2) and amputation (HR 4.5, 95% CI 2.2–9.5) compared to those who did not have revascularization [37]. These findings should be considered when managing these patients and included in shared decision-making discussions. It is critically important to disclose that intervention carries a risk of limb loss; the specific likelihood of limb loss with revascularization versus that likelihood without revascularization has not been clearly delineated.

Conclusion

Intermittent claudication is a symptomatic manifestation of PAD. Management should be tailored to establishing a baseline thorough history and physical, patient education and shared decision-making, maximizing medical management, and implementing exercise therapy. The natural history of claudication does not include limb loss; progression to chronic limb-threatening ischemia occurs in a very small subset of patients. The indication for revascularization is to improve quality of life and physical function, not to reduce the risk of limb loss. Close follow-up to assure medical compliance, monitoring of the quality of life, and implementing risk reduction strategies to optimize the overall vascular health of the patient are essential.

References

1. Adou C, Magne J, Gazere N, Aouida M, Chastaingt L, Aboyans V. Global epidemiology of lower extremity artery disease in the 21st century (2000-21): a systematic review and meta-analysis. Eur J Prev Cardiol. 2024;31(7):803–11.
2. Collaborators GBDPAD. Global burden of peripheral artery disease and its risk factors, 1990-2019: a systematic analysis for the global burden of disease study 2019. Lancet Glob Health. 2023;11(10):e1553–e65.
3. Criqui MH, Matsushita K, Aboyans V, Hess CN, Hicks CW, Kwan TW, et al. Lower extremity peripheral artery disease: contemporary epidemiology, management gaps, and future directions: a scientific statement from the American Heart Association. Circulation. 2021;144(9):e171–e91.
4. Yost M. The current U.S. prevalence of peripheral artery disease. Vasc Dis Manag. 2023;20(4):E67–73.
5. Matsushita K, Sang Y, Ning H, Ballew SH, Chow EK, Grams ME, et al. Lifetime risk of lower-extremity peripheral artery disease defined by Ankle-Brachial Index in the United States. J Am Heart Assoc. 2019;8(18):e012177.
6. Writing Committee M, Gornik HL, Aronow HD, Goodney PP, Arya S, Brewster LP, et al. 2024 ACC/AHA/AACVPR/APMA/ABC/SCAI/SVM/SVN/SVS/SIR/VESS guideline for the Management of Lower Extremity Peripheral Artery Disease: a report of the American College of Cardiology/American Heart Association joint Committee on clinical practice guidelines. J Am Coll Cardiol. 2024;83(24):2497–604.
7. Hirsch AT, Hartman L, Town RJ, Virnig BA. National health care costs of peripheral arterial disease in the Medicare population. Vasc Med. 2008;13(3):209–15.
8. McDermott MM, Greenland P, Liu K, Guralnik JM, Criqui MH, Dolan NC, et al. Leg symptoms in peripheral arterial disease: associated clinical characteristics and functional impairment. JAMA. 2001;286(13):1599–606.
9. Hirsch AT, Criqui MH, Treat-Jacobson D, Regensteiner JG, Creager MA, Olin JW, et al. Peripheral arterial disease detection, awareness, and treatment in primary care. JAMA. 2001;286(11):1317–24.

10. Schorr EN, Treat-Jacobson D. Methods of symptom evaluation and their impact on peripheral artery disease (PAD) symptom prevalence: a review. Vasc Med. 2013;18(2):95–111.
11. Newman AB, Naydeck BL, Sutton-Tyrrell K, Polak JF, Kuller LH, Cardiovascular Health Study Research G. The role of comorbidity in the assessment of intermittent claudication in older adults. J Clin Epidemiol. 2001;54(3):294–300.
12. McDermott MM, Guralnik JM, Ferrucci L, Tian L, Liu K, Liao Y, et al. Asymptomatic peripheral arterial disease is associated with more adverse lower extremity characteristics than intermittent claudication. Circulation. 2008;117(19):2484–91.
13. Nordanstig J, Behrendt CA, Baumgartner I, Belch J, Back M, Fitridge R, et al. Editor's choice - European Society for Vascular Surgery (ESVS) 2024 clinical practice guidelines on the management of asymptomatic lower limb peripheral arterial disease and intermittent claudication. Eur J Vasc Endovasc Surg. 2024;67(1):9–96.
14. Selvin E, Erlinger TP. Prevalence of and risk factors for peripheral arterial disease in the United States: results from the National Health and nutrition examination survey, 1999–2000. Circulation. 2004;110(6):738–43.
15. Alahdab F, Wang AT, Elraiyah TA, Malgor RD, Rizvi AZ, Lane MA, et al. A systematic review for the screening for peripheral arterial disease in asymptomatic patients. J Vasc Surg. 2015;61(3 Suppl):42S–53S.
16. Aboyans V, Criqui MH, Abraham P, Allison MA, Creager MA, Diehm C, et al. Measurement and interpretation of the ankle-brachial index: a scientific statement from the American Heart Association. Circulation. 2012;126(24):2890–909.
17. Tehan PE, Bray A, Chuter VH. Non-invasive vascular assessment in the foot with diabetes: sensitivity and specificity of the ankle brachial index, toe brachial index and continuous wave Doppler for detecting peripheral arterial disease. J Diabetes Complicat. 2016;30(1):155–60.
18. Aday AW, Kinlay S, Gerhard-Herman MD. Comparison of different exercise ankle pressure indices in the diagnosis of peripheral artery disease. Vasc Med. 2018;23(6):541–8.
19. Ankle Brachial Index C, Fowkes FG, Murray GD, Butcher I, Heald CL, Lee RJ, et al. Ankle brachial index combined with Framingham risk score to predict cardiovascular events and mortality: a meta-analysis. JAMA. 2008;300(2):197–208.
20. Diehm C, Allenberg JR, Pittrow D, Mahn M, Tepohl G, Haberl RL, et al. Mortality and vascular morbidity in older adults with asymptomatic versus symptomatic peripheral artery disease. Circulation. 2009;120(21):2053–61.
21. McDermott MM, Liu K, Ferrucci L, Criqui MH, Greenland P, Guralnik JM, et al. Physical performance in peripheral arterial disease: a slower rate of decline in patients who walk more. Ann Intern Med. 2006;144(1):10–20.
22. Dittman JM, Amendola MF, Lavingia KS. Medical optimization of the peripheral artery disease patient. Semin Vasc Surg. 2022;35(2):113–23.
23. Society for Vascular Surgery Lower Extremity Guidelines Writing Group, Conte MS, Pomposelli FB, Clair DG, Geraghty PJ, McKinsey JF, et al. Society for Vascular Surgery practice guidelines for atherosclerotic occlusive disease of the lower extremities: management of asymptomatic disease and claudication. J Vasc Surg. 2015;61(3 Suppl):2S–41S.
24. Sagris M, Katsaros I, Giannopoulos S, Rosenberg RD, Altin SE, Rallidis L, et al. Statins and statin intensity in peripheral artery disease. Vasa. 2022;51(4):198–211.
25. Grundy SM, Stone NJ, Bailey AL, Beam C, Birtcher KK, Blumenthal RS, et al. 2018 AHA/ACC/AACVPR/AAPA/ABC/ACPM/ADA/AGS/APhA/ASPC/NLA/PCNA guideline on the Management of Blood Cholesterol: a report of the American College of Cardiology/American Heart Association task force on clinical practice guidelines. Circulation. 2019;139(25):e1082–e143.
26. Gallagher KA, Mills JL, Armstrong DG, Conte MS, Kirsner RS, Minc SD, et al. Current status and principles for the treatment and prevention of diabetic foot ulcers in the cardiovascular patient population: a scientific statement from the American Heart Association. Circulation. 2024;149(4):e232–e53.
27. McDermott MM. Lower extremity manifestations of peripheral artery disease: the pathophysiologic and functional implications of leg ischemia. Circ Res. 2015;116(9):1540–50.

28. Lane R, Harwood A, Watson L, Leng GC. Exercise for intermittent claudication. Cochrane Database Syst Rev. 2017;12(12):CD000990.
29. Hageman D, Fokkenrood HJ, Gommans LN, van den Houten MM, Teijink JA. Supervised exercise therapy versus home-based exercise therapy versus walking advice for intermittent claudication. Cochrane Database Syst Rev. 2018;4(4):CD005263.
30. Fakhry F, Rouwet EV, den Hoed PT, Hunink MG, Spronk S. Long-term clinical effectiveness of supervised exercise therapy versus endovascular revascularization for intermittent claudication from a randomized clinical trial. Br J Surg. 2013;100(9):1164–71.
31. Woo K, Siracuse JJ, Klingbeil K, Kraiss LW, Osborne NH, Singh N, et al. Society for Vascular Surgery appropriate use criteria for management of intermittent claudication. J Vasc Surg. 2022;76(1):3–22 e1.
32. O'Banion LA, Saadi S, Hasan B, Nayfeh T, Simons JP, Murad MH, et al. Lack of patient-centered evaluation of outcomes in intermittent claudication literature. J Vasc Surg. 2023;78(3):828–36.
33. Fakhry F, Spronk S, van der Laan L, Wever JJ, Teijink JA, Hoffmann WH, et al. Endovascular revascularization and supervised exercise for peripheral artery disease and intermittent claudication: a randomized clinical trial. JAMA. 2015;314(18):1936–44.
34. Abaraogu UO, Abaraogu OD, Dall PM, Tew G, Stuart W, Brittenden J, et al. Exercise therapy in routine management of peripheral arterial disease and intermittent claudication: a scoping review. Ther Adv Cardiovasc Dis. 2020;14:1753944720924270.
35. Kim TI, Kiwan G, Mohamedali A, Zhang Y, Dardik A, Guzman RJ, et al. Multiple Reinterventions for claudication are associated with progression to chronic limb-threatening ischemia. Ann Vasc Surg. 2021;72:166–74.
36. Sorber R, Dun C, Kawaji Q, Abularrage CJ, Black JH 3rd, Makary MA, et al. Early peripheral vascular interventions for claudication are associated with higher rates of late interventions and progression to chronic limb threatening ischemia. J Vasc Surg. 2023;77(3):836–47 e3.
37. Madabhushi V, Davenport D, Jones S, Khoudoud SA, Orr N, Minion D, et al. Revascularization of intermittent claudicants leads to more chronic limb-threatening ischemia and higher amputation rates. J Vasc Surg. 2021;74(3):771–9.

Contemporary Health Disparities in the Diagnosis and Management of Claudication

6

Amber B. Kernodle, Nkiruka Arinze, Brandi M. Mize, and Olamide Alabi

Introduction

Peripheral artery disease (PAD) disproportionately affects non-Hispanic Black individuals in the United States (US) with prevalence estimates of 7.9% (95% CI: 5.2–10.6) that are 2- to three-fold greater than non-Hispanic White individuals and Mexican Americans [1–7]. In a study leveraging data from large, multi-racial, community based studies and included understudied racial minority groups, PAD prevalence increased with every decade of life, but more rapidly for non-Hispanic Black men as well as non-Hispanic Black and Hispanic women (Fig. 6.1) [3]. Simulations based on similar community-based cohorts estimate a 30% lifetime risk of PAD among Black individuals as compared to 20% among White and Hispanic populations with the risk varying and being graded according to sex and the number of traditional cardiovascular risk factors [6]. For example, a Black man with a history of smoking, heart disease or stroke, and diabetes mellitus has a 70% lifetime risk of PAD. The San Diego Population Study that intentionally oversampled women and ethnic minorities found that Asian populations have a PAD prevalence similar to White populations [8].

PAD is a spectrum of disease states that can range from no symptoms at all to a degree of arterial insufficiency that becomes limb-threatening. Intermittent claudication, the least aggressive, symptomatic form of PAD, is characterized by exertional leg pain that is relieved with a short period of rest. Treatment for intermittent

A. B. Kernodle
Department of Vascular and Endovascular Surgery, Brigham and Women's Hospital, Boston, MA, USA
e-mail: akernodle@mgb.org

N. Arinze · B. M. Mize · O. Alabi (✉)
Division of Vascular Surgery and Endovascular Therapy, Department of Surgery, Emory University School of Medicine, Atlanta, GA, USA
e-mail: brandi.michelle.mize@emory.edu; olamide.alabi@emory.edu; akernodle@mgb.org

W. P. Robinson III, J. P. Simons (eds.), *The Patient-Centered Approach to Claudication*, https://doi.org/10.1007/978-3-032-02460-2_6

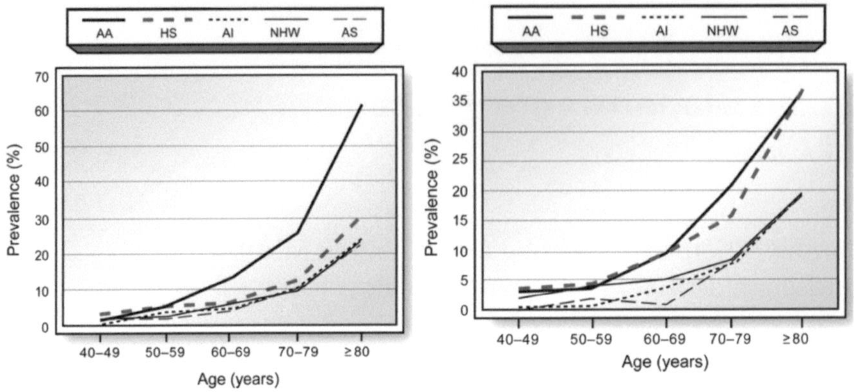

Fig. 6.1 Ethnic-specific prevalence of peripheral artery disease in men and women. (Ref. [3])

claudication aims to maintain or improve mobility and function and/or health-related quality of life. Current guidelines recommend smoking cessation, guideline-directed medical therapy, supervised and home-based exercise therapy for patients with intermittent claudication. Surgical management is generally reserved for patients with severely debilitating and lifestyle-limiting claudication after a trial of supervised exercise therapy plus optimal medical therapy for 6 months [9, 10]. Racial, ethnic, and sex minorities with claudication have proven to represent vulnerable groups of patients with published examples of under-, over-, and mistreatment of intermittent claudication [11], worse outcomes for same procedures with similar underlying PAD stage [12, 13], and higher than expected rates of progression to chronic limb-threatening ischemia and subsequent limb loss [14].

This chapter focuses on racial, ethnic, and sex disparities in the presentation and management of intermittent claudication. The National Institute on Minority Health and Health Disparities (NIHMD) defines a health disparity as an avoidable or preventable health difference that adversely affects socially disadvantaged populations in comparison to a reference population, with "social disadvantage" being largely attributable to discrimination and being underserved in health care. This chapter centers social epidemiologic definitions that conceptualize race as a sociopolitical construct, rather than a biological construct, and ethnicity as being a distinct and separate construct from race that might include shared culture, history, traditions, and language, for example. Sex is a fixed, binary biological variable and is based on genetic and physiologic characteristics. Gender refers to the socially constructed norms that impose and determine roles, relationships, and positional power for all people across their lifetime [15, 16]. Further, the chapter centers social epidemiologic theories that use social, economic, and structural inequality across time in nested hierarchies to understand root causes of health disparities rather than defaulting to inherent, biologic racial/ethnic difference logical fallacies. More specifically, this chapter reviews [1] high burden of medical comorbidities that mediate the relationship between race/ethnicity and incident intermittent claudication, [2] social disadvantage as measured by individual and area-level measures of socioeconomic status and its relationship to intermittent claudication, [3] barriers to timely health-care access that lead to delayed presentation of PAD among racial and female minority populations, and [4] relatively high volume and inappropriate use of endo-vascular interventions in racial minorities with intermittent claudication. In the final sections of the chapter, the NIHMD Research Framework is leveraged to highlight knowledge gaps and future directions [17].

Traditional Cardiovascular Risk Factors *Partially* Explain the Relationship Between Race and Ethnicity Differences in PAD Prevalence

Racial and ethnic minority populations have a higher prevalence of traditional cardiovascular risk factors that lead to PAD, and the historic presumption and research focus of race-based disparities mechanisms have been based on this rudimentary assumption. It is true that in many studies of incident PAD procedures, there are differences in the distribution of chronic comorbid conditions according to race. In a cohort of Black and White individuals presenting for their first revascularization procedure for PAD, the prevalence of diabetes mellitus, hypertension, and renal dysfunction and dialysis dependence was higher among Black individuals compared to White individuals; while smoking prevalence, and, presumably, aortoiliac disease, was higher among White individuals [18, 19]. However, this basic, reductive mechanistic assumption that comorbidity differences explain racial and ethnic differences in PAD has been tempered by several large population-based, epidemiologic studies. Using National Health and Nutrition Examination Survey (NHANES) data, within each traditional cardiovascular risk factor category that included age, diabetes mellitus, smoking, kidney disease, hypertension, and hypercholesterolemia, there was a higher prevalence of PAD among some racial and ethnic minority populations as compared to White populations with complex interactions observed according to race and gender [20]. Black men have a higher PAD prevalence as compared to White men across all risk factor categories. For example, the PAD prevalence for Black men with diabetes mellitus was 18.75% as compared to 10.97% among White men. Using this dataset, Mexican American populations with a history of diabetes mellitus, smoking, or hypercholesterolemia had lower PAD prevalence than both White and Black populations. In a cross-sectional study of the Multiethnic Study of Atherosclerosis (MESA), after adjustment for traditional and "novel" risk factors (e.g., interleukin-6, fibrinogen, D-dimer, and homocysteine), Black individuals had a higher odds of PAD than White individuals (odds ratio = 1.47, 95% CI: 1.07–2.02), suggesting that differences in risk factors, alone, do not explain racial disparities [21]. Unmeasured factors that might explain the difference include socioeconomic resources, access to healthcare resources, social disadvantage and bias, discrimination and differential treatment by providers, proceduralists, and surgeons (Fig. 6.2).

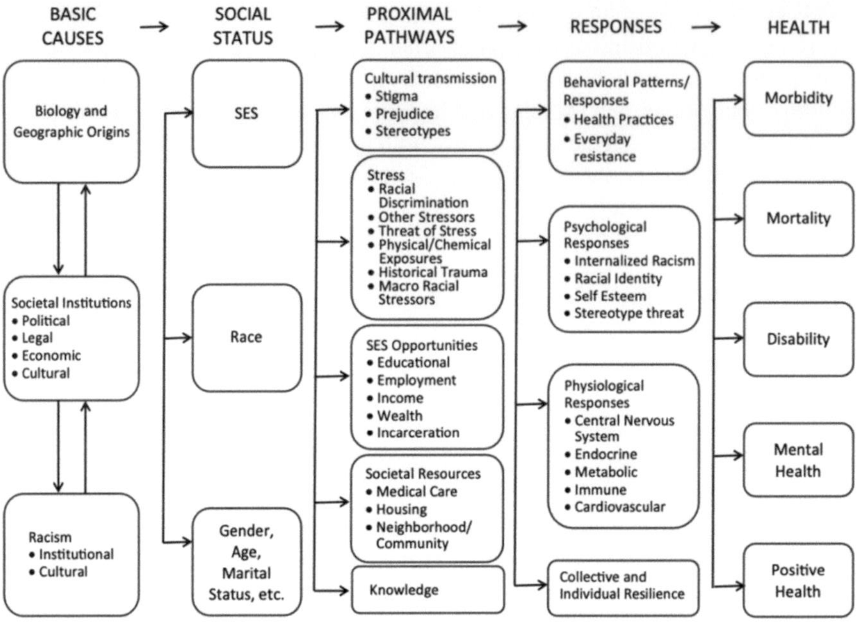

Fig. 6.2 A framework for the study of racism and health. (Ref. [22]

Socioeconomic Status Is a Key Driver of Racial and Ethnicity Differences in PAD Prevalence

In the social epidemiologic theory, fundamental social causes that explain health disparities, knowledge, power, prestige, and beneficial social connections allow one to avoid and/or protect themselves from morbidity, and to maintain or improve health [23, 24]. The interplay between race and socioeconomic resources and position shapes access to knowledge and power to affect one's health, and studies that have incorporated social determinants of health in PAD have found social determinants to be a key driver in explaining race-based PAD disparities. In a study using National Health and Nutrition Examination Survey (NHANES) data, the Black versus White population difference in cardiovascular-related mortality was attenuated in regression models that adjusted for both traditional cardiovascular risk factors and social determinants of health, such as unemployment, low family income, food insecurity, and lack of home ownership. The age- and sex-adjusted hazard ratio of Black-White difference in cardiovascular disease mortality was 1.5 (95% CI: 1.34–1.77) and decreased to 1.04 (95% CI: 0.9–1.21) or no difference [25], suggesting that both medical comorbidities and social determinants of health explain race-based disparities seen in cardiovascular disease-related mortality. The attenuation of racial disparities after adjustment for socioeconomic risk factors, such as education and income, has been replicated across other studies with low socioeconomic status explaining race-based disparities in mobility loss and walking distance among similar clinical profiles [26]. It might be that socioeconomic status, which is directly correlated with access to green space and neighborhood walkability [27, 28], contribute to race-based differences in symptomatic PAD.

Underdiagnosis of Symptomatic PAD in Racial and Ethnic Minorities

Despite the higher prevalence of PAD in racial and ethnic minority populations, observational studies have found that racial and ethnic minorities are less likely to present with claudication and more often present with chronic limb threatening ischemia as compared to White patients with PAD [29, 30]. Barriers to healthcare access, screening failures, or relatively lower baseline functional status due to comorbidities that mask PAD may all be reasons why Black patients with claudication are recognized and diagnosed less often than White patients. In a study that screened patients over the age of 50 for PAD in primary care clinics using ankle-brachial index and surveys that ascertained symptoms of intermittent claudication, walking difficulty, medical history, and quality of life, intermittent claudication was a rare finding among those diagnosed with PAD [2]. The low prevalence of classic claudication symptoms, also replicated in other population-based studies [31], might be the result of measurement bias, as questionnaires of variable sensitivity and specificity to capture both typical and atypical claudication symptoms have been used in research [32]. The failure to capture and/or diagnose intermittent claudication is also apparent in the clinical setting with primary care physician having little awareness of PAD prevalence, insufficient training to recognize PAD based on early diagnostic clues, and being constrained by time and space, limiting diagnosis and management during annual evaluations [33]. In the PAD Awareness, Risk and Treatment New Resources for Survival program, which was a multi-center, cross-sectional study that captured physician and patient awareness of PAD in patients who were defined as having PAD in the medical record, ABI measurement, or history of revascularization procedure, 83% of patients with PAD had prior knowledge of their diagnosis, but only 49% of their physicians recognized their diagnosis at the time of screening [31]. Currently, the United States Preventative Services Task Force does not recommend screening with ABI in asymptomatic populations, but given measurement bias and provider awareness concerns, some have advocated for screening interventions as a method to address healthcare disparities.

Differential Medical and Procedural Management of Intermittent Claudication

The Society for Vascular Surgery (SVS), in accordance with existing American Heart Association/American College of Cardiology guidelines, created practice guidelines for treatment strategies in patients with PAD [34, 35]. Despite clinical practice guidelines, racial and ethnic minorities have less access to and success with smoking cessation and supervised exercise therapy programs, are less often prescribed optimal medical therapy [36], are subject to inappropriate procedures, and have worse revascularization outcomes [37].

The association between smoking and social disadvantage is a long-standing finding across epidemiologic studies [38, 39]. Using a nationally representative sample of US adults from the National Survey of Drug Use and Health, current every day smoking prevalence was highest in adults with less than a high school diploma as compared to higher educational attainment groups, and higher in non-Hispanic White populations as compared to non-Hispanic Black, Asian, and Hispanic populations (White = 41.6% [95% CI: 49.9–43.3], Black = 37% [95% CI: 33.9–40.1], Asian = 12.5% [95% CI: 8.1–18.7], and Hispanic = 17% [95% CI: 15.8–18.7]). When stratified by gender, Asian and Hispanic women who have relatively lower socioeconomic status, uniquely, have a lower prevalence of current everyday smoking [40]. Smoking status according to race and ethnicity varies according to vascular pathology, PAD symptomatology, and across studies. However, in a systematic review including 49 PAD-specific studies, smoking was more common in Black and indigenous populations as compared to White populations [41]. Race-based differences in smoking cessation have also been observed. Black individuals have been found to be less likely to receive smoking cessation assistance [42, 43], more likely to fail attempts at cessation [44], and have lower quit rates compared to White individuals [43] ultimately placing them at higher risk of development of PAD and disease progression. In a retrospective study of patients with symptomatic PAD at a single, public, inner-city hospital, there was no difference in medical management and provider referrals to multidisciplinary smoking cessation program according to race, which might reflect the positive and diligent practice patterns of the providers and environment at this facility [45]. Despite referrals, however, patients who were insured more often quit smoking as compared to uninsured patients with the conclusion that this finding might be related to frequency of healthcare visits, health insurance coverage limitations, and financial constraints. When patients with symptomatic PAD are stratified according to insurance status (i.e., private, Medicare, Medicaid, and uninsured), there is no difference in smoking based on insurance status at a single institution, but patients who are insured are more likely to be successful in quitting smoking than uninsured patients. Even patients who are newly insured have higher success with smoking cessation with newly insured patients having a 40% higher odds of quitting smoking and triple the odds of having a prescription for smoking cessation aid [46]. Consistent with fundamental social causes theory of health disparities, disparities in smoking cessation observations demonstrated that individuals with resources, knowledge, and power are better equipped to change health behaviors and patients who are facing social disadvantage and discrimination may not be able to change health behaviors as easily.

While the Center for Medicare & Medicaid Services covers supervised exercise therapy for beneficiaries with intermittent claudication, in an early study following the implementation of this coverage in 2017, race, sex, and socioeconomic differences were observed with Black individuals, women, and dual Medicaid-Medicare enrollment were less likely to be prescribed supervised exercise therapy as ascertained by CPT codes [47]. In a cross-sectional study of patients with PAD across the Chicagoland area and in the surrounding suburbs being seen at Northwestern Memorial Hospital between 2019 and 2022, Black participants were more likely to have been recommended supervised exercise therapy than White participants, but were less likely to receive an actual referral for supervised exercise therapy [48]. Compared to non-Black individuals, Black participants were more likely to be willing to participate in supervised exercise therapy (79.6% vs 65.8%, p = 0.001), but were less willing or able to pay the $11 copay per exercise session for a total of 36 sessions (34.8% vs 47.3%, p = 0.017) [48]. Reasons for lower prescriptions for supervised exercise therapy in racial and ethnic minority populations with claudication are not well studied, but could reflect provider bias, patient counseling and education missteps, and/or financial, transportation, or other neighborhood-level barriers affecting attendance and adherence to supervised exercise therapy programs.

Guideline-directed, or optimal medical therapy (OMT) is underutilized in the general population with PAD [49, 50], with well-documented racial and ethnic disparities seen in large-scale epidemiologic studies of patients with cardiovascular risk factors [51]. There are few studies, however, that focus on disparities in OMT use in patients with claudication, alone. In a state-wide, registry-based, retrospective cohort study of patients undergoing open revascularization for claudication between 2012 and 2021, less than 50% of the study population was on OMT, which was defined as antiplatelet, statin and angiotensin-converting enzyme inhibitors or angiotensin II receptor therapy, prior to surgery and there was no difference according to race or insurance status [52]. In contrast to this study's findings and using a different study population, the Best Endovascular versus Best Surgical Therapy in Patients with CLTI (BEST-CLI) randomized controlled trial that compared the effectiveness of endovascular versus open revascularization in patients with CLTI, found racial disparities in OMT use at trial entry before randomization. Specifically, only 25% of patients met the four components of OMT that included hypertension control, smoking abstinence, lipid management, and use of an antiplatelet. In a regression model adjusted for age, sex, geographic location, and comorbidity, fewer Black participants met OMT criteria as compared to White participants (−0.14%, 95% CI: −0.26 - -0.02) [53]. The qualitative differences in disparities in OMT use comparing patients with claudication to CLTI might reflect differences in study populations and/or methodology, and definitions of OMT. It is uncertain if differences in OMT use explain health disparities in PAD incidence and intervention outcomes and if interventions that target disparate OMT use alone would lead to a meaningful reduction in health disparities.

Racial and ethnic disparities in the surgical management of claudication have also been studied with evidence that racial and ethnic minorities with claudication undergo revascularization less often than White populations with claudication. When they do undergo revascularization, they are subject to endovascular procedures not supported by clinical practice guidelines and with worse limb outcomes [54]. Among patients undergoing their first vascular procedure, as captured within the VQI, Black patients undergoing revascularization were more likely to have an indication of chronic limb-threatening ischemia compared to claudication, compared to White patients [18]. In a state-wide registry study that did not differentiate between intermittent claudication and CLTI, the anatomic distribution of PAD and subsequent interventions have also been found to differ according to race, with White individuals being almost 4 times more likely to undergo surgical management for aortoiliac disease but less likely to undergo infra-popliteal artery interventions, compared to Black patients [55]. Using a multi-level framework to conceptualize procedure rates for intermittent claudication, factors for relatively lower procedure rates among racial and ethnic minorities might include patient disease awareness (individual-level), provider judgement in assessment of symptoms and willingness to provide care (interpersonal/provider-level) and/or healthcare access barriers (community/policy-level), among others [56].

When focusing on endovascular interventions for intermittent claudication alone, complex interactions are observed between race, income, geography, proceduralist specialty, and practice setting. In a cross-sectional cohort study of Medicare beneficiaries with an incident intermittent claudication diagnosis, endovascular intervention in the femoral-popliteal artery segment was highest among Black individuals with relatively lower income with the crude peripheral vascular intervention (PVI) rate for Black individuals with median household incomes less than $48,000 being 20 per 1000 patients with claudication. In adjusted models, this PVI rate was significantly higher compared to White individuals in the same income category (OR 1.30, 95% CI 1.20–1.40) [11]. Higher income was protective with negligible race-specific differences observed at higher incomes. In a similar study population, Black race was associated with 47% higher odds of tibial intervention for claudication, and interventions were more often performed by proceduralists who practice in high-volume and high-reimbursement settings, raising suspicion for provider-driven overuse and mistreatment as a key driver of health disparities in claudication outcomes [57].. Using data from the PINC AI Healthcare database, which is an all-payer database from geographically diverse hospitals across the United States, Black patients were more likely than White patients to undergo femoral-popliteal artery atherectomy and had a 13% higher rate of reintervention compared to White patients [58].

Downstream health outcome disparities, such as amputation, are the culmination of differential medical and surgical management of claudication arising from the unequal distribution of knowledge, power, and resources in the United States. Socially disadvantaged individuals with claudication in the United States have the worst limb outcomes. In a VQI-based study of procedures for claudication (that did not stratify by open versus endovascular intervention), Black and Hispanic patients had a higher 1-year adjusted cumulative incidence of major amputation compared to White patients, 1.59 (95% CI, 1.17–2.15) and 1.34 (95% CI, 0.81–2.21), respectively [12]. Low-income, Black patients with claudication have the highest amputation risk at three years despite similar comorbidity burden as White patients with claudication of similar socioeconomic status [59]. Early endovascular intervention for claudication, in particular, has been highlighted in the literature for subsequent poor outcomes and progression to chronic limb-threatening ischemia [14]. The major adverse limb event-free survival at 1 year is 79.2% among Black individuals versus 83.8% among White individuals, $p < 0.001$ [60].

Heterogeneity in Disparities in Hispanic Populations Might Represent "Hispanic Paradox"

While differences in Black versus White populations have been extensively studied, Hispanic populations, other racial groups in the United States (e.g., American Indian and Native Hawaiian or Pacific Islander, etc.), and Middle Eastern or North African (MENA) populations are less often represented, possibly due to relatively small numbers in large-scale studies. Consistent with fundamental social causes theory, some Hispanic ethnic minorities in the United States face similar social barriers and have a similar distribution of PAD-related risk factors and health outcomes that mirror those of Black racial minorities in some studies. Reports suggest that Hispanic patients with PAD present with more severe disease, have lower rates of revascularization attempts, and have higher rates of lower extremity amputation [30, 61–63]. Among those that undergo revascularization for PAD, Loja et al. showed that within a year of revascularization, Hispanic patients had a hazard ratio for amputation of 1.69 compared to White patients ($p < 0.0001$) [54]. In a more contemporary cohort that included a study population of patients with claudication that was 24.3% Hispanic, Luna et al. reported that Hispanic patients had lower odds of revascularization (surgical: OR, 0.62; 95% CI 0.57–0.67; endovascular: OR, 0.94; 95% CI, 0.89–0.996) but higher odds of amputation (minor amputation: OR, 1.25, 95% CI 1.20–1.31; major amputation: OR, 1.08, 95% CI 1.03–1.14) [63].

There are some notable findings among Hispanic populations that have been highlighted in rare studies that reflect the heterogeneity of the populations defined as "Hispanic" in research, the unique mechanisms of disparities according to ethnicity, and differentiate the "minority" experience in the United States from that of Black populations. While Hispanic individuals may share a common language, they are a heterogenous group in terms of ancestry, country of origin, migrant status, and degree of acculturation [64, 65]. The first notable difference among Hispanic populations, which might not be anticipated based on their "minority" status in the United States, is that Hispanic individuals have been found to have a similar prevalence of PAD compared to White individuals [2, 3, 7]. When the Hispanic population is stratified according to generation status (i.e., individuals who were not born in the United States versus individuals with a parent not born in the United States), and self-identification as Mexican, Puerto Rican, Cuban, Dominican, Central American, or Other, important differences emerge. Using data from the Hispanic Community Study - Study of Latinos (HCHS-SOL), which is the most comprehensive long-term study of health and disease of United States-based Hispanic populations, Cuban Americans had the highest age- and gender-adjusted PAD prevalence as compared to Mexican Americans and the highest among other groups within the Hispanic population [66]. Using the HCHS-SOL study population, OMT use among patients with PAD, 77% of whom reported claudication, varied within the Hispanic population. Specifically, patients who self-identified as Dominican, Cuban, or Puerto Rican were more likely than Mexican Americans to use anti-platelet or statin therapy, and there were no differences according to generation status [67]. Health insurance status attenuated differences between groups across some medication subclasses suggesting that socioeconomic status explains some of the differences between Mexican Americans and other groups within the Hispanic population. The observation that some Hispanic populations have similar or better health outcomes to White populations in the United States despite being socially disadvantaged has been described as the "Hispanic paradox". There are several explanations of the "Hispanic paradox" in the literature that include the Hispanic population being made up of the healthiest immigrants from their countries of origin, measurement bias in ethnicity classification, and protection afforded by social cohesion and connection, for example [68, 69]. It might be that when using coarse categorizations of ethnicity, at the population level, Hispanic populations look very similar to White populations. The limited available data suggests that more nuanced data that includes ethnicity dimensions, such as country of origin, ancestry, and acculturation, and its interaction with socioeconomic variables, may better delineate the heterogeneity in PAD prevalence and outcomes among the Hispanic population and divergence from other socially disadvantaged groups in the United States.

Unique Mechanisms of Claudication Health Disparities Among Women

Historically, it has been thought that the prevalence of PAD is lower in women compared to men, however, this assertion has been challenged over the years. In a systematic review incorporating women of various ages and risk factor distribution, PAD prevalence ranged from 3 to 29% [70]. The relationship between sex-related hormones, such as estrogen and progesterone, and hormone replacement therapies have also been investigated as modifiable risk factors for incident PAD [71, 72]. The Risk of Arterial Thrombosis In relation to Oral Contraceptives (RATIO) study that used a case-control study design found that women aged 18–49 who reported oral contraceptive use had a higher odds of PAD [73]. Given the increase in risk of PAD in women after menopause, two large trials: the HERS trial and the Women's Health Initiative (WHI) sought to investigate the role of hormone replacement therapy on PAD and CAD risk [71, 72]. The HERS trial and WHI trial have demonstrated no benefit from hormone replacement therapy against PAD and coronary artery disease [71]. However, in the Rotterdam study, there was a decrease in PAD with greater than one year of use of hormone replacement therapy [74]. The WHI looked at the effect of estrogen with progestin or estrogen alone on peripheral vascular events and there was no significantly different incidence of PAD in women with and without treatment identified [72]. In summary, there is insufficient evidence to suggest clear hormonal mechanisms among women.

A fact that has been true across studies in women is that women more often have asymptomatic cardiovascular disease, and present with atypical claudication symptoms [75]. In a cohort of women older than age 55 and sampled from 3 general internal medicine practices in the Chicago area, women with intermittent claudication were more often debilitated by the pain and more often have to stop exertion with the onset of symptoms as compared to men who reporting being able to "carry on" or work through their pain [76]. Further, on objective measures documented in this study, women had slower walking velocities after adjustment for age, height, race, comorbidities, and leg symptoms and strength. In a community-based setting that examined the association in walking cadence to strides per minute and as time to ischemia, as measured by calf muscle hemoglobin oxygen saturation, women with intermittent claudication were found to ambulate slower and to reach ischemia sooner [77]. The effect of intermittent claudication on women extended beyond just walking impairment and affected other activities of daily living. Women with PAD more often report fear of falls, less activity outside of their homes, more often have tandem walk errors, and rate their health as poor as compared to women without PAD [78].

Future Directions for Claudication Health Disparities Research

There is a preponderance of research describing the burden of PAD, medical and procedural treatments for PAD, and health outcomes according to race. This body of literature is not well balanced with the knowledge and study of sociopolitical determinants of health, which leads to incomplete understanding as well as sometimes misleading conclusions and misdirected resources and/or solutions [79]. While our knowledge of racial, ethnic, and sex disparities has increased over the years, there is still much to uncover in understanding these differences. The data that we currently have largely stems from observational studies that use secondary data sources, rarely separates populations with intermittent claudication and CLTI, uses imprecise and basic definitions of complex social constructs, and imputes socioeconomic data using census-based resources. This leads to bias and a severely limited understanding of potential intervention targets. Several opportunities exist in improving PAD-specific research and care by improving the following: [1] broadening research into sociopolitical determinants of health that affect PAD care, [2] employing advanced epidemiologic methods to determine causality, [3] improving representation in randomized controlled trials (RCTs) and pragmatic implementation trials, and [4] incorporating patient reported outcome measures (PROMs) into symptomatic PAD evaluation.

Broadening Investigation into Sociopolitical Determinants of Health Effecting PAD Care

Most of the literature in evaluating socioeconomic status in patients with PAD utilizes insurance status, education level, household income or residential unit composite measures, such as the area-deprivation index or the social vulnerability index, all of which use the same underlying data sources and essentially assess the same determinant (Fig. 6.3). There are many unstudied sociopolitical determinants that may play a key role in claudication disparities, such as occupational status, transportation, food insecurity, built environment that might account for access to sidewalks and public gyms, healthcare workforce diversity and/or discrimination, to name a few [80]. Using the NIHMD Research Framework [17], the greatest research gaps are in the study of community and societal level influences (Fig. 6.3). Future research in these knowledge gap areas might include examining the influence of social networks on PAD-related health and its potential as a protective or resiliency factor (which has been described in other disease states to account for trends in Hispanic populations), structural racism that is encoded in policies and laws and its pervasive effects on contemporary disease prevalence, provider behaviors, patient entrustment, and longitudinal outcomes, and/or embodiment hypotheses whereby everyday racism and stress leads to differences in allostatic load and epigenetic changes to individuals and various communities, for example.

Next-Generation Health Disparities Research Employs Social Epidemiologic Theory and Advanced Methods

Most of the literatureof health disparities in the diagnosis and management of claudication is descriptive, includes prevalence studies and risk factor analyses, and demonstrates the statistical association between variables, such as race and PAD outcomes, and not causality. Further, nearly all studies lack variable definitions,

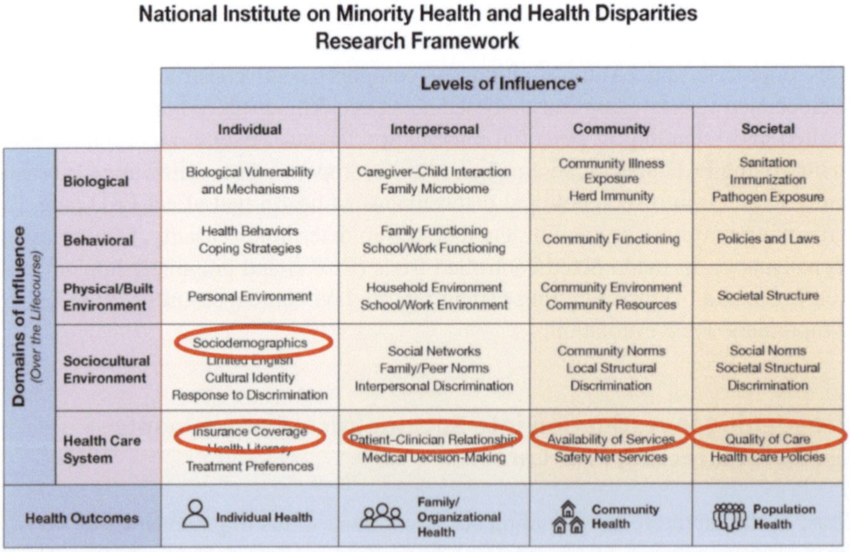

Fig. 6.3 Scope of health disparities research according to NIHMD Research Framework

conceptual framework, and modeling approaches that are grounded in social epidemiologic theory. In a conceptual framework of generations of health disparities research that includes (a) first-generation research that focuses detection, identification, and documentation of disparities according to vulnerable populations; (b) second-generation research that seeks to identify causal relationships that underlie health disparities; (c) third-generation research involving the development and implementation of interventions to directly address health disparities; and (d) community-engaged research that shifts away from individualistic and biomedical models to multi-level determinants with a public health focus [81], the majority of PAD health disparities research represents first-generation, with some second-generation, research. Each observational study that aims to study health disparities should start with a causal diagram. In a guidance document on how to create causal diagrams, social epidemiologists put forth the following recommendations for more rigorous and informative health disparities research [82], [1] in lieu of "race" variable and to avoid "race" being interpreted as a biologic variable, the diagram should include a variable that reflects membership in a societally imposed marginalized group caused by historical and/or contemporary institutional processes, [2] explicitly state that "race" is socially constructed, [3] depict health determinants as operating on multiple levels, [4] include both historical and contemporary institutional forces shaping structural differences, and [5] include the downstream biologic determinants of health outcomes under study (e.g., stress, access to healthcare, quality of health care). Uncommon methods in the current PAD literature that would be examples of third- and fourth-generation health disparities research include mediation analysis, decomposition methods, instrumental variable analysis, natural experiments, multi-level models, agent-based modeling, network analysis, and community-based participatory research for example [83].

Improving Reporting and Representation in RCTs

Causal methods, such as randomized controlled trials (RCTs), lack racial, ethnic, and sex minority population representation, despite higher PAD prevalence and greater need. Hoel et al. reviewed aortic aneurysm repair, carotid revascularization, and lower extremity revascularization RCTs conducted in the United States and published between 1983 and 2007. Of the 52 studies meeting inclusion criteria, ethnicity was reported in 21% of the studies and in 5 of the 13 studies (38.5%) that focused specifically on lower extremity revascularization. They found that race/ethnicity was more commonly reported in large (> 280 patients), multi-center, government-funded RCTs [84]. Castro-Dominguez et al. reviewed all PAD-specific RCTs cited in the 2016 AHA/ACC treatment guidelines for lower extremity PAD. There were 79 of 409 references meeting the inclusion criteria. Of these, only 27% of the studies reported racial and ethnic distribution with North American trials reporting this metric more frequently than European trials (61.9% versus 4.4%). The pooled proportion of Black patients was 3.2% compared to the proportion of Black patients with PAD in the United States which was estimated to be 15.9% in this study [85]. In another contemporary systematic review, Long et al. examined diversity in RCTs focused on lower-extremity endovascular PAD interventions. Their group found that, of the 14 RCT publications that met all inclusion criteria, only 4 reported on racial and ethnic status while all 14 publications reported on age and sex [86]. To help improve reporting, we recommend several interventions. The use of standard race and ethnicity categories such as those used by the Office of Management and Budget and expansion of gender categories as well as ethnic categorization schemes that allow for the capture of country of origin, ancestry, and acculturation will allow for a more granular community-based examination of race, ethnicity, and sex disparities in claudication and PAD at large. Often when reporting demographics, ethnicity and race are used interchangeably which discounts and weakens the evidence of studies being performed with regards to generalizability. There must be diverse study team investigators and research staff as well as continued education with research staff regarding differences in race and ethnicity. Long et al. also suggested patient-provider concordance as a potential solution to improving representation of racial and ethnic minorities and females into RCTs [86]. Therefore, increasing diversity of principal investigators (i.e., more women and individuals that identify as racial and ethnic minorities) may improve engagement in research among patients from these same groups.

Incorporating PROMs into Clinical Research and Practice

Although guidelines exist regarding the management of PAD, a key component of treatment is shared decision-making between the physician and patient; documenting conduct of this process and/or lack thereof will be an important treatment variable in the population with PAD. In a study of 281 PAD patients experiencing claudication, the number one treatment goal for patients was improved quality of life (31.3%) [87]. In a similar survey of 150 patients with claudication, Powell et al. showed that the majority (62.0%) of patients' primary treatment goals were to increase walking distance or duration without stopping while 23.0% of the patients had goals of performing a specific activity, commonly a sport or outdoor recreational activity [88]. Because there are varying degrees of disability experienced by patients with claudication depending on their activity level and lifestyle, improving quality of life can mean many different things to patients affected by claudication. Incorporating PROMs into clinical practice, as an adjunct to objective measures of PAD disease burden, will help physicians to understand the patient experience, their longitudinal journey with their condition, and their subjective views regarding their care. The peripheral artery questionnaire (PAQ), vascular quality of life questionnaire (VascuQOL), and walking impairment questionnaire (WIQ) meet quality standards for internal consistency in questionnaire subdomains and summary scores making them good resources to use to measure PROMs [89]. While they are commonly used in trials, it is important to incorporate the use of PROMs in clinical practice to better understand our patients' goals of care and quality of life, especially in racial and ethnic minorities that have disproportionate access to and differential provision of claudication management.

Conclusions

Health disparities in the management of claudication among race, ethnic, and sex minority groups are well-documented, and the best available evidence points toward provider-level decision-making, and social and public policies that shape how, when, and where patients get care as key drivers of health disparities. Minority populations with claudication in the United States do not receive care that is in accordance with clinical practice guidelines, and future claudication-specific health disparities research will hopefully incorporate more granular populations and socio-political determinants of health, employ epidemiologic methods that establish causality and propose intervention targets, and study interventions via natural experiments, decomposition methods, RCTs, or community-based efforts that center minority populations.

References

1. Zheng ZJ, Rosamond WD, Chambless LE, Nieto FJ, Barnes RW, Hutchinson RG, et al. Lower extremity arterial disease assessed by ankle-brachial index in a middle-aged population of African Americans and whites: the atherosclerosis risk in communities (ARIC) study. Am J Prev Med. 2005;29(5 Suppl 1):42–9.
2. Collins TC, Petersen NJ, Suarez-Almazor M, Ashton CM. The prevalence of peripheral arterial disease in a racially diverse population. Arch Intern Med. 2003;163(12):1469–74.
3. Allison MA, Ho E, Denenberg JO, Langer RD, Newman AB, Fabsitz RR, et al. Ethnic-specific prevalence of peripheral arterial disease in the United States. Am J Prev Med. 2007;32(4):328–33.
4. Criqui MH, Aboyans V. Epidemiology of peripheral artery disease. Circ Res. 2015;116(9):1509–26.
5. Kalbaugh CA, Kucharska-Newton A, Wruck L, Lund JL, Selvin E, Matsushita K, et al. Peripheral artery disease prevalence and incidence estimated from both outpatient and inpatient settings among Medicare fee-for-service beneficiaries in the atherosclerosis risk in communities (ARIC) study. J Am Heart Assoc 2017;6(5).
6. Matsushita K, Sang Y, Ning H, Ballew SH, Chow EK, Grams ME, et al. Lifetime risk of lower-extremity peripheral artery disease defined by ankle-brachial index in the United States. J Am Heart Assoc. 2019;8(18):e012177.
7. Selvin E, Erlinger TP. Prevalence of and risk factors for peripheral arterial disease in the United States: results from the National Health and nutrition examination survey, 1999-2000. Circulation. 2004;110(6):738–43.
8. Criqui MH, Vargas V, Denenberg JO. Ethnicity and peripheral arterial disease: the San Diego population study. J Vasc Surg. 2006;43(6):1312–3.
9. Conte MS, Pomposelli FB, Clair DG, Geraghty PJ, McKinsey JF, Mills JL, et al. Society for Vascular Surgery practice guidelines for atherosclerotic occlusive disease of the lower extremities: management of asymptomatic disease and claudication. J Vasc Surg. 2015;61(3 Suppl):2S–41S.

10. Woo K, Siracuse JJ, Klingbeil K, Kraiss LW, Osborne NH, Singh N, et al. Society for Vascular Surgery appropriate use criteria for management of intermittent claudication. J Vasc Surg. 2022;76(1):3–22 e21.
11. Hicks CW, Wang P, Bruhn WE, Abularrage CJ, Lum YW, Perler BA, et al. Race and socioeconomic differences associated with endovascular peripheral vascular interventions for newly diagnosed claudication. J Vasc Surg. 2020;72(2):611–621.e615.
12. Kalbaugh CA, Witrick B, Sivaraj LB, McGinigle KL, Lesko CR, Cykert S, et al. Non-Hispanic Black and Hispanic patients have worse outcomes than White patients within similar stages of peripheral artery disease. J Am Heart Assoc. 2022;11(1):e023396.
13. Krawisz AK, Natesan S, Wadhera RK, Chen S, Song Y, Yeh RW, et al. Differences in comorbidities explain Black-White disparities in outcomes after Femoropopliteal endovascular intervention. Circulation. 2022;146(3):191–200.
14. Sorber R, Dun C, Kawaji Q, Abularrage CJ, Black JH 3rd, Makary MA, et al. Early peripheral vascular interventions for claudication are associated with higher rates of late interventions and progression to chronic limb threatening ischemia. J Vasc Surg. 2023;77(3):836–847.e833.
15. Mauvais-Jarvis F, Bairey Merz N, Barnes PJ, Brinton RD, Carrero JJ, DeMeo DL, et al. Sex and gender: modifiers of health, disease, and medicine. Lancet. 2020;396(10250):565–82.
16. Shannon G, Jansen M, Williams K, Cáceres C, Motta A, Odhiambo A, et al. Gender equality in science, medicine, and global health: where are we at and why does it matter? Lancet. 2019;393(10171):560–9.
17. Alvidrez J, Castille D, Laude-Sharp M, Rosario A, Tabor D. The National Institute on Minority Health and Health Disparities research framework. Am J Public Health. 2019;109(S1):S16–s20.
18. Soden PA, Zettervall SL, Deery SE, Hughes K, Stoner MC, Goodney PP, et al. Black patients present with more severe vascular disease and a greater burden of risk factors than white patients at time of major vascular intervention. J Vasc Surg. 2018;67(2):549–556.e543.
19. Alasaad M, Zaitoun A, Szpunar S, Lalonde T, Rosman HS, Mehta RH, et al. Association of race with long-term outcomes in patients undergoing popliteal and infra-popliteal percutaneous peripheral arterial interventions. Cardiovasc Revasc Med. 2019;20(8):649–53.
20. Eraso LH, Fukaya E, Mohler ER 3rd, Xie D, Sha D, Berger JS. Peripheral arterial disease, prevalence and cumulative risk factor profile analysis. Eur J Prev Cardiol. 2014;21(6):704–11.
21. Allison MA, Criqui MH, McClelland RL, Scott JM, McDermott MM, Liu K, et al. The effect of novel cardiovascular risk factors on the ethnic-specific odds for peripheral arterial disease in the multi-ethnic study of atherosclerosis (MESA). J Am Coll Cardiol. 2006;48(6):1190–7.
22. Williams DR, Mohammed SA. Racism and health I: pathways and scientific evidence. Am Behav Sci. 2013;57(8):1152.
23. Link BG, Phelan J. Social conditions as fundamental causes of disease. J Health Soc Behav. 1995;36:80–94.
24. Phelan JC, Link BG, Diez-Roux A, Kawachi I, Levin B. "Fundamental causes" of social inequalities in mortality: a test of the theory. J Health Soc Behav. 2004;45(3):265–85.
25. He J, Bundy JD, Geng S, Tian L, He H, Li X, et al. Social, behavioral, and metabolic risk factors and racial disparities in cardiovascular disease mortality in U.S. adults: an observational study. Ann Intern Med. 2023;176(9):1200–8.
26. McDermott MM, Polonsky TS, Kibbe MR, Tian L, Zhao L, Pearce WH, et al. Racial differences in functional decline in peripheral artery disease and associations with socioeconomic status and education. J Vasc Surg. 2017;66(3):826–34.
27. Schüle SA, Hilz LK, Dreger S, Bolte G. Social inequalities in environmental resources of green and blue spaces: a review of evidence in the WHO European region. Int J Environ Res Public Health 2019;16(7).
28. Chudyk AM, McKay HA, Winters M, Sims-Gould J, Ashe MC. Neighborhood walkability, physical activity, and walking for transportation: a cross-sectional study of older adults living on low income. BMC Geriatr. 2017;17(1):82.
29. Lee MH, Li B, Feridooni T, Li PY, Shakespeare A, Samarasinghe Y, et al. Racial and ethnic differences in presentation severity and postoperative outcomes in vascular surgery. J Vasc Surg. 2023;77(4):1274–1288.e1214.

30. Eslami MH, Zayaruzny M, Fitzgerald GA. The adverse effects of race, insurance status, and low income on the rate of amputation in patients presenting with lower extremity ischemia. J Vasc Surg. 2007;45(1):55–9.
31. Hirsch AT, Criqui MH, Treat-Jacobson D, Regensteiner JG, Creager MA, Olin JW, et al. Peripheral arterial disease detection, awareness, and treatment in primary care. JAMA. 2001;286(11):1317–24.
32. Schorr EN, Treat-Jacobson D. Methods of symptom evaluation and their impact on peripheral artery disease (PAD) symptom prevalence: a review. Vasc Med. 2013;18(2):95–111.
33. Grant C, Cuddeback JK, Alabi O, Hicks CW, Sadik K, Ciemins EL. Perspectives on lower extremity peripheral artery disease: a qualitative study of early diagnosis and treatment and the impact of health disparities. Popul Health Manag. 2023;26(6):387–96.
34. Conte MS, Pomposelli FB. Society for Vascular Surgery Practice guidelines for atherosclerotic occlusive disease of the lower extremities management of asymptomatic disease and claudication. Introduction. J Vasc Surg. 2015;61(3 Suppl):1s.
35. Gerhard-Herman MD, Gornik HL, Barrett C, Barshes NR, Corriere MA, Drachman DE, et al. 2016 AHA/ACC guideline on the Management of Patients with Lower Extremity Peripheral Artery Disease: a report of the American College of Cardiology/American Heart Association task force on clinical practice guidelines. J Am Coll Cardiol. 2017;69(11):e71–e126.
36. Meadows TA, Bhatt DL, Hirsch AT, Creager MA, Califf RM, Ohman EM, et al. Ethnic differences in the prevalence and treatment of cardiovascular risk factors in US outpatients with peripheral arterial disease: insights from the reduction of atherothrombosis for continued health (REACH) registry. Am Heart J. 2009;158(6):1038–45.
37. O'Donnell TFX, Powell C, Deery SE, Darling JD, Hughes K, Giles KA, et al. Regional variation in racial disparities among patients with peripheral artery disease. J Vasc Surg. 2018;68(2):519–26.
38. Barbeau EM, Krieger N, Soobader MJ. Working class matters: socioeconomic disadvantage, race/ethnicity, gender, and smoking in NHIS 2000. Am J Public Health. 2004;94(2):269–78.
39. Okechukwu CA, Krieger N, Chen J, Sorensen G, Li Y, Barbeau EM. The association of workplace hazards and smoking in a U.S. multiethnic working-class population. Public Health Rep. 2010;125(2):225–33.
40. Garrett BE, Martell BN, Caraballo RS, King BA. Socioeconomic differences in cigarette smoking among sociodemographic groups. Prev Chronic Dis. 2019;16:E74.
41. Lee MH, Li B, Feridooni T, Li PY, Shakespeare A, Samarasinghe Y, et al. Racial and ethnic differences in presentation severity and postoperative outcomes in vascular surgery. J Vasc Surg. 2023;77(4):1274–1288 e1214.
42. Bailey SR, Heintzman J, Jacob RL, Puro J, Marino M. Disparities in smoking cessation assistance in US primary care clinics. Am J Public Health. 2018;108(8):1082–90.
43. Fu SS, Kodl MM, Joseph AM, Hatsukami DK, Johnson EO, Breslau N, et al. Racial/ethnic disparities in the use of nicotine replacement therapy and quit ratios in lifetime smokers ages 25 to 44 years. Cancer Epidemiol Biomarkers Prev. 2008;17(7):1640–7.
44. Piper ME, Cook JW, Schlam TR, Jorenby DE, Smith SS, Bolt DM, et al. Gender, race, and education differences in abstinence rates among participants in two randomized smoking cessation trials. Nicotine Tob Res. 2010;12(6):647–57.
45. Huen KH, Chowdhury R, Shafii SM, Brewster LP, Arya S, Duwayri Y, et al. Smoking cessation is the least successful outcome of risk factor modification in uninsured patients with symptomatic peripheral arterial disease. Ann Vasc Surg. 2015;29(1):42–9.
46. Bailey SR, Hoopes MJ, Marino M, Heintzman J, O'Malley JP, Hatch B, et al. Effect of gaining insurance coverage on smoking cessation in community health centers: a cohort study. J Gen Intern Med. 2016;31(10):1198–205.
47. Divakaran S, Carroll BJ, Chen S, Shen C, Bonaca MP, Secemsky EA. Supervised exercise therapy for symptomatic peripheral artery disease among medicare beneficiaries between 2017 and 2018: participation rates and outcomes. Circ Cardiovasc Qual Outcomes. 2021;14(8):e007953.

48. Cetlin MD, Polonsky T, Ho K, Zhang D, Tian L, Zhao L, et al. Barriers to participation in supervised exercise therapy reported by people with peripheral artery disease. J Vasc Surg. 2023;77(2):506–14.
49. Berger JS, Ladapo JA. Underuse of prevention and lifestyle counseling in patients with peripheral artery disease. J Am Coll Cardiol. 2017;69(18):2293–300.
50. Pande RL, Perlstein TS, Beckman JA, Creager MA. Secondary prevention and mortality in peripheral artery disease: National Health and nutrition examination study, 1999 to 2004. Circulation. 2011;124(1):17–23.
51. Dorsch MP, Lester CA, Ding Y, Joseph M, Brook RD. Effects of race on statin prescribing for primary prevention with high atherosclerotic cardiovascular disease risk in a large healthcare system. J Am Heart Assoc. 2019;8(22):e014709.
52. Howard R, Albright J, Powell C, Osborne N, Corriere M, Laveroni E, et al. Underutilization of medical management of peripheral artery disease among patients with claudication undergoing lower extremity bypass. J Vasc Surg. 2022;76(4):1037–1044.e1032.
53. Menard MT, Jaff MR, Farber A, Rosenfield K, Conte MS, White CJ, et al. Baseline modern medical management in the BEST-CLI trial. J Vasc Surg. 2023;78(3):711–718.e715.
54. Loja MN, Brunson A, Li CS, Carson JG, White RH, Romano PS, et al. Racial disparities in outcomes of endovascular procedures for peripheral arterial disease: an evaluation of California hospitals, 2005-2009. Ann Vasc Surg. 2015;29(5):950–9.
55. Brothers TE, Robison JG, Sutherland SE, Elliott BM. Racial differences in operation for peripheral vascular disease: results of a population-based study. Cardiovasc Surg. 1997;5(1):26–31.
56. Purnell TS, Calhoun EA, Golden SH, Halladay JR, Krok-Schoen JL, Appelhans BM, et al. Achieving health equity: closing the gaps in health care disparities, interventions and research. Health Aff (Millwood). 2016;35(8):1410–5.
57. Bose S, Dun C, Sorber R, Stonko DP, Solomon AJ, Black JH 3rd, et al. Practice patterns surrounding the use of tibial interventions for claudication in the medicare population. J Vasc Surg. 2023;77(2):454–462.e451.
58. Altin SE, Parise H, Hess CN, Rosenthal NA, Julien HM, Curtis JP. Co-morbidity differences associated with long-term amputation and repeat revascularization rates after femoropopliteal artery intervention for intermittent claudication by sex, race, and ethnicity. Am J Cardiol. 2024;226:40–9.
59. Arya S, Binney Z, Khakharia A, Brewster LP, Goodney P, Patzer R, et al. Race and socioeconomic status independently affect risk of major amputation in peripheral artery disease. J Am Heart Assoc 2018;7(2).
60. Semaan DB, Abdul-Malak OM, Avgerinos ED, Chaer RA, Madigan MC, Siracuse JJ, et al. Racial disparities in treatment indications and outcomes for limb ischemia. Ann Vasc Surg. 2023;96:89–97.
61. Rowe VL, Weaver FA, Lane JS, Etzioni DA. Racial and ethnic differences in patterns of treatment for acute peripheral arterial disease in the United States, 1998–2006. J Vasc Surg. 2010;51(4 Suppl):21s–6s.
62. Holman KH, Henke PK, Dimick JB, Birkmeyer JD. Racial disparities in the use of revascularization before leg amputation in medicare patients. J Vasc Surg. 2011;54(2):420–426.e421.
63. Luna P, Harris K, Castro-Dominguez Y, Algara M, Severiche-Mena C, Smolderen KG, et al. Risk profiles, access to care, and outcomes in Hispanics hospitalized for lower extremity peripheral artery disease. J Vasc Surg. 2023;77(1):216–224 e215.
64. Lin SS, Kelsey JL. Use of race and ethnicity in epidemiologic research: concepts, methodological issues, and suggestions for research. Epidemiol Rev. 2000;22(2):187–202.
65. González Burchard E, Borrell LN, Choudhry S, Naqvi M, Tsai HJ, Rodriguez-Santana JR, et al. Latino populations: a unique opportunity for the study of race, genetics, and social environment in epidemiological research. Am J Public Health. 2005;95(12):2161–8.
66. Allison MA, Gonzalez F 2nd, Raij L, Kaplan R, Ostfeld RJ, Pattany MS, et al. Cuban Americans have the highest rates of peripheral arterial disease in diverse Hispanic/Latino communities. J Vasc Surg. 2015;62(3):665–72.

67. Hua S, Isasi CR, Kizer JR, Matsushita K, Allison MA, Tarraf W, et al. Underuse of cardiovascular medications in individuals with known lower extremity peripheral artery disease: HCHS/SOL. J Am Heart Assoc. 2020;9(16):e015451.
68. Teruya SA, Bazargan-Hejazi S. The immigrant and hispanic paradoxes: a systematic review of their predictions and effects. Hisp J Behav Sci. 2013;35(4):486–509.
69. Fernandez J, García-Pérez M, Orozco-Aleman S. Unraveling the hispanic health paradox. J Econ Perspect. 2023;37(1):145–68.
70. Higgins JP, Higgins JA. Epidemiology of peripheral arterial disease in women. J Epidemiol. 2003;13(1):1–14.
71. Grady D, Herrington D, Bittner V, Blumenthal R, Davidson M, Hlatky M, et al. Cardiovascular disease outcomes during 6.8 years of hormone therapy: heart and estrogen/progestin replacement study follow-up (HERS II). JAMA. 2002;288(1):49–57.
72. Hsia J, Criqui MH, Rodabough RJ, Langer RD, Resnick HE, Phillips LS, et al. Estrogen plus progestin and the risk of peripheral arterial disease: the Women's Health Initiative. Circulation. 2004;109(5):620–6.
73. Van Den Bosch MAAJ, Kemmeren JM, Tanis BC, Mali WPTM, Helmerhorst FM, Rosendaal FR, et al. The RATIO study: oral contraceptives and the risk of peripheral arterial disease in young women. J Thromb Haemost. 2003;1(3):439–44.
74. Jelani QU, Petrov M, Martinez SC, Holmvang L, Al-Shaibi K, Alasnag M. Peripheral arterial disease in women: an overview of risk factor profile, clinical features, and outcomes. Curr Atheroscler Rep. 2018;20(8):40.
75. Patel T, Baydoun H, Patel NK, Tripathi B, Nanavaty S, Savani S, et al. Peripheral arterial disease in women: the gender effect. Cardiovasc Revasc Med. 2020;21(3):404–8.
76. McDermott MM, Greenland P, Liu K, Criqui MH, Guralnik JM, Celic L, et al. Sex differences in peripheral arterial disease: leg symptoms and physical functioning. J Am Geriatr Soc. 2003;51(2):222–8.
77. Gardner AW, Parker DE, Montgomery PS, Khurana A, Ritti-Dias RM, Blevins SM. Gender differences in daily ambulatory activity patterns in patients with intermittent claudication. J Vasc Surg. 2010;52(5):1204–10.
78. Vogt MT, Cauley JA, Kuller LH, Nevitt MC. Functional status and mobility among elderly women with lower extremity arterial disease: the study of osteoporotic fractures. J Am Geriatr Soc. 1994;42(9):923–9.
79. Zenk SN, Simoni JM, Pérez-Stable EJ. Prioritizing research on social determinants of health—"yes, and…". JAMA Intern Med. 2024;185:253.
80. Duran DG, Perez-Stable EJ. Novel approaches to advance minority health and health disparities research. Am J Public Health. 2019;109(S1):S8–s10.
81. Thomas SB, Quinn SC, Butler J, Fryer CS, Garza MA. Toward a fourth generation of disparities research to achieve health equity. Annu Rev Public Health. 2011;32:399–416.
82. Howe CJ, Bailey ZD, Raifman JR, Jackson JW. Recommendations for using causal diagrams to study racial health disparities. Am J Epidemiol. 2022;191(12):1981–9.
83. Jeffries N, Zaslavsky AM, Diez Roux AV, Creswell JW, Palmer RC, Gregorich SE, et al. Methodological approaches to understanding causes of health disparities. Am J Public Health. 2019;109(S1):S28–33.
84. Hoel AW, Kayssi A, Brahmanandam S, Belkin M, Conte MS, Nguyen LL. Under-representation of women and ethnic minorities in vascular surgery randomized controlled trials. J Vasc Surg. 2009;50(2):349–54.
85. Castro-Dominguez Y, Mena-Hurtado C, Algara M, Obas V, Ahmed Z, Romain G, et al. Representativeness of peripheral artery disease randomized clinical trials supporting current guidelines. Am J Cardiol. 2023;201:166–9.
86. Long C, Williams AO, McGovern AM, Jacobsen CM, Hargens LM, Duval S, et al. Diversity in randomized clinical trials for peripheral artery disease: a systematic review. Int J Equity Health. 2024;23(1):29.
87. Smolderen KG, Romain G, Gosch K, Arham A, Provance JB, Spertus JA, et al. Patient knowledge and preferences for peripheral artery disease treatment. Vasc Med. 2023;28(5):397–403.

88. Powell CA, Kim GY, Edwards SN, Aalami O, Treat-Jacobson D, Byrnes ME, et al. Characterizing patient-reported claudication treatment goals to support patient-centered treatment selection and measurement strategies. J Vasc Surg. 2023;77(2):465–473 e465.
89. Rymer JA, Narcisse D, Cosiano M, Tanaka J, McDermott MM, Treat-Jacobson DJ, et al. Patient-reported outcome measures in symptomatic, non-limb-threatening peripheral artery disease: a state-of-the-art review. Circ Cardiovasc Interv. 2022;15(1):e011320.

7 Risk Factors for Claudication and Management to Modify Them

Ramprakash Devadoss and Alvaro Alonso

Introduction

Of the various etiologies of lower extremity peripheral artery disease (PAD), atherosclerosis is by far the most prevalent. The prevalence of atherosclerotic PAD is estimated to be approximately 5% at age 40, and 12% at age 70 [30]. PAD is the third leading cause of atherosclerotic morbidity, following coronary heart disease and stroke [23]. Patients with PAD have a high cardiovascular mortality risk that exceeds that of other cardiovascular conditions and many malignancies [5, 37]. The five-year cumulative incidence of clinical progression from asymptomatic PAD to claudication is 7%, and from claudication to critical limb-threatening ischemia (CLTI) is 21%. All patients with PAD are at high risk of major adverse cardiovascular events (MACE), cerebrovascular disease, and major adverse limb events (MALE). The five-year cumulative incidence of cardiovascular mortality is greater than 13% in patients with symptomatic PAD, which is considered very high risk. Patients who develop MALE have a poor prognosis, with a three-fold increase in the risk of death and a 200-fold increase in subsequent amputations [48].

Common risk factors associated with PAD include older age, diabetes, tobacco smoking, hypertension, and dyslipidemia. Other associated risk factors for PAD include African American race, obesity, systemic inflammation, elevated homocysteine, elevated lipoprotein (a), metabolic syndrome, chronic kidney disease, and sedentary lifestyle—Fig. 7.1 [39, 55, 63].

The strongest conventional risk factors associated with the development of lower extremity PAD are diabetes and smoking, which result in an exponential increase in risk in certain ethnic groups, such as African Americans [23, 27, 72].

Structured exercise, pharmacological and revascularization therapies for claudication, as well as smoking cessation are discussed at length in separate chapters of

R. Devadoss · A. Alonso (✉)
UMass Chan Medical School, UMass Memorial Medical Center, Worcester, MA, USA
e-mail: Ramprakash.Devadoss@umassmemorial.org; Alvaro.Alonso@umassmed.edu

W. P. Robinson III, J. P. Simons (eds.), *The Patient-Centered Approach to Claudication*, https://doi.org/10.1007/978-3-032-02460-2_7

Fig. 7.1 Approximate range of odds ratios for risk factors for symptomatic peripheral arterial disease. (Reprinted from: Norgren et al. [55], Copyright, 2007, with permission from Elsevier)

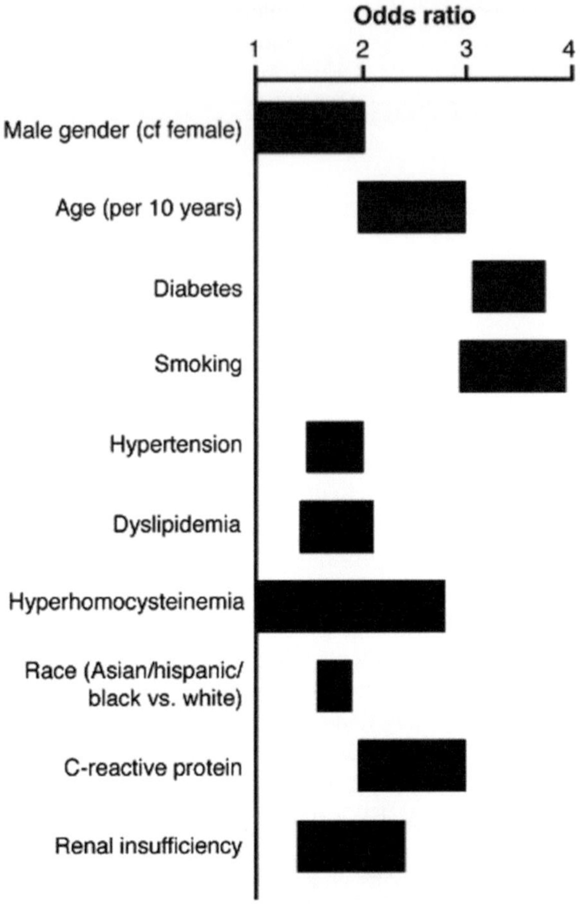

this book. Our objective in this chapter is to provide an overview of the management of cardiovascular risk factors and cardiovascular event reduction via risk factor modification therapies and antithrombotic therapies in patients with PAD, providing specific information in patients with claudication where available.

Diabetes Mellitus

The prevalence of PAD in patients with diabetes is 20%–30% [48]. Even though only about half of patients with diabetes have symptomatic PAD—often masked due to concurrent peripheral neuropathy and decreased pain sensitivity, individuals with diabetes still experience a two- to three-fold greater risk of developing claudication compared with individuals without diabetes [22]. Diabetes not only promotes atherosclerosis, but outcomes in patients with diabetes, including progression to CLTI, amputation and cardiovascular morbidity and mortality are also worse in patients with diabetes. The interrelation between diabetes, PAD, and neuropathy is also associated with the development of diabetic foot ulcers [13, 34, 64]. Therefore, screening and aggressive treatment of diabetes is paramount to improve MALE and MACE risk in patients with PAD [32, 48].

Type 1 Diabetes

In the Diabetes Control and Complications Trial (DCCT), there was a non-significant trend toward a reduction in the incidence of claudication, peripheral revascularization, or amputation in patients with type 1 diabetes treated with intensive insulin therapy. There was, however, a significant reduction in microvascular complications (retinopathy, albuminuria, neuropathy) [67]. This landmark trial sets the benchmark for optimal insulin therapy in these patients.

Type 2 Diabetes

In the UK Prospective Diabetes Study (UKPDS), there was no reduction in amputation risk in patients with type 2 diabetes who had more aggressive glucose control with sulfonylurea or insulin therapy despite reductions in microvascular complications [71]. However, a 10-year follow-up report of the UKPDS demonstrated a significant reduction in MACE [38].

The thiazolidinedione, pioglitazone, was evaluated in the Prospective Pioglitazone Clinical trial in macrovascular events, which showed no difference in need for revascularization or leg amputation in patients with PAD, however there was a significant decrease in all-cause mortality, non-fatal myocardial infarction, and stroke in high-risk type 2 diabetes patients [28].

Treatment with metformin in patients with type 2 diabetes was associated with decreased MACE and MALE in the HOME and DIAPA studies [43].

Dipeptidyl peptidase 4 inhibitors (DPP4i) have not been proven to decrease MACE; however, retrospective data suggests there may be a lower risk for development of PAD and lower risk of amputation in patients treated with these agents [18, 77].

Recent randomized controlled trials have demonstrated a consistent reduction in MACE among patients with PAD and type 2 diabetes treated with glucagon-like peptide-1 receptor agonists (GLP1RA) or sodium glucose cotransporter-2 inhibitors (SGLT2i). GLP1RA are thought to decrease adverse events through anti-atherogenic activity, whereas SGLT2i are thought to modulate the cardiovascular system through endothelial function improvements and hemodynamic effects [32, 77].

Regarding SGLT2i use in patients with PAD, there was an initial concern, specifically with canagliflozin, which was associated with an increased risk of—mostly minor—amputations in the CANVAS trial (6.3 versus 3.4 placebo per 1000 patient years; $P < 0.001$); however, these findings were not reproduced in the CREDENCE trial, and a meta-analysis of 30 trials, leading to the removal of the black box warning for canagliflozin by the FDA in 2020 [17, 35, 53, 59]. A subgroup analysis of patients with PAD at baseline (n = 1462; 20.8%) in EMPA-REG OUTCOME showed superior limb outcomes in patients treated with empagliflozin versus placebo [79].

Investigations on the effects of GLP1RA treatment on limb events have suggested improved outcomes. A post hoc analysis of the LEADER trial found that liraglutide was associated with reduced risk for amputation compared with placebo [26].

There are no randomized comparisons between GLPP1RA and SGLT2i, however observational data suggests there might be a greater reduction in MALE and all-cause mortality in patients treated with GLP1RA compared to SGLT2i [46, 75].

According to the 2023 American Diabetes Association Standards of Care in Diabetes, treatment should be chosen based on cardiovascular risk stratification. The main objective, which is a reduction in cardiovascular and cardiorenal risk, can be achieved using either SGLT2i or GLP1RA. The choice of the exact drug is made depending on comorbidities: SGLT2 inhibitors are preferred to GLP1RA in patients with documented heart failure or chronic kidney disease. In subjects with atherosclerotic cardiovascular disease or high cardiovascular risk, the guidelines do not prioritize one agent class over another. Combination therapy can be considered in patients who have not reached target hemoglobin A1C levels [29].

Contemporary PAD guidelines recommend a target hemoglobin A1C level of <7% and tight glycemic control. For patients with type 2 diabetes, this should be preferably achieved with agents with proven cardiovascular benefits such as SGLT2i and GLP-1RA, adding metformin or other glucose-lowering agents as necessary [32, 48].

Lipid-Lowering Therapy

In addition to low-density lipoprotein (LDL) cholesterol elevations, increases in total cholesterol, apolipoprotein B, lipoprotein(a) levels and triglyceride-rich lipoproteins as well as low high-density lipoprotein have been associated with the development of PAD [23].

Dyslipidemia is often undertreated and inadequately controlled in patients with PAD compared to patients with coronary disease [41, 44].

Contemporary guidelines recommend an LDL reduction of ≥50% and an LDL cholesterol goal of <55 mg/dL to obtain a reduction in MACE in patients at very high risk of future atherosclerotic events, such as individuals with a history of myocardial infarction, ischemic stroke, or symptomatic PAD [47].

Statins

Statins have been demonstrated to decrease MACE, MALE, and improve walking distance in patients with PAD [3, 44, 51, 58]. It is recommended to treat patients with PAD with high-intensity statin, i.e., atorvastatin dose ≥40 mg daily or rosuvastatin dose ≥20 mg daily [32, 48].

Ezetimibe

Ezetimibe, particularly when combined with statins, is particularly useful when target LDL cholesterol has not been achieved or in patients who are intolerant to statins [15, 52]. A sub-analysis of the IMPROVE-IT trial showed a consistent reduction in MACE in patients with PAD treated with ezetimibe plus statin [11]. No data exists to support the use of ezetimibe to decrease MALE.

Proprotein Convertase Subtilisin/Kexin Type 9 Inhibitors

Proprotein convertase subtilisin/kexin type 9 (PCSK9i), reduce CV events in patients with symptomatic atherosclerotic disease with an LDL cholesterol >70 mg/dL [62]. Adding a PCSK9i to statins further reduces MACE and MALE risk in patients with PAD and improves walking distance in patients with claudication [20].

Inclisiran, a PCSK9i administered at baseline, 3 months, and every 6 months thereafter, has been demonstrated to decrease the risk of MACE by 26% [61]. The role of inclisiran in patients with PAD is currently being investigated.

Bempedoic Acid

Bempedoic acid, an adenosine triphosphate-citrate lyase inhibitor which works upstream of statins in cholesterol metabolism, has been demonstrated to decrease MACE in statin-intolerant patients with atherosclerosis, including patients with symptomatic PAD [54].

Hypertriglyceridemia

Fibrates have not demonstrated improvements in MACE in patients with PAD [50, 74].

Icosapent ethyl improved MACE in the REDUCE-IT trial, however this study did not report PAD as an outcome [8].

Antihypertensive Therapy

Hypertension is the most common cardiovascular risk factor [45]. Elevated blood pressure is associated with increased risk for PAD and is present in about half of patients diagnosed with PAD [21].

Any antihypertensive agent can be used to control blood pressure in these patients. However, angiotensin-converting enzyme inhibitors (ACEI) and angiotensin receptor blockers (ARB) are a preferred first line therapy, as supported by two randomized trials: HOPE and ONTARGET [33, 56]. Ramipril, specifically, appears to decrease the risk of MACE in patients with PAD [57]. In addition, a meta-analysis suggested that optimal antihypertensive treatment may improve walking distance in patients with PAD [65].

Clinical practice guidelines recommend treating high blood pressure to a goal <130/80 mmHg to maximize cardiovascular event reduction [76]. European guidelines acknowledge that certain groups, such as patients older than 85 years of age, those with orthostasis or clinical frailty, might benefit from a more lenient target of <140/90 mmHg [49].

Antithrombotic Therapy

Antiplatelet therapy with either aspirin or clopidogrel is indicated to reduce the risk of MACE in patients with symptomatic PAD [32, 48].

The Antithrombotic Trialists' Collaboration meta-analysis showed a 22% reduction of MACE in patients with cardiovascular disease who received antiplatelet therapies (aspirin, clopidogrel, or ticlopidine)—including patients with PAD. In this meta-analysis, there was a 23% reduction of MACE specifically in patients with claudication. When considering aspirin as the antiplatelet agent, a dose of 75–150 mg daily conferred a greater proportional reduction in vascular events compared to higher doses of aspirin [2]. In addition to MACE reduction, antiplatelet therapy may also reduce the risk of MALE: a meta-analysis of 54 randomized trials in patients with claudication found that aspirin compared to placebo reduced the risk of arterial occlusion [31].

Clopidogrel as a single antiplatelet agent was associated with an 8.7% relative risk reduction in MACE compared to aspirin in the CAPRIE trial, which evaluated patients with atherosclerotic cardiovascular disease, including patients with symptomatic PAD [16].

As for other P2Y12 inhibitors, in the EUCLID trial, single antiplatelet therapy with ticagrelor was not superior to clopidogrel [6]. Prasugrel has not been studied specifically for PAD indications.

The role of dual antiplatelet therapy [e.g., aspirin plus clopidogrel or other more potent antiplatelet agents (e.g., vorapaxar)] in patients with claudication and no recent revascularization is uncertain and is associated with an increased risk of bleeding [10, 12, 14].

Dual antithrombotic therapy with aspirin and vascular-dose rivaroxaban (2.5 mg twice daily) in patients with PAD is more effective than aspirin alone in reducing MACE, MALE, and preventing acute limb ischemia, however at the expense of an increase in major bleeding. The COMPASS PAD trial included patients across the entire spectrum of PAD, including patients with claudication, previous revascularization, amputation, and CLTI. Rivaroxaban plus aspirin resulted in a 4.2% absolute risk reduction in MALE, MACE, and major amputation, with a 2% increase in major bleeding. The subsets of patients with the greatest event reduction were those with high-risk presentations (such as CLTI, prior amputation, prior revascularization) or high-risk comorbidities (kidney disease, heart failure, diabetes, or polyvascular disease). The net clinical benefit of rivaroxaban plus aspirin in patients with claudication alone in the absence of high-risk presentations or comorbidities is less clear, with a MACE/MALE risk reduction of 1% and major bleeding increase of 0.8% [42]. The use of bleeding risk assessment tools such as the OAC3PAD score has been proposed by two European guideline groups to help inform decisions regarding rivaroxaban use [4, 48, 70]. In terms of symptom improvement, the recently published COMPASS Claudication trial suggested an improvement in total walking distance measured by a 6-minute walk test in patients treated with aspirin plus rivaroxaban compared to aspirin alone, which warrants further exploration [60].

Despite its widespread use, use of dual antiplatelet therapy (DAPT) after endovascular revascularization is supported by limited data, and largely extrapolated from coronary interventions [66, 69]. Short DAPT duration for 1–3 months post-revascularization is not associated with reduced MACE but seems to improve vessel patency without a significant increase in major bleeding [19, 40, 68]. The combination of aspirin and rivaroxaban initiated post-revascularization was associated with a lower incidence of MALE and MACE compared to aspirin alone in the VOYAGER-PAD trial [9]. It should be noted that triple antithrombotic therapy (aspirin plus clopidogrel plus rivaroxaban) is associated with a significant increase in bleeding when administered for more than one-month post-revascularization [36].

Other Risk Factors

Lipoprotein (a)

Lipoprotein (a) [Lp(a)] is an LDL particle with an added apolipoprotein(a) attached to the apolipoprotein(b) component of the LDL particle. An individual's Lp(a) level is >80% genetically determined. In the general population, Lp(a) levels greater than 50 mg/dL are associated with an increased risk for the development of PAD, myocardial infarction, carotid atherosclerosis, ischemic stroke, aortic valve stenosis, and cardiovascular mortality [23, 78]. Some guidelines recommend a once in a lifetime screening for Lp(a) levels, particularly in individuals with a personal or family history of premature atherosclerotic cardiovascular disease, those with familial hypercholesterolemia with a family history of elevated Lp(a) [48, 78]. Increased levels of Lp(a) may be considered a risk-enhancing factor. Statins do not decrease Lp(a) levels, but the addition of PCSK9i or even apheresis are treatment options for these individuals [78].

Homocysteine

Despite an association between elevated homocysteine levels and the development of atherosclerosis and PAD, it remains unclear whether treatment for hyperhomocysteinemia would result in improved outcomes in patients with PAD [1].

Nonconventional Risk Factors and Risk Amplifiers

Chronic inflammation, defined as elevated C-reactive protein and interleukin-6 levels, is observed in patients with PAD. Elevated fibrinogen levels have been identified as a risk factor for PAD. Infection with the human immunodeficiency virus, air pollution, heavy metal and lead exposure, depression, as well as the presence of microvascular disease such as retinopathy have been implicated in the development or progression of PAD [23]. Cannabis use has been associated with the development of PAD, thromboangiitis, and increased complications after bypass revascularization [7, 24, 25, 73]. The role of these nonconventional risk factors continues to be the focus of investigations and is beyond the purpose of this chapter.

However, it is important to mention the role of risk amplifiers, which are factors that further increase the risk of MACE and MALE in patients with PAD. These include older age, ongoing smoking, chronic kidney disease, and end-stage kidney disease, the presence of polyvascular disease and of microvascular disease. It is recommended that these are considered and incorporated when developing patient-centered treatment recommendations [32]. Likewise, social determinants of health have been associated with disparities in outcomes in PAD patients that may be relevant to the comprehensive treatment of these patients—Figs. 7.2 and 7.3 [32].

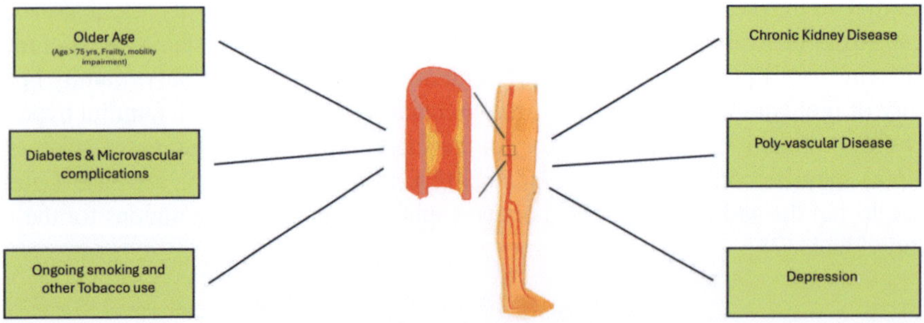

Fig. 7.2 Peripheral artery disease-related risk amplifiers increase risk of major adverse cardiac and limb events

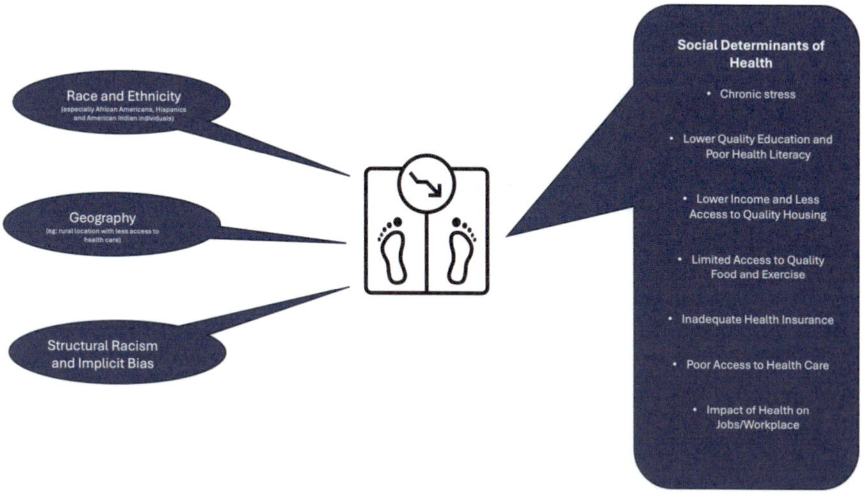

Fig. 7.3 Factors influencing health disparities in patients with peripheral artery disease

Practical Approach

The following points provide a summary and practical guidance for the evaluation and management of risk factors in patients with claudication.

- History. Personal and family history of cardiovascular disease, familial hypercholesterolemia, and Lp(a) elevation.
- Physical exam. Complete vascular examination. Bilateral arm blood pressure measurement.
- Ankle-Brachial Index and adjunctive vascular testing as indicated.
- Laboratory evaluation. Lipid profile (including Lp(a) once in a lifetime), fasting glucose or hemoglobin A1C, kidney function, liver function, and electrolytes.
- Antiplatelet therapy with aspirin or clopidogrel in all patients with symptomatic PAD (e.g., claudication).
- Dual antithrombotic therapy (aspirin plus PAD-dosed rivaroxaban) in selected high-risk individuals and in patients post-revascularization and low bleeding risk.
- If triple antithrombotic therapy is used after revascularization, it should be limited to <1 month.
- If type 2 diabetes, prefer GLP1RA or SGLT2 inhibitors, with additional agents added if needed.
- If type 1 diabetes, intensive insulin therapy.
- Any diabetes, treatment to goal hemoglobin A1C < 7%.
- High intensity statin to target LDL < 55. If statin not at goal, or statin intolerant, add ezetimibe. If LDL not at goal on these therapies, or if elevated Lp(a), add PCSK9i.

- Other lipid lowering therapies such as inclisiran, bempedoic acid, or icosapent ethyl can be considered.
- Smoking cessation education, pharmacotherapy, and referral to smoking cessation programs.
- Evaluation for social determinants of health and risk enhancers.

References

1. Andras A, Stansby G, Hansrani M. Homocysteine lowering interventions for peripheral arterial disease and bypass grafts. Cochrane Database Syst Rev. 2013;2013(7):CD003285. https://doi.org/10.1002/14651858.CD003285.pub2.
2. Antithrombotic Trialists' Collaboration. Collaborative meta-analysis of randomised trials of antiplatelet therapy for prevention of death, myocardial infarction, and stroke in high risk patients. BMJ. 2002;324(7329):71–86. https://doi.org/10.1136/bmj.324.7329.71.
3. Aung PP, Maxwell HG, Jepson RG, et al. Lipid-lowering for peripheral arterial disease of the lower limb. Cochrane Database Syst Rev. 2007;2007(4):CD000123. https://doi.org/10.1002/14651858.CD000123.pub2.
4. Behrendt C, Kreutzburg T, Nordanstig J, et al. The OAC(3)-PAD risk score predicts major bleeding events one year after hospitalisation for peripheral artery disease. Eur J Vasc Endovasc Surg. 2022;63(3):503–10. https://doi.org/10.1016/j.ejvs.2021.12.019.
5. Belch JJF, Brodmann M, Baumgartner I, et al. Lipid-lowering and anti-thrombotic therapy in patients with peripheral arterial disease: European atherosclerosis society/European Society of Vascular Medicine Joint Statement. Atherosclerosis. 2021;338:55–63. https://doi.org/10.1016/j.atherosclerosis.2021.09.022.
6. Berger JS, Abramson BL, Lopes RD, et al. Ticagrelor versus clopidogrel in patients with symptomatic peripheral artery disease and prior coronary artery disease: insights from the EUCLID trial. Vasc Med. 2018;23(6):523–30. https://doi.org/10.1177/1358863X18775594.
7. Bergere G, Toquet C, Hoffmann C, et al. Effect of cannabis consumption on characteristics and evolution of thromboangitis obliterans. Vasa. 2021;50(4):301–5. https://doi.org/10.1024/0301-1526/a000948.
8. Bhatt DL, Steg PG, Miller M, et al. Cardiovascular risk reduction with Icosapent ethyl for hypertriglyceridemia. N Engl J Med. 2019;380(1):11–22. https://doi.org/10.1056/NEJMoa1812792.
9. Bonaca MP, Bauersachs RM, Anand SS, et al. Rivaroxaban in peripheral artery disease after revascularization. N Engl J Med. 2020;382(21):1994–2004. https://doi.org/10.1056/NEJMoa2000052.
10. Bonaca MP, Bhatt DL, Storey RF, et al. Ticagrelor for prevention of ischemic events after myocardial infarction in patients with peripheral artery disease. J Am Coll Cardiol. 2016;67(23):2719–28. https://doi.org/10.1016/j.jacc.2016.03.524.
11. Bonaca MP, Gutierrez JA, Cannon C, et al. Polyvascular disease, type 2 diabetes, and long-term vascular risk: a secondary analysis of the IMPROVE-IT trial. Lancet Diabetes Endocrinol. 2018;6(12):934–43. https://doi.org/10.1016/S2213-8587(18)30290-0.
12. Bonaca MP, Scirica BM, Creager MA, et al. Vorapaxar in patients with peripheral artery disease: results from TRA2degreesP-TIMI 50. Circulation. 2013;127(14):1522–6. https://doi.org/10.1161/CIRCULATIONAHA.112.000679.
13. Brand FN, Abbott RD, Kannel WB. Diabetes, intermittent claudication, and risk of cardiovascular events. The Framingham Study Diabetes. Diabetes. 1989;38(4):504–9. https://doi.org/10.2337/diab.38.4.504.
14. Cacoub PP, Bhatt DL, Steg PG, et al. Patients with peripheral arterial disease in the CHARISMA trial. Eur Heart J. 2009;30(2):192–201. https://doi.org/10.1093/eurheartj/ehn534.

15. Cannon CP, Blazing MA, Giugliano RP, et al. Ezetimibe added to statin therapy after acute coronary syndromes. N Engl J Med. 2015;372(25):2387–97. https://doi.org/10.1056/NEJMoa1410489.
16. CAPRIE Steering Committee. A randomised, blinded, trial of clopidogrel versus aspirin in patients at risk of ischaemic events (CAPRIE). CAPRIE Steering Committee. Lancet. 1996;348(9038):1329–39. https://doi.org/10.1016/s0140-6736(96)09457-3.
17. Center for Drug Evaluation and Research (2024) FDA removes boxed warning about risk of leg and foot amputations for the diabetes medicine canagliflozin (Invokana, Invokamet, Invokamet XR). FDA.
18. Chang C, Chen Y, Hsu C, et al. Dipeptidyl peptidase-4 inhibitors, peripheral arterial disease, and lower extremity amputation risk in diabetic patients. Am J Med. 2017;130(3):348–55. https://doi.org/10.1016/j.amjmed.2016.10.016.
19. Cho S, Lee Y, Ko Y, et al. Optimal strategy for antiplatelet therapy after endovascular revascularization for lower extremity peripheral artery disease. JACC Cardiovasc Interv. 2019;12(23):2359–70. https://doi.org/10.1016/j.jcin.2019.08.006.
20. Clavijo LC, Caro J, Choi J, et al. The addition of evolocumab to maximal tolerated statin therapy improves walking performance in patients with peripheral arterial disease and intermittent claudication (Evol-PAD study). Cardiovasc Revasc Med. 2023;55:1–5. https://doi.org/10.1016/j.carrev.2023.04.020.
21. Clement DL, De Buyzere ML, Duprez DA. Hypertension in peripheral arterial disease. Curr Pharm Des. 2004;10(29):3615–20. https://doi.org/10.2174/1381612043382819.
22. Criqui MH, Aboyans V. Epidemiology of peripheral artery disease. Circ Res. 2015;116(9):1509–26. https://doi.org/10.1161/CIRCRESAHA.116.303849.
23. Criqui MH, Matsushita K, Aboyans V, et al. Lower extremity peripheral artery disease: contemporary epidemiology, management gaps, and future directions: a scientific statement from the American Heart Association. Circulation. 2021;144(9):e171–91. https://doi.org/10.1161/CIR.0000000000001005.
24. Dakour-Aridi H, Arora M, Nejim B, et al. Association between drug use and in-hospital outcomes after Infrainguinal bypass for peripheral arterial occlusive disease. Ann Vasc Surg. 2019;58:122–133.e4. https://doi.org/10.1016/j.avsg.2018.12.070.
25. Desbois AC, Cacoub P. Cannabis-associated arterial disease. Ann Vasc Surg. 2013;27(7):996–1005. https://doi.org/10.1016/j.avsg.2013.01.002.
26. Dhatariya K, Bain SC, Buse JB, et al. The impact of liraglutide on diabetes-related foot ulceration and associated complications in patients with type 2 diabetes at high risk for cardiovascular events: results from the LEADER trial. Diabetes Care. 2018;41(10):2229–35. https://doi.org/10.2337/dc18-1094.
27. Ding N, Sang Y, Chen J, et al. Cigarette smoking, smoking cessation, and long-term risk of 3 major atherosclerotic diseases. J Am Coll Cardiol. 2019;74(4):498–507. https://doi.org/10.1016/j.jacc.2019.05.049.
28. Dormandy JA, Charbonnel B, Eckland DJA, et al. Secondary prevention of macrovascular events in patients with type 2 diabetes in the PROactive study (PROspective pioglitAzone clinical trial in macrovascular events): a randomised controlled trial. Lancet. 2005;366(9493):1279–89. https://doi.org/10.1016/S0140-6736(05)67528-9.
29. ElSayed NA, Aleppo G, Aroda VR, et al. 9. Pharmacologic approaches to glycemic treatment: standards of care in diabetes-2023. Diabetes Care. 2023;46(Suppl 1):S140–57. https://doi.org/10.2337/dc23-S009.
30. Fowkes FGR, Rudan D, Rudan I, et al. Comparison of global estimates of prevalence and risk factors for peripheral artery disease in 2000 and 2010: a systematic review and analysis. Lancet. 2013;382(9901):1329–40. https://doi.org/10.1016/S0140-6736(13)61249-0.
31. Girolami B, Bernardi E, Prins MH, et al. Antithrombotic drugs in the primary medical management of intermittent claudication: a meta-analysis. Thromb Haemost. 1999;81(5):715–22.
32. Gornik HL, Aronow HD, Goodney PP, et al. 2024 ACC/AHA/AACVPR/APMA/ABC/SCAI/SVM/SVN/SVS/SIR/VESS guideline for the management of lower extremity peripheral artery disease: a report of the American College of Cardiology/American Heart Association

Joint Committee on clinical practice guidelines. Circulation. 2024;149(24):e1313–410. https://doi.org/10.1161/CIR.0000000000001251.
33. Heart Outcomes Prevention Evaluation Study Investigators, Yusuf S, Sleight P, et al. Effects of an angiotensin-converting-enzyme inhibitor, ramipril, on cardiovascular events in high-risk patients. N Engl J Med. 2000;342(3):145–53. https://doi.org/10.1056/NEJM200001203420301.
34. Herzstein J, Weinroth LA. Arteriosclerotic peripheral vascular disease in diabetes. Arch Intern Med (Chic). 1945;76(1):34–8. https://doi.org/10.1001/archinte.1945.00210310042005.
35. Heyward J, Mansour O, Olson L, et al. Association between sodium-glucose cotransporter 2 (SGLT2) inhibitors and lower extremity amputation: a systematic review and meta-analysis. PLoS One. 2020;15(6):e0234065. https://doi.org/10.1371/journal.pone.0234065.
36. Hiatt WR, Bonaca MP, Patel MR, et al. Rivaroxaban and aspirin in peripheral artery disease lower extremity revascularization: impact of concomitant clopidogrel on efficacy and safety. Circulation. 2020;142(23):2219–30. https://doi.org/10.1161/CIRCULATIONAHA.120.050465.
37. Hirsch AT, Gotto AMJ. Undertreatment of dyslipidemia in peripheral arterial disease and other high-risk populations: an opportunity for cardiovascular disease reduction. Vasc Med. 2002;7(4):323–31. https://doi.org/10.1191/1358863x02vm453ra.
38. Holman RR, Paul SK, Bethel MA, et al. 10-year follow-up of intensive glucose control in type 2 diabetes. N Engl J Med. 2008;359(15):1577–89. https://doi.org/10.1056/NEJMoa0806470.
39. Housley E, Leng GC, Donnan PT, et al. Physical activity and risk of peripheral arterial disease in the general population: edinburgh artery study. J Epidemiol Community Health. 1993;47(6):475–80. https://doi.org/10.1136/jech.47.6.475.
40. Ipema J, Welling RHA, Bakker OJ, et al. Short-term clinical outcomes of single versus dual antiplatelet therapy after infrainguinal endovascular treatment for peripheral arterial disease. J Clin Med. 2020;9(11):3515. https://doi.org/10.3390/jcm9113515.
41. Kaasenbrood L, Boekholdt SM, van der Graaf Y, et al. Distribution of estimated 10-year risk of recurrent vascular events and residual risk in a secondary prevention population. Circulation. 2016;134(19):1419–29. https://doi.org/10.1161/CIRCULATIONAHA.116.021314.
42. Kaplovitch E, Eikelboom JW, Dyal L, et al. Rivaroxaban and aspirin in patients with symptomatic lower extremity peripheral artery disease: a subanalysis of the COMPASS randomized clinical trial. JAMA Cardiol. 2021;6(1):21–9. https://doi.org/10.1001/jamacardio.2020.4390.
43. Kooy A, de Jager J, Lehert P, et al. Long-term effects of metformin on metabolism and microvascular and macrovascular disease in patients with type 2 diabetes mellitus. Arch Intern Med. 2009;169(6):616–25. https://doi.org/10.1001/archinternmed.2009.20.
44. Kumbhani DJ, Steg PG, Cannon CP, et al. Statin therapy and long-term adverse limb outcomes in patients with peripheral artery disease: insights from the REACH registry. Eur Heart J. 2014;35(41):2864–72. https://doi.org/10.1093/eurheartj/ehu080.
45. Lawes CMM, Vander Hoorn S, Rodgers A, et al. Global burden of blood-pressure-related disease, 2001. Lancet. 2008;371(9623):1513–8. https://doi.org/10.1016/S0140-6736(08)60655-8.
46. Lin DS, Yu A, Lo H, et al. Major adverse cardiovascular and limb events in people with diabetes treated with GLP-1 receptor agonists vs SGLT2 inhibitors. Diabetologia. 2022;65(12):2032–43. https://doi.org/10.1007/s00125-022-05772-9.
47. Lloyd-Jones DM, Morris PB, Ballantyne CM, et al. 2022 ACC expert consensus decision pathway on the role of nonstatin therapies for LDL-cholesterol lowering in the management of atherosclerotic cardiovascular disease risk: a report of the American College of Cardiology Solution Set Oversight Committee. J Am Coll Cardiol. 2022;80(14):1366–418. https://doi.org/10.1016/j.jac22.07.006.
48. Mazzolai L, Teixido-Tura G, et al. 2024 ESC guidelines for the management of peripheral arterial and aortic diseases. Eur Heart J. 2024;45(36):3538–700. https://doi.org/10.1093/eurheartj/ehae179.
49. McEvoy JW, McCarthy CP, Brouwers S, et al. 2024 ESC guidelines for the management of elevated blood pressure and hypertension. Eur Heart J. 2024;45(38):3912–4018. https://doi.org/10.1093/eurheartj/ehae178.

50. Meade T, Zuhrie R, Cook C, et al. Bezafibrate in men with lower extremity arterial disease: randomised controlled trial. BMJ. 2002;325(7373):1139. https://doi.org/10.1136/bmj.325.7373.1139.
51. Mohler ER 3rd, Hiatt WR, Creager MA. Cholesterol reduction with atorvastatin improves walking distance in patients with peripheral arterial disease. Circulation. 2003;108(12):1481–6. https://doi.org/10.1161/01.CIR.0000090686.57897.F5.
52. Murphy SA, Cannon CP, Blazing MA, et al. Reduction in total cardiovascular events with ezetimibe/simvastatin post-acute coronary syndrome: the IMPROVE-IT trial. J Am Coll Cardiol. 2016;67(4):353–61. https://doi.org/10.1016/j.jacc.2015.10.077.
53. Neal B, Perkovic V, Matthews DR. Canagliflozin and cardiovascular and renal events in type 2 diabetes. N Engl J Med. 2017;377(21):2099. https://doi.org/10.1056/NEJMc1712572.
54. Nissen SE, Lincoff AM, Brennan D, et al. Bempedoic acid and cardiovascular outcomes in statin-intolerant patients. N Engl J Med. 2023;388(15):1353–64. https://doi.org/10.1056/NEJMoa2215024.
55. Norgren L, Hiatt WR, Dormandy JA, et al. Inter-society consensus for the management of peripheral arterial disease (TASC II). J Vasc Surg. 2007;45(Suppl S):5. https://doi.org/10.1016/j.jvs.2006.12.037.
56. ONTARGET Investigators, Yusuf S, Teo KK, et al. Telmisartan, ramipril, or both in patients at high risk for vascular events. N Engl J Med. 2008;358(15):1547–59. https://doi.org/10.1056/NEJMoa0801317.
57. Ostergren J, Sleight P, Dagenais G, et al. Impact of ramipril in patients with evidence of clinical or subclinical peripheral arterial disease. Eur Heart J. 2004;25(1):17–24. https://doi.org/10.1016/j.ehj.2003.10.033.
58. Pastori D, Farcomeni A, Milanese A, et al. Statins and major adverse limb events in patients with peripheral artery disease: a systematic review and meta-analysis. Thromb Haemost. 2020;120(5):866–75. https://doi.org/10.1055/s-0040-1709711.
59. Perkovic V, Jardine MJ, Neal B, et al. Canagliflozin and renal outcomes in type 2 diabetes and nephropathy. N Engl J Med. 2019;380(24):2295–306. https://doi.org/10.1056/NEJMoa1811744.
60. Ramacciotti E, Volpiani GG, Britto KF, et al. Rivaroxaban for patients with intermittent claudication. NEJM Evid. 2024;3(9):EVIDoa2400021. https://doi.org/10.1056/EVIDoa2400021.
61. Ray KK, Raal FJ, Kallend DG, et al. Inclisiran and cardiovascular events: a patient-level analysis of phase III trials. Eur Heart J. 2023;44(2):129–38. https://doi.org/10.1093/eurheartj/ehac594.
62. Sabatine MS, Giugliano RP, Keech AC, et al. Evolocumab and clinical outcomes in patients with cardiovascular disease. N Engl J Med. 2017;376(18):1713–22. https://doi.org/10.1056/NEJMoa1615664.
63. Selvin E, Erlinger TP. Prevalence of and risk factors for peripheral arterial disease in the United States: results from the National Health and nutrition examination survey, 1999–2000. Circulation. 2004;110(6):738–43. https://doi.org/10.1161/01.CIR.0000137913.26087.F0.
64. Semple R. Diabetes and peripheral arterial disease; a clinical study. Lancet. 1953;1(6770):1064–8. https://doi.org/10.1016/s0140-6736(53)92200-4.
65. Shahin Y, Barnes R, Barakat H, et al. Meta-analysis of angiotensin converting enzyme inhibitors effect on walking ability and ankle brachial pressure index in patients with intermittent claudication. Atherosclerosis. 2013;231(2):283–90. https://doi.org/10.1016/j.atherosclerosis.2013.09.037.
66. Strobl FF, Brechtel K, Schmehl J, et al. Twelve-month results of a randomized trial comparing mono with dual antiplatelet therapy in endovascularly treated patients with peripheral artery disease. J Endovasc Ther. 2013;20(5):699–706. https://doi.org/10.1583/13-4275MR.1.
67. The Diabetes Control and Complications Trial Research Group. Effect of intensive diabetes management on macrovascular events and risk factors in the diabetes control and complications trial. Am J Cardiol. 1995;75(14):894–903. https://doi.org/10.1016/s0002-9149(99)80683-3.
68. Thott O, Granath F, Malmstedt J, et al. Editor's choice – dual antiplatelet therapy improves outcome in diabetic patients undergoing endovascular Femoropopliteal stenting for critical

limb ischaemia. Eur J Vasc Endovasc Surg. 2017;53(3):403–10. https://doi.org/10.1016/j.ejvs.2016.12.014.

69. Tsai S, Li Y, Lee C, et al. Mono or dual antiplatelet therapy for treating patients with peripheral artery disease after lower extremity revascularization: a systematic review and meta-analysis. Pharmaceuticals (Basel). 2022;15(5):596. https://doi.org/10.3390/ph15050596.
70. Twine CP, Kakkos SK, Aboyans V, et al. Editor's choice – European Society for Vascular Surgery (ESVS) 2023 clinical practice guidelines on antithrombotic therapy for vascular diseases. Eur J Vasc Endovasc Surg. 2023;65(5):627–89. https://doi.org/10.1016/j.ejvs.2023.03.042.
71. UK Prospective Diabetes Study Group. Intensive blood-glucose control with sulphonylureas or insulin compared with conventional treatment and risk of complications in patients with type 2 diabetes (UKPDS 33). UK Prospective Diabetes Study (UKPDS) Group. Lancet. 1998;352(9131):837–53.
72. Virani SS, Alonso A, Benjamin EJ, et al. Heart disease and stroke Statistics-2020 update: a report from the American Heart Association. Circulation. 2020;141(9):e139–596. https://doi.org/10.1161/CIR.0000000000000757.
73. Vyas H, Jain H, et al. Impact of marijuana use on prevalence and interventions in peripheral artery disease. J Soc Cardiovasc Angiogr Interv. 2023;2(3):Suppl 100817. https://doi.org/10.1016/j.jscai.2023.100817.
74. Wang D, Liu B, Tao W, et al. Fibrates for secondary prevention of cardiovascular disease and stroke. Cochrane Database Syst Rev. 2015;2015(10):CD009580. https://doi.org/10.1002/14651858.CD009580.pub2.
75. Werkman NCC, Driessen JHM, Stehouwer CDA, et al. The use of sodium-glucose co-transporter-2 inhibitors or glucagon-like peptide-1 receptor agonists versus sulfonylureas and the risk of lower limb amputations: a nation-wide cohort study. Cardiovasc Diabetol. 2023;22(1):160–2. https://doi.org/10.1186/s12933-023-01897-2.
76. Whelton PK, Carey RM, Aronow WS, et al. 2017 ACC/AHA/AAPA/ABC/ACPM/AGS/APhA/ASH/ASPC/NMA/PCNA guideline for the prevention, detection, evaluation, and Management of High Blood Pressure in adults: executive summary: a report of the American College of Cardiology/American Heart Association Task Force on Clinical Practice Guidelines. Hypertension. 2018;71(6):1269–324. https://doi.org/10.1161/HYP0000000000000066.
77. Wilcox T, De Block C, Schwartzbard AZ, et al. Diabetic agents, from metformin to SGLT2 inhibitors and GLP1 receptor agonists: JACC focus seminar. J Am Coll Cardiol. 2020;75(16):1956–74. https://doi.org/10.1016/j.jacc.2020.02.056.
78. Wilson DP, Jacobson TA, Jones PH, et al. Use of lipoprotein(a) in clinical practice: a biomarker whose time has come. A scientific statement from the National Lipid Association. J Clin Lipidol. 2019;13(3):374–92. https://doi.org/10.1016/j.jacl.2019.04.010.
79. Zinman B, Wanner C, Lachin JM, et al. Empagliflozin, cardiovascular outcomes, and mortality in type 2 diabetes. N Engl J Med. 2015;373(22):2117–28. https://doi.org/10.1056/NEJMoa1504720.

Defining and Choosing Outcome Measures for Managing Claudication

8

M. Libby Weaver and Caitlin W. Hicks

Patient-centered care emphasizes patient preferences and values in the development of a clinical care plan. This care model requires consideration of traditional disease-specific clinical outcomes alongside important health-related quality-of-life measures. Objective measures assessing intervention efficacy and durability and pre- and post-intervention functionality, in combination with subjective patient-reported outcome measures (PROMs), allow physicians to measure both the durability of a treatment or intervention and how that treatment impacts a patient's overall quality of life [1]. In the case of intermittent claudication (IC), a condition in which revascularization does not confer significant limb salvage or mortality benefit, identifying pertinent short- and long-term outcomes that also consider a patient's functional status and quality of life is an evolving process [2–4]. The purpose of this chapter is to provide contemporary insights regarding short- and long-term objective and subjective outcome measures that are most relevant to the care of patients with IC.

Limb-Based Outcome Measures

Limb-based outcome measures focus on limb-centered outcomes after an intervention performed for PAD. Progression to chronic limb-threatening ischemia (CLTI) and major lower extremity amputation are long-term clinical outcome measures traditionally used to evaluate the efficacy of medical and surgical interventions for

M. L. Weaver (✉)
Division of Vascular Surgery, University of Utah Spencer Fox Eccles School of Medicine, Salt Lake City, UT, USA
e-mail: libby.weaver@hsc.utah.edu

C. W. Hicks
Division of Vascular Surgery and Endovascular Therapy, Johns Hopkins University School of Medicine, Baltimore, MD, USA
e-mail: chicks11@jhmi.edu

W. P. Robinson III, J. P. Simons (eds.), *The Patient-Centered Approach to Claudication*, https://doi.org/10.1007/978-3-032-02460-2_8

PAD. Patients diagnosed with IC are not at a significantly higher risk of progression to CLTI or amputation compared to patients with asymptomatic PAD [2, 3]. However, recent research suggests that patients who undergo early peripheral vascular interventions (PVI) for IC without adequate medical optimization (aspirin, statin, and cilostazol therapy) and lifestyle modification (smoking cessation and supervised exercise therapy), or who undergo non-guideline compliant revascularization strategies, progress to CLTI and need for amputation at higher rates than patients who are appropriately optimized prior to intervention [5–8]. Additionally, studies show that isolated tibial-level intervention on index peripheral vascular intervention (PVI) for IC is associated with higher rates of both major and minor amputation [9]. Although patients with IC may have promising results in terms of symptom resolution and functional improvement in the short term, it is important to consider the long-term implications of inappropriate early or aggressive interventional treatment of IC. Therefore, although a diagnosis of IC does not significantly increase a patient's risk for amputation or progression to CLTI, it remains necessary to monitor nuances of how various treatment plans might alter the natural history of this disease process by continuing to study limb-based outcomes including progression to CLTI, minor amputation, and major amputation.

Lesion-Based Outcome Measures

Lesion-based outcomes focus on the anatomy, technique, patency, and reintervention rates for an intervention performed on lower extremity arterial lesions. Historically, primary, primary-assisted, and secondary patency of endovascular and open interventions have been the most frequency utilized outcome measures to report on the technical success of interventions for peripheral artery disease (PAD) of all severities [10]. Additional anatomic details including lesion severity and location, as well as technical approach (i.e., open vs endovascular; balloon angioplasty vs atherectomy, etc.) are also useful metrics in understanding expected outcomes of interventions performed for the treatment of IC. Finally, target-lesion revascularization (TLR) is a common endpoint used in device trials.

Patency of interventions is useful to understand the durability of various intervention types in the treatment of IC. Primary patency refers to the durability of a procedure without requiring re-interventions. Primary-assisted patency refers to the durability of a procedure with additional re-interventions to maintain patency (i.e., angioplasty of a stenosis). Secondary patency refers to overall durability after thrombosis of a primary intervention requiring surgical salvage. The Society for Vascular Surgery objective performance measures and clinical practice guidelines emphasize the importance of patency, stating any PVI or surgical treatment for IC "should provide a reasonable likelihood of sustained benefit to the patient" defined as a "greater than 50% likelihood of clinical efficacy for at least 2 years" [11]. Patency is a useful measure to compare durability of various procedure types in the setting of IC. However, it does not provide information regarding a patient's functional outcome as a result of the intervention.

Anatomical location of interventions for IC, as well as lesion severity, remain important as the technical approach at different anatomic levels may have variable patency outcomes. For example, patients with IC undergoing iliac intervention in the setting of TransAtlantic Inter-Society Consensus (TASC) A/B lesions may experience optimal patency with self-expanding bare metal stent placement, whereas those with TASC C/D lesions may experience better patency with covered stents [2]. Alternatively, femoral lesions are typically best treated with open revascularization [2]. Finally, tibial-level interventions have repeatedly demonstrated poor long-term outcomes in patients with IC [5, 9, 12]. Thus, recent major societal guidelines and appropriateness criteria applicable to the treatment of IC advise against isolated tibial-level intervention [2, 13]. The major limitation of these measures, again, is the lack of association with functional outcomes.

TLR is commonly utilized as an outcome measure in device trials to determine performance of a given revascularization technique at a clinically significant lesion. However, TLR neglects to account for either durability of an intervention or functional outcomes. Therefore, TLR as an outcome measure in IC is of limited use and is not recommended [14].

In summary, lesion-based outcomes are objective and relatively straightforward data points to collect, as patency can be monitored during routine surveillance with non-invasive imaging studies. Duplex ultrasound, in combination with ankle-brachial indices, provides measurable data points to objectively track the patency of revascularization interventions. Lesion-based outcome measures are useful when selecting the preferred revascularization technique for patients with IC who are undergoing intervention. They are also a useful way to measure both short- and long-term technical outcomes in a quantifiable manner. The major limitation of lesion-based outcome measures is that these measures do not provide information on a patient's functional or symptomatic response to therapy, which is of utmost importance in the treatment of IC. Therefore, although lesion-based outcomes are useful metrics for understanding the strengths and weaknesses of various technical strategies for revascularization of PAD, alternative patient-centered outcome measures may be of higher utility [1, 15].

Major Adverse Limb Event

Major adverse limb event (MALE) is a combined limb- and lesion-based outcome that is defined as either major (above ankle) amputation or reintervention or revision of a revascularization procedure [16]. As with all limb- and lesion-based end points, MALE does not account for functional outcomes of the patient. However, it is a comprehensive outcome that captures both the durability of revascularization procedure, as well as the long-term potential of a procedure to alter the natural course of disease in a patient with IC.

Patient-Based Outcome Measures

Patient-based outcome measures evaluate the symptomatic and functional responses patients experience in response to a treatment. Patient-centered outcomes for IC can be measured both objectively and subjectively and are inherently more patient-centered than either lesion- or limb-based outcome measures.

Objective patient-based outcome measures utilize functional status metrics. Several outcome measures exist to evaluate the pre- and post-intervention functional status of a patient presenting with IC. These are important tools given patients are known to inaccurately estimate and recall their own walking distances [17]. The most commonly implemented and studied of objective patient-based outcome measures include treadmill testing and the 6-minute walk test. Treadmill exercise testing can be performed under one of two accepted protocols for the evaluation of IC. The constant-load protocol sets the patient at a standard speed (usually 2 miles per hour (mph)) and grade (10–12%) and measures the distance of ambulation until a drop in ankle-brachial index is observed. A more commonly used treadmill protocol is the graded test, whereby the patient begins walking at 2 mph and 0% grade, and the grade is increased by 2% every 2 minutes until the patient can no longer ambulate due to claudication-induced pain [18]. Each of these tests can be used for diagnostic purposes or for measuring treatment response, though the graded protocol with measurement of absolute claudication distance has the highest reliability of the two [19]. Significant limitations with treadmill testing include use of a gait that may not be typical in everyday life, and a learned improvement that occurs with sequential testing, which may improve results even when no intervention has been applied [20].

The 6-minute walk test is an additional objective measure of function used to measure outcomes of medical or invasive interventions on patients with IC. This patient-based outcome measure has been shown to be highly sensitive and reliable in measuring improvement in walking endurance as a response to treatment, and even predictive of mortality rates and loss of mobility in patients with PAD who do not undergo interventions [20, 21]. There is a single protocol for the 6-minute walk test during which patients are instructed to walk up and down a 100-foot hallway for 6 minutes with the goal of covering as much distance as possible during that time. Patients are instructed not to speak during the test, unless expressing symptom onset, and the administrator timing the test calls out each one-minute interval. Besides a stopwatch, no other equipment is necessary to administer this examination. In studies evaluating the utility of the 6-minute walk test, patients in the lowest quartile of distance walked during a baseline 6-minute walk test are found to have higher all-cause and cardiovascular-related mortality compared to those in the highest quartile of distance at baseline, even when corrected for other relevant variables such as smoking or ankle brachial index [20]. Additionally, patients with IC followed for 2 years without medical or invasive intervention that had the largest declines in their six-minute walk test difference were found to have higher all-cause and cardiovascular mortality, as well as higher mobility loss. Improvement in the 6-minute walk test distance has been observed in response to medical therapy for IC, with a small meaningful change defined as 20 meters and a large meaningful changed defined as 50 meters between baseline and follow-up tests [20]. Six-minute walk test performance is also associated with quality of life assessments [22]. The 6-minute walk test is safe to administer. In a series of 7900 consecutive tests, only one adverse event of a fall with resulting forearm fracture occurred. Treadmill tests, on the other hand, have been associated with arrhythmias, and not all patients can tolerate the balance required to ambulate on a treadmill [23].

Patient-reported outcome measures (PROMs) are perhaps the most important patient-centered outcome measures in the management of IC. Surgeons have been the leaders of implementation of PROMs for over a century. In 1918, Ernest Codman described an outcomes registry system that would holistically include both clinical and patient-reported outcomes. He called the system the “End-Result System”, stating “modern medicine is continually fighting a battle to teach people the difference between treating symptoms and pathological condition. When this step is taken by our great hospitals, true clinical science will begin” [24]. Dr. Codman’s ideas were considered outlandish at the time. However, the perceived benefit of PROMs has evolved over time, particularly with regard to treatment of non-life-threatening pathologies such as IC. PROMs are even taken under consideration in the Federal Drug Administration (FDA) regulation of drug and device development, and have been used to help distinguish high-value from low-value care [25].

PROMs allow physicians to measure both how a disease process impacts a patient’s quality of life (QOL) and how subsequent treatments will impact QOL. PROMs are delivered in two formats. Multi-attribute utility instruments (MAUIs) incorporate both physical and psychological domains and are most valuable for chronic disease processes. Visual analogue scales (VASs) are typically utilized acutely to understand benefits from an intervention, such as a revascularization procedure [26]. PROMs tools can be general QOL assessments or disease-specific. Generic PROMs tools are useful in that they may be generalized across multiple patient populations, healthcare settings, and datasets. However, disease-specific PROMs tools target symptoms and functional capacity most relevant to a given pathology, often making them more useful in a clinical setting [1]. Development and implementation of a PROMs tools requires a rigorous 5-phase process to ensure efficacy and feasibility of tool use. First, relevant QOL symptoms for a given disease are identified. Second, related symptoms are categorized into domains. Once the relevant domains are developed, a pre-test is performed and the tool is revised as appropriate. The finalized tool is then implemented into generalized clinical practices. Finally, validation of the PROMs tool is performed [26].

PROMs have demonstrated utility in both pre- and post-intervention phases of care, as well as in the short and long-term in patients with claudication. For example, general PROMs have demonstrated similar functional and social domain outcomes in patients with IC, regardless of whether they underwent surgical or medical therapy, up to 7 years post-intervention [27]. Despite their utility in quantifying the patients’ experience and treatment response, a recent survey of vascular surgeons revealed only 23% use PROMs in their clinical practice, despite there being 31 PROMs available for vascular disease processes. This cohort of surgeons felt that patients with IC benefit most from inclusion of PROMs instruments as part of their care [1].

There are currently 14 PROMs developed for the evaluation of PAD, 7 of which are specific to IC. Each PROM instrument has strengths and weaknesses, and selecting the most appropriate for physicians to implement in their own practice depends on the goals and resources of that practice [1] (Table 8.1). A multidisciplinary review of available PAD PROMs considered content and construct validity, reliability, sensitivity, use in research, and ease of administration to identify preferred PROMs for IC [28]. A subsequent Delphi consensus with an international multidisciplinary panel of physicians convened to determine the optimal PROM instrument for use in registries and trials [29]. The consensus of each of these manuscripts is that there is not one independent "best" PROM instrument for either clinical practice or research purposes, and that multiple tools may be combined for optimal utility. For the purposes of this chapter, we will outline those PROMs instruments found to have the most robust validity evidence, have established minimally clinically important differences (MCID), are most practical to administer, and are most useful for trials and registries.

VascuQoL and VascuQoL-6

The original VascuQoL contains 25 questions and was first published in 2001. Although the average time to complete the VascuQoL is less than 10 min, a subsequent abbreviated version of this PROM containing only 6 questions (VascuQoL-6) has been used and validated and is the most commonly used PROM instrument in PAD trials and registries to date. Each tool was developed with both physician and patient input. The content for each version of the VascuQoL includes pain, activities, symptoms, emotional, and social domains [30]. Scores for the full-length VascuQoL may be calculated by subdomain or as a summary score [28]. VascuQoL has extensive content and construct validity evidence, although notably most populations in which validation was performed included patients with both IC and CLTI, whereas other tools have been validated in purely IC patient populations [31–34]. The reliability and sensitivity of the VascuQoL and VascuQoL-6 have both been shown to be high when utilized both pre- and post-revascularization. MCID has been defined in patients with IC post-revascularization for VascuQoL-6 (meaning statistically significant changes seen in patient scores across time correlate with clinically meaningful differences). A 2-point difference between pre- and post-revascularization scores is considered suggestive, while 4 4-point difference is considered certain, of a clinically significant change in patient condition in either direction [31].

A Delphi Consensus published in the European Journal of Vascular and Endovascular Surgery on behalf of the European Society for Vascular Surgery concluded with a recommendation for the use of VascuQoL-6 for trials and registry data, along with 12 additional items felt to be important in assessing QOL in patients with IC. The purpose of the recommendation was to include relevant and holistic

Table 8.1 Peripheral arterial disease-related patient-reported outcome measures (PROM)

PROM	Year	No. of items	Domains	Time to complete, min	Validated	Advantages	Disadvantages
CSI—Vascular [3, 4]	2016	5	Symptoms	5	Yes	Assess specific symptoms, as opposed to global symptoms; designed and validated for assessment of outcomes to treatment	Limited testing in diverse populations; study was not designed for optimal evaluation of CSI sensitivity to change (responsiveness to change in patient's symptoms)
CLAU-S [5–7]	1995	47	Everyday life, pain, effect on social activities, illness-specific fears, psychological impact	5	Yes	Strongly associated with objective measures of PAD severity	Functional assessment with limited use as global QOL tool
ECQ [8, 9]	1992	6	Identification of claudication	Not reported	Yes	Tantamount to WHO/Rose but more specific	Not a true QOL assessment

(continued)

Table 8.1 (continued)

PROM	Year	No. of items	Domains	Time to complete, min	Validated	Advantages	Disadvantages
FLeQKI [10, 11]	2007	35	Comorbidity, effect on physical activities, effect on social activities, pain, psychological impact	Not reported	Yes	Correlate with SF-36	Only validated in German
Intermittent Claudication Questionnaire [12–15]	2002	16	Pain, effect on physical activities, effect on social activities, psychological impact	3.7	No	Brief	Requires further validation
Peripheral Artery Disease Quality of Life Questionnaire [16, 17]	2012	38	Social relationships and interactions, self-concept and feelings, symptoms, effect on physical activities, psychological impact, positive adaptation	<10	Yes	Demonstrates physical and emotional consequences of PAD on patient QOL	Limited testing in diverse populations, distinct age and race subgroups, and impact of intervention on disease progression
Peripheral Artery Questionnaire [18, 19]	2004	20	Symptoms, change in symptoms, effect on physical activities, effect on social activities, treatment satisfaction, overall QOL	Not reported	Yes	Holistic assessment of QOL and treatment effect	Less comprehensive than other PAD-specific QOL tools

Peripheral Artery Occlusive Disease 86-Item Questionnaire [12, 13, 16–23]	1995	86	Functional status, pain, general complaints, mood, anxiety, social life, evaluation of treatment for PAD	20	Yes	Extensive	Length limits adherence
PBI-PAD [24, 25]	2018	12	Everyday life, working life, therapy, leisure time, body, psychological impact	Not reported	Yes	Calculates pre- and post differences	Feasibility; 2 questionnaires over 3 months
Sickness Impact Profile—Intermittent Claudication [26–30]	1975	12	Sleep and rest, home management, ambulation, mobility, social interaction and alertness, behavior	Not reported		Brief; uses simple scoring scheme	Largely bereft in clinical spaces
VascuQoL [31–34]	2001	25	Pain, symptoms, effect on physical activities, effect on social activities, psychological impact	9	Yes	Highlights PAD treatment effects on QOL	Relationship with functional status is lacking

(continued)

Table 8.1 (continued)

PROM	Year	No. of items	Domains	Time to complete, min	Validated	Advantages	Disadvantages
VascuQoL-6 [35]	2014	6	Pain, symptoms, effect on physical activities, effect on social activities, psychological impact	1.4	Yes	Derived from VascuQoL but shorter	Limited comprehensiveness
WHO/Rose Questionnaire [8, 36, 37]	1962	8	Identification of claudication	Not reported	Yes	Global utilization; endorsed by WHO	Not a true QOL assessment
Walking Impairment Questionnaire [34, 38–41]	1990	22	Pain, distance, walking speed, stair climbing	5	Yes	Strong correlation with objective measures of PAD severity	Functional tool only, not a global assessment of QOL

CLAU-S Claudication Scale, *CSI* Claudication Symptom Instrument, *ECQ* Edinburgh Claudication Questionnaire, *PAD* peripheral artery disease, *PBIPAD* Patient Benefit Index for Peripheral Arterial Disease, *QOL* quality of life, *SF-36* Short Form-36, *WHO* World Health Organization

PROMs domains while standardizing measured outcomes across clinical trials and registries on an international level. The additional domains that the group recommended adding to the VascuQoL-6 include perceived improvement following treatment, impact of IC on ability to walk and distance walked, compliance with treatment plan, and satisfaction with treatment, among others [29] (Table 8.2).

Table 8.2 Overview of the 18 consensus items regarding their clinical relevance and practicability in this modified Delphi study on patient-reported outcomes for registries and trials including patients with intermittent claudication (IC)

Item name	VascuQoL-6	Clinical relevance—%	Practicability—%	Description
Intensity of IC[a]	2x Yes	93	87	Intensity of claudication pain in activities of daily living by indicating frequency and subjective severity
Degree of walking impairment due to PAOD[a]	Yes	94	85	Degree of walking impairment due to PAOD in activities of daily living
Limitation of everyday functioning (disease related)[a]	Yes	94	81	Limitation of everyday functioning due to PAOD/IC (physical or emotional)
Limitation of social activities due to PAOD[a]	Yes	91	76[b]	Limitation of social activities due to PAOD/IC (physical problems or emotional problems)
Improvement of IC after treatment[a]		94	93	Improvement of claudication pain in daily activities after intervention or surgery
Smoking[a]		100	94	Former and actual quantification of exposure to nicotine
Physical training/exercise[a]		94	83	Participation in physical training or regular exercise (e.g., incl. long walks)
Compliance with medication[a]		94	72[b]	Degree to which a patient correctly follows medical advice about medication
Presence of IC in daily living[c]		87	96	Presence of claudication pain in activities of daily living

(continued)

Table 8.2 (continued)

Item name	VascuQoL-6	Clinical relevance—%	Practicability—%	Description
Dissatisfaction with actual IC		81	57[b]	Presence of dissatisfaction/annoyance caused by claudication pain during daily activities
Presence of post-treatment pain/symptoms or other complications		85	85	Presence of pain/symptoms after a treatment for IC (e.g., wound pain, numbness, discomfort, superficial nerve pain, neuralgia), or other complications (e.g., disorder of wound healing)
Poorly healing wounds/ulcers		87	85	Leg or foot wounds heal poorly (e.g., it takes more than a few weeks to heal)
Presence of walking impairment due to PAOD[c]		85	83	Presence of walking impairment caused by PAOD such as claudication, post-treatment pain, or post-treatment wound
Impact of walking impairment due to PAOD		83	69[b]	Negative effects of walking impairment due to PAOD in daily life, e.g., isolation, dependency, embarrassment, depression, lifestyle change
Limitation of walking distance due to IC		89	81	Limitation of walking distance at normal speed on level ground due to IC
Limitation of work capacity due to PAOD		80	65[b]	Limitation of work capacity due to PAOD/IC, because of physical or emotional problems
Satisfaction with current treatment (PAOD)		80	83	Satisfaction with current treatment regarding PAOD
Perception of IC-related QoL		81	65[b]	Subjective perception of IC-related quality of life (e.g., impact of IC on QoL)

PAOD peripheral arterial occlusive disease, *QoL* quality of life

[a] High-rated items (> 90% agreement)

[b] Failed to reach consensus for practicability

[c] These items regarding "presence of" are already covered in VascuQoL-6 (when asking for "intensity of IC" or "degree of walking impairment")

Peripheral Artery Questionnaire (PAQ)

The PAQ is a holistic PROM that includes 20 questions [35]. Similar to the VascuQoL, it was developed with both patient and clinician input, and both subdomain and composite scores can be calculated. Reliability and sensitivity are high pre- and post-treatment. PAQ has also demonstrated good correlation with generic (i.e., non-disease-specific) PROMs instruments. MCID have also been established for PAQ, including MCID determined utilizing patient perspectives, whereby a 10-point change is considered clinically meaningful [36]. The primary limitation of PAQ is that it is somewhat less comprehensive than other IC-specific PROMs.

Walking Impairment Questionnaire (WIQ)

The WIQ is a PROM focused solely on functional impairment. It has 22 domains and takes an average of 5 minutes to complete, making it a highly feasible tool [37]. Like other high-quality instruments, patient input was utilized during development. Although certain objective measures such as ankle-brachial indices have not correlated well with many PROMs, ABI has been found to correlate with the WIQ distance and speed domain scores [38]. While VascuQoL and PAQ are more frequently used PROMs following revascularization interventions, the WIQ has been used in randomized controlled trials comparing various surgical, medical, and lifestyle modification treatments [39–49]. It should be noted that the VascuQoL, PAQ, and WIQ PROMs are all available in multiple languages and have been validated across a range of patient populations.

Limitations of PROMs

Obvious limitations of PROMs include resource utilization and patient and physician buy-in. Tools for easy and reliable collection and archiving of patient responses must be available to implement a PROM into one's clinical practice. Additionally, patients must complete many forms when visiting a physician's clinic and may not be willing to fill out an additional questionnaire. However, the Society for Vascular Surgery Quality Improvement Committee has made available free resources for effective implementation into a clinical practice [50]. Additionally, many other surgical specialties now use PROMs as standards of care in their practice, especially orthopedic surgery and oncology services. Patients perceive PROMs as useful in improving patient-physician communication and enhancing patient-centric care [51].

It is notable that the PROMs do not always correlate with objective outcome measures, and therefore must be used in a complementary fashion to other outcome measures, rather than independently. For example, in the CLEVER trial, which compared optimal medical therapy, primary stent placement, supervised exercise therapy, and combined stenting with supervised exercise therapy, discordance was observed between objective outcome measures and PROMs. Specifically, treadmill walking distance was best improved with supervised exercise therapy compared to revascularization or medical therapies, while PROMs scores were most improved in those patients undergoing endovascular revascularization [39]. Consistent with these findings, six-minute walk distances and PROMs scores have demonstrated poor correlation in a meta-analysis of trials examining results of supervised exercise therapy in patients with PAD [52]. Therefore, the results of PROMs are best used to guide patient-centered treatment plan development, and as adjunctive data to evaluate response post-treatment, along with objective outcomes measures described above.

Value of Healthcare

Although healthcare costs should not prohibit patients from receiving needed care, the costs of care relative to the benefit provided may be an important outcome to consider in patients with IC. High Value Care (HVC) is defined as "the best care for the patient, with the optimal results for the circumstances, delivered at the right price" [53] This can, perhaps, be thought of mathematically as the sum of quality of care and achievement of patient's goals of care per dollar spent. Resource utilization applied to the treatment of patients with IC is currently very high. Medicare expenditures on interventions for claudication cost as much as $266 million annually, and 90% of this cost covers procedures that are not guideline-directed and are not only not beneficial, but may be harmful, to patients [54]. These costs do not account for the multiple downstream procedures a patient may require, particularly when receiving inappropriate care upfront [6, 55]. Therefore, understanding the *value* of care as an outcome measure in the treatment of IC is of utmost importance. However, measuring said "value" of care is a complex endeavor that requires a formal cost effectiveness analysis, which requires specific quality of life instruments to calculate the quality-adjusted life years (QALY) of two potential interventions. Finances, resources, valid patient-reported outcomes, and objective outcomes surrounding the care of patients with IC must be considered to optimally determine the value of care provided in the treatment of IC.

Conclusion

In summary, the application of multiple objective and subjective outcome measures is important in the treatment of IC. Emphasis on the impact of various treatment choices on the natural evolution of the disease, patient function, and quality of life, as well as ensuring appropriate durability of interventions, allows for meaningful shared decision making between patient and provider. PROMs are important outcome measures that are often overlooked and underreported in the clinical setting but can provide meaningful information to both patient and provider. Although standardization of PROMs used in the evaluation of patients with IC may be useful for research purposes, physicians should incorporate the specific PROM that most practically aligns with their clinical practice and resources.

References

1. Hicks CW, Vavra AK, Earl Goldsborough III, Rebuffatti M, Almeida J, Duwayri YM, et al. Current status of patient-reported outcome measures in vascular surgery. J Vasc Surg. 2021;74(5):1693.
2. Nordanstig J, Behrendt CA, Baumgartner I, Belch J, Bäck M, Fitridge R, et al. Editor's choice – European Society for Vascular Surgery (ESVS) 2024 clinical practice guidelines on the management of asymptomatic lower limb peripheral arterial disease and intermittent claudication. Eur J Vasc Endovasc Surg. 2024;67(1):9–96.
3. Kumakura H, Kanai H, Hojo Y, Iwasaki T, Ichikawa S. Long-term survival and fate of the leg in de novo intermittent claudication. Eur Heart J Qual Care Clin Outcomes. 2017;3(3):208–15.
4. Tan LT, McDermott KM, Hicks CW. Overview and comparison of contemporary Society for Vascular Surgery, American Heart Association/American College of Cardiology, and European Society for Vascular Surgery guidelines for the management of patients with intermittent claudication. Semin Vasc Surg. 2024;37(2):188–209.
5. Bose S, Dun C, Solomon AJ, Black JH, Conte MS, Kalbaugh CA, et al. Infrapopliteal peripheral vascular interventions for claudication are performed frequently in the USA and are associated with poor long term outcomes. Eur J Vasc Endovasc Surg. 2024;S1078-5884(24):00490–8.
6. Sorber R, Dun C, Kawaji Q, Abularrage CJ, Black JH, Makary MA, et al. Early peripheral vascular interventions for claudication are associated with higher rates of late interventions and progression to chronic limb threatening ischemia. J Vasc Surg. 2023;77(3):836–847.e3.
7. Kawaji Q, Dun C, Walsh C, Sorber RA, Stonko DP, Abularrage CJ, et al. Index atherectomy peripheral vascular interventions performed for claudication are associated with more reinterventions than non-atherectomy interventions R1WC: 380/3505. J Vasc Surg. 2022;76(2):489–498.e4.
8. Hicks CW, Holscher CM, Wang P, Black JH, Abularrage CJ, Makary MA. Overuse of early peripheral vascular interventions for claudication. J Vasc Surg. 2020;71(1):121–130.e1.
9. Axley JC, McFarland GE, Novak Z, Scali ST, Patterson MA, Pearce BJ, et al. Factors associated with amputation after peripheral vascular intervention for intermittent claudication. Ann Vasc Surg. 2020;62:133–41.
10. Conte MS, Bradbury AW, Kolh P, White JV, Dick F, Fitridge R, et al. Global vascular guidelines on the management of chronic limb-threatening ischemia. J Vasc Surg. 2019;69(6S):3S–125S.e40.
11. Conte MS, Pomposelli FB, Clair DG, Geraghty PJ, McKinsey JF, Mills JL, et al. Society for vascular surgery practice guidelines for atherosclerotic occlusive disease of the lower extremities: management of asymptomatic disease and claudication. J Vasc Surg. 2015;61(3):2S–41S.e1.
12. Levin SR, Farber A, Osborne NH, Beck AW, McFarland GE, Rybin D, et al. Tibial bypass in patients with intermittent claudication is associated with poor outcomes. J Vasc Surg. 2021;73(2):564–571.e1.
13. Woo K, Siracuse JJ, Klingbeil K, Kraiss LW, Osborne NH, Singh N, et al. Society for vascular surgery appropriate use criteria for management of intermittent claudication. J Vasc Surg. 2022;76(1):3–22.e1.
14. Conte MS. Data, guidelines, and practice of revascularization for claudication. J Vasc Surg. 2017;66(3):911–5.
15. Harris LM. Importance of patient-related outcomes for assessment of claudication. J Vasc Surg. 2024;80(3):791.

16. Conte MS, Geraghty PJ, Bradbury AW, Hevelone ND, Lipsitz SR, Moneta GL, et al. Suggested objective performance goals and clinical trial design for evaluating catheter-based treatment of critical limb ischemia. J Vasc Surg. 2009;50(6):1462–1473.e3.
17. Watson CJ, Phillips D, Hands L, Collin J. Claudication distance is poorly estimated and inappropriately measured. Br J Surg. 1997;84(8):1107–9.
18. Hiatt WR, Rogers RK, Brass EP. The treadmill is a better functional test than the 6-minute walk test in therapeutic trials of patients with peripheral artery disease. Circulation. 2014;130(1):69–78.
19. Nicolaï SPA, Viechtbauer W, Kruidenier LM, Candel MJJM, Prins MH, Teijink JAW. Reliability of treadmill testing in peripheral arterial disease: a meta-regression analysis. J Vasc Surg. 2009;50(2):322–9.
20. McDermott MM, Guralnik JM, Criqui MH, Liu K, Kibbe M, Ferrucci L. The six-minute walk is a better outcome measure than treadmill walking tests in therapeutic trials of patients with peripheral artery disease. Circulation. 2014;130(1):61.
21. Sandberg A, Cider Å, Jivegård L, Nordanstig J, Wittboldt S, Bäck M. Test-retest reliability, agreement, and minimal detectable change in the 6-minute walk test in patients with intermittent claudication. J Vasc Surg. 2020;71(1):197–203.
22. Golledge J, Yip L, Fernando ME, Pinchbeck J, Rowbotham S, Jenkins J, et al. Relationship between requirement to stop during a six-minute walk test and health-related quality of life, physical activity and physical performance amongst people with intermittent claudication. Ann Vasc Surg. 2021;76:363–9.
23. Dewey FE, Kapoor JR, Williams RS, Lipinski MJ, Ashley EA, Hadley D, et al. Ventricular arrhythmias during clinical treadmill testing and prognosis. Arch Intern Med. 2008;168(2):225–34.
24. Codman EA. The classic: a study in hospital efficiency: as demonstrated by the case report of first five years of private hospital. Clin Orthop Relat Res. 2013;471(6):1778.
25. The evolution and use of patient-reported outcomes in regulatory decision making [Internet]. [cited 2024 Nov 3]. Available from: https://www.raps.org/News-and-Articles/News-Articles/2023/3/The-evolution-and-use-of-patient-reported-outcomes.
26. Athanasiou T, Patel V, Darzi A, editors. Patient reported outcomes and quality of life in surgery [internet]. Cham: Springer; 2023. [cited 2024 Nov 3]. Available from: https://link.springer.com/10.1007/978-3-031-27597-5.
27. Holeman TA, Chester C, Hales JB, Zhang Y, Johnson CE, Brooke BS. Long-term patient-reported outcomes among patients undergoing revascularization vs medical therapy for intermittent claudication. J Vasc Surg. 2024;80(2):466–477.e4.
28. Rymer JA, Narcisse D, Cosiano M, Tanaka J, McDermott MM, Treat-Jacobson DJ, et al. Patient-reported outcome measures in symptomatic, non–limb-threatening peripheral artery disease: a state-of-the-art review. Circ Cardiovasc Interv. 2022;15(1):e011320.
29. Arndt H, Nordanstig J, Bertges DJ, Budtz-Lilly J, Venermo M, Espada CL, et al. A Delphi consensus on patient reported outcomes for registries and trials including patients with intermittent claudication: recommendations and reporting standard. Eur J Vasc Endovasc Surg. 2022;64(5):526–33.
30. Morgan MBF, Crayford T, Murrin B, Fraser SCA. Developing the vascular quality of life questionnaire: a new disease-specific quality of life measure for use in lower limb ischemia. J Vasc Surg. 2001;33(4):679–87.
31. Larsen ASF, Reiersen AT, Jacobsen MB, Kløw NE, Nordanstig J, Morgan M, et al. Validation of the vascular quality of life questionnaire—6 for clinical use in patients with lower limb peripheral arterial disease. Health Qual Life Outcomes. 2017;15:184.
32. Kumlien C, Nordanstig J, Lundström M, Pettersson M. Validity and test retest reliability of the vascular quality of life Questionnaire-6: a short form of a disease-specific health-related quality of life instrument for patients with peripheral arterial disease. Health Qual Life Outcomes. 2017;15:187.
33. Correia M d A, Andrade-Lima A, de Oliveira PLM, Domiciano RM, Domingues WJR, Wolosker N, et al. Translation and validation of the Brazilian-Portuguese short version of

vascular quality of life questionnaire in peripheral artery disease patients with intermittent claudication symptoms. Ann Vasc Surg. 2018;51:48–54.e1.
34. Nordanstig J, Wann-Hansson C, Karlsson J, Lundström M, Pettersson M, Morgan MBF. Vascular quality of life questionnaire-6 facilitates health-related quality of life assessment in peripheral arterial disease. J Vasc Surg. 2014;59(3):700–707.e1.
35. Spertus J, Jones P, Poler S, Rocha-Singh K. The peripheral artery questionnaire: a new disease-specific health status measure for patients with peripheral arterial disease. Am Heart J. 2004;147(2):301–8.
36. Peri-Okonny PA, Wang J, Gosch KL, Patel MR, Shishehbor MH, Safley DL, et al. Establishing thresholds for minimal clinically important differences for the peripheral artery disease questionnaire. Circ Cardiovasc Qual Outcomes. 2021;14(5):e007232.
37. McDermott MM, Liu K, Guralnik JM, Martin GJ, Criqui MH, Greenland P. Measurement of walking endurance and walking velocity with questionnaire: validation of the walking impairment questionnaire in men and women with peripheral arterial disease. J Vasc Surg. 1998;28(6):1072–81.
38. Banerjee S, Badhey N, Lichtenwalter C, Varghese C, Brilakis ES. Relationship of walking impairment and ankle-brachial index assessments with peripheral arterial translesional pressure gradients. J Invasive Cardiol. 2011;23(9):352–6.
39. Murphy TP, Cutlip DE, Regensteiner JG, Mohler ER, Cohen D, Reynolds MR, et al. Supervised exercise vs primary stenting for claudication due to aortoiliac peripheral artery disease: 6-month outcomes from the CLEVER study. Circulation. 2011;125(1):130.
40. Murphy TP, Reynolds MR, Cohen DJ, Regensteiner JG, Massaro JM, Cutlip DE, et al. Correlation of patient-reported symptom outcomes and treadmill test outcomes after treatment for aortoiliac claudication. J Vasc Interv Radiol. 2013;24(10):1427–35. quiz 1436
41. Gray WA, Feiring A, Cioppi M, Hibbard R, Gray B, Khatib Y, et al. S.M.A.R.T. self-expanding nitinol stent for the treatment of atherosclerotic lesions in the superficial femoral artery (STROLL): 1-year outcomes. J Vasc Interv Radiol. 2015;26(1):21–8.
42. Jiang Y, Fan J, Li Y, Wu G, Wang Y, Yang J, et al. Rapid reduction in plaque inflammation by sonodynamic therapy inpatients with symptomatic femoropopliteal peripheral artery disease:A randomized controlled trial. Int J Cardiol. 2021;325:132–9.
43. McDermott MM, Spring B, Tian L, Treat-Jacobson D, Ferrucci L, Lloyd-Jones D, et al. Effect of low-intensity vs high-intensity home-based walking exercise on walk distance in patients with peripheral artery disease: the LITE randomized clinical trial. JAMA. 2021;325(13):1266–76.
44. McDermott MM, Spring B, Berger JS, Treat-Jacobson D, Conte MS, Creager MA, et al. Effect of a home-based exercise intervention of wearable technology and telephone coaching on walking performance in peripheral artery disease: the HONOR randomized clinical trial. JAMA. 2018;319(16):1665–76.
45. Liao CJ, Song SH, Li T, Zhang Y, de Zhang W. Randomized controlled trial of orchid drug-coated balloon versus standard percutaneous transluminal angioplasty for treatment of femoropopliteal artery in-stent restenosis. Int Angiol. 2019;38(5):365–71.
46. Teichgräber U, Lehmann T, Aschenbach R, Scheinert D, Zeller T, Brechtel K, et al. Drug-coated balloon angioplasty of Femoropopliteal lesions maintained superior efficacy over conventional balloon: 2-year results of the randomized EffPac trial. Radiology. 2020;295(2):478–87.
47. Rundback J, Chandra P, Brodmann M, Weinstock B, Sedillo G, Cawich I, et al. Novel laser-based catheter for peripheral atherectomy: 6-month results from the Eximo Medical B-Laser™ IDE study. Catheter Cardiovasc Interv. 2019;94(7):1010–7.
48. Angle JF, Gasparetto A, Yokoi H, Jaff MR, Popma JJ, Piegari GN, et al. Three-year efficacy and safety of the misago peripheral stent for superficial femoral artery disease: final results from the OSPREY trial. J Vasc Interv Radiol. 2020;31(6):978–85.
49. Schroë H, Holden AH, Goueffic Y, Jansen SJ, Peeters P, Keirse K, et al. Stellarex drug-coated balloon for treatment of femoropopliteal arterial disease-the ILLUMENATE global study: 12-month results from a prospective, multicenter, single-arm study. Catheter Cardiovasc Interv. 2018;91(3):497–504.

50. PROs Toolkits | Society for Vascular Surgery [Internet]. [cited 2024 Dec 15]. Available from: https://vascular.org/vascular-specialists/practice-and-quality/quality/pros-toolkits.
51. Aiyegbusi OL, Isa F, Kyte D, Pankhurst T, Kerecuk L, Ferguson J, et al. Patient and clinician opinions of patient reported outcome measures (PROMs) in the management of patients with rare diseases: a qualitative study. Health Qual Life Outcomes. 2020;18(1):177.
52. Thangada ND, Zhang D, Tian L, Zhao L, Rejeski WJ, Ho KJ, et al. Home-based walking exercise and supervised treadmill exercise in patients with peripheral artery disease: an individual participant data meta-analysis. JAMA Netw Open. 2023;6(9):e2334590.
53. Korenstein D. Charting the route to high value care: the role of medical education. JAMA. 2015;314(22):2359.
54. Dun C, Stonko DP, Bose S, Keegan AC, McDermott KM, Rumalla KC, et al. Trends and factors associated with peripheral vascular interventions for the treatment of claudication from 2011 to 2022: a National Medicare Cohort Study. J Am Heart Assoc. 2024;13(14):e033463.
55. McCready RA, Brown OW, Kiell CS, Goodson SF. Revascularization for claudication: changing the natural history of a benign disease! J Vasc Surg. 2024;79(1):159–66.

Pharmacologic Therapy to Improve Functional and Limb Outcomes

9

Aishwarya Raja and Eric A. Secemsky

Introduction

Contemporary pharmacologic therapies for patients with peripheral artery disease (PAD) focus on improving functional capacity and reducing the risk of major adverse cardiovascular and cerebrovascular events (MACCE) and major adverse limb events (MALE) (Table 9.1). Few pharmacotherapies are available that decrease lower extremity symptoms secondary to claudication. However, as the majority of patients with PAD die due to cardiovascular events versus limb-related events, reducing global cardiovascular risks remains the priority for treatment. For instance, the rate of the MACCE, which includes myocardial infarction (MI), stroke, and cardiovascular death, is higher in the PAD population as demonstrated by trials like Examining Use of Ticagrelor in Peripheral Artery Disease (EUCLID) in which 44% of patients had concomitant cerebrovascular and/or coronary artery disease (CAD), and the majority of deaths were cardiovascular in etiology [1]. Thus, it is important to remember that PAD is a marker for systemic atherosclerosis [2]. Nonetheless, this population is also at elevated risk for MALE, such as acute limb ischemia, chronic limb-threatening ischemia [CLTI] (the most severe disease manifestation of PAD),

A. Raja
Massachusetts General Hospital, Boston, MA, USA

Interventional Cardiology and Vascular Research, Richard A. and Susan F. Smith Center for Outcomes Research, Beth Israel Deaconess Medical Center, Boston, MA, USA

E. A. Secemsky (✉)
Interventional Cardiology and Vascular Research, Richard A. and Susan F. Smith Center for Outcomes Research, Beth Israel Deaconess Medical Center, Boston, MA, USA

Vascular Intervention, Interventional Cardiology and Vascular Research, Richard A. and Susan F. Smith Center for Outcomes Research, Beth Israel Deaconess Medical Center, Boston, MA, USA

Harvard Medical School, Boston, MA, USA
e-mail: esecemsk@bidmc.harvard.edu

W. P. Robinson III, J. P. Simons (eds.), *The Patient-Centered Approach to Claudication*, https://doi.org/10.1007/978-3-032-02460-2_9

Table 9.1 Optimal medical therapy for PAD

Class	Goal	2024 AHA/ACC PAD Guideline class recommendations
Antiplatelet and antithrombotic therapy	Reduce cerebrovascular, coronary, and peripheral artery thrombotic risk	In patients with symptomatic PAD, single antiplatelet therapy is recommended to reduce the risk of MACE (**Class 1**). In patients with symptomatic PAD, single antiplatelet therapy with clopidogrel alone (75 mg daily) is recommended to reduce the risk of MACCE (**Class 1**). In patients with symptomatic PAD, single antiplatelet therapy with aspirin alone (range, 75-325 mg daily) is recommended to reduce the risk of MACCE (**Class 1**). In patients with symptomatic PAD, low-dose rivaroxaban (2.5 mg twice daily) combined with low-dose aspirin is effective to reduce the risk of MACCE and MALE (**Class 1**). After endovascular or surgical revascularization for PAD, antiplatelet therapy is recommended **(Class 1**). After endovascular or surgical revascularization for PAD, low-dose rivaroxaban (2.5 mg twice daily) combined with low-dose aspirin is recommended to reduce the risk of MACCE and MALE (**Class 1**). After endovascular revascularization for PAD, dual antiplatelet therapy with a P2Y12 antagonist and low-dose aspirin is reasonable for at least 1 to 6 months **(Class 2a**). After endovascular or surgical revascularization in patients with PAD who require full-intensity anticoagulation for another indication and are not at high risk for bleeding, adding single antiplatelet therapy is reasonable (**Class 2a**). In patients with asymptomatic PAD, single antiplatelet therapy is reasonable to reduce the risk of MACCE (**Class 2a**). In patients with symptomatic PAD without recent revascularization, the benefit of dual antiplatelet therapy is uncertain (**Class 2b**). In patients with symptomatic PAD, the benefit of vorapaxar added to existing antiplatelet therapy is uncertain (**Class 2b**). After surgical revascularization for PAD with a prosthetic graft, dual antiplatelet therapy with a P2Y12 antagonist and low-dose aspirin may be reasonable for at least 1 month **(Class 2b**). In patients with PAD without another indication (eg, atrial fibrillation), full-intensity oral anticoagulation should not be used to reduce the risk of MACCE and MALE (**Class 3: harm**).

Lipid-lowering therapy	Reduce cardiovascular risk and target LDL-C to <70 mg/dL	In patients with PAD, treatment with high-intensity statin therapy is indicated, with an aim of achieving a ≥ 50% reduction in low-density lipoprotein cholesterol (LDL-C) level (**Class 1**). In patients with PAD who are on maximally tolerated statin therapy and have an LDL-C level of ≥ 70 mg/dL, it is reasonable to add PCSK9 inhibitor therapy (**Class 2a**). In patients with PAD who are on maximally tolerated statin therapy and have an LDL-C level of ≥ 70 mg/dL, it is reasonable to add ezetimibe therapy (**Class 2a**).
Antihypertensive therapy	Reduce cardiovascular risk and target blood pressure < 130/80 mmHg	In patients with PAD and hypertension, antihypertensive therapy should be administered to reduce the risk of MACCE (**Class 1**). In patients with PAD and hypertension, a systolic blood pressure goal of < 130 mm Hg and a diastolic blood pressure goal of < 80 mm Hg is recommended (**Class 1**). In patients with PAD and hypertension, the selective use of angiotensin-converting (ACE) inhibitors or angiotensin-receptor blockers is recommended to reduce the risk of MACCE (**Class 1**).
Diabetes therapy	Target A1c to <7% to reduce microvascular and macrovascular complications	In patients with PAD and type 2 diabetes, use of glucagon-like peptide-1 agonists (liraglutide and semaglutide) and sodium-glucose cotransporter-2 (SGLT-2) inhibitors (canagliflozin, dapagliflozin, and empagliflozin) is effective to reduce the risk of MACCE (**Class 1**). In patients with PAD and diabetes, glycemic control may be beneficial to improve limb outcomes (**Class 2b**).
Claudication medications	Improve functional status and reduce symptom burden	In patients with claudication, cilostazol is recommended to improve leg symptoms and increase walking distance (**Class 1**). In patients with PAD, cilostazol may be useful to reduce restenosis after endovascular therapy for femoropopliteal disease (**Class 2b**). In patients with PAD and congestive heart failure of any severity, cilostazol should not be administered (**Class 3: harm**). In patients with chronic symptomatic PAD, pentoxifylline is not recommended for treatment of claudication (**Class 3: no benefit**). In patients with chronic symptomatic PAD, chelation therapy is not recommended for treatment of claudication (**Class 3: no benefit**).

peripheral revascularization, and major lower extremity amputation [2]. It is important to recognize that the majority of the published literature includes mixed cohorts of PAD; that is, cohorts include both patients with claudication and those with CLTI. While it may be appropriate for MACCE to be studied in this heterogenous patient population, limb-specific outcomes may be better studied in separate analyses.

Current medical treatments have been shown to reduce the risk of major cardiovascular and limb-related events in patients with PAD. However, there is marked underutilization of these risk-reducing therapies among patients with PAD relative to patients with CAD [3]. Multiple studies have shown that this trend is likely driven by factors like poor disease awareness, racial and ethnic disparities, delays in diagnosis, fragmentation of care, and lack of education about optimal treatment in this population [4, 5]. A 2017 retrospective study on ~2000 patient visits to office-based or hospital-affiliated outpatient settings from 2005 to 2012 demonstrated that only 36% of visits reported antiplatelet use, 33% statin use, and 28% angiotensin-converting enzyme inhibitor or angiotensin receptor blocker use [6]. Notably, a clinical history of CAD was associated with significantly higher use of all these risk-reducing therapies, further supporting the notion that there is a significant treatment gap among patients with PAD.

Overall, existing data suggest that raising awareness about optimal medical management strategies for PAD will be critical in order to improve outcomes in this patient population. This chapter will elaborate on guideline-directed pharmacotherapy for PAD and its association with reducing the overall risk of MACCE and MALE, as well as the risk of progression to more symptomatic and limb-threatening disease.

Antiplatelet and Anticoagulant Therapies in PAD

The role of antithrombotic therapy in PAD involves both antiplatelet and anticoagulant therapy (Fig. 9.1). Among patients with CAD, cerebrovascular disease, or symptomatic PAD, the role of antithrombotic therapy to prevent MACCE has been well-established [7–11]. In patients with PAD who have undergone recent revascularization procedures (i.e., within 6 months), these therapies have also been shown to reduce the occurrence of recurrent symptoms and MALE [12, 13]. Finally, their use in patients with asymptomatic PAD and those without a history of recent revascularization is not as well supported due to the elevated risks of bleeding. Overall, the decision to initiate antiplatelet therapy, anticoagulant therapy, or both should be weighed against potential risks.

Antithrombotic Therapy in Symptomatic PAD

Among patients with symptomatic PAD, single antiplatelet therapy has been shown to reduce the risk of MACCE and has a Class I recommendation by the 2024 AHA/ACC PAD guideline (Table 9.1) [14]. Aspirin at a dose of 81-100 mg has remained the antiplatelet of choice in the PAD population [7–9]. However, trials have

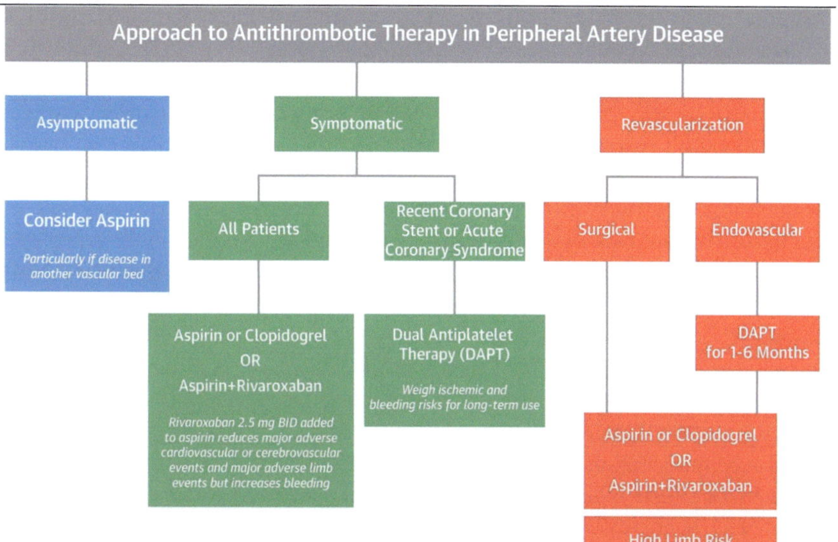

↑ Ischemic Risk	↑ Bleeding Risk	↑ Limb Risk
Prior MI	Anticoagulation	Prosthetic bypass
Diabetes	Prior bleeding	Below-knee bypass
Older age	Older age	Suboptimal conduit
Chronic kidney disease	Chronic kidney disease	Poor arterial run-off
Heart failure	Anemia	Extensive lesions
Current smoker	Low body weight	Tissue loss

Fig. 9.1 Antithrombotic approaches to PADAbbreviations: BID = 2 times per day; MI = myocardial infarctionReprinted from Hussain et al. [105]

demonstrated that P2Y12 inhibitors, such as clopidogrel and ticagrelor, are also efficacious among PAD patients at reducing cardiovascular event rates. For instance, in the Clopidogrel versus Aspirin in Patients at Risk of Ischemic Events (CAPRIE) trial examining 19,185 patients randomized to receive either clopidogrel 75 milligrams daily or aspirin 325 milligrams daily, single antiplatelet therapy with clopidogrel was noted to have improved efficacy for prevention of MACCE, with similar rates of bleeding [10]. In the EUCLID trial, which randomized 13,885 patients to receive monotherapy with ticagrelor 90 milligrams twice daily or clopidogrel 75 milligrams once daily, ticagrelor was not shown to be superior to clopidogrel, although rates of adverse events in the ticagrelor group were higher [1]. A recent meta-analysis of trials in patients with CAD, cerebrovascular disease, or PAD also demonstrated that aspirin and P2Y12 inhibitors had similar efficacy [11].

Although platelet inhibition is important in reducing thrombotic-related cardiovascular events, recent data have also promoted the role of addressing the coagulation cascade in parallel, termed dual pathway inhibition. This may be particularly relevant to the management of PAD. An analysis of 239 arteries from limbs of patients who underwent amputation for CLTI found that 73% had chronic thrombotic occlusions, more often without significant atherosclerosis [15]. This suggests that thromboembolic or in-situ thrombosis may contribute to the progression to CLI, and the use of antithrombotic agents may slow this process. The 2017 Cardiovascular Outcomes for People Using Anticoagulation Strategies (COMPASS) trial, which randomized 27,395 participants with stable atherosclerotic vascular disease to receive low dose rivaroxaban plus aspirin (100 milligrams once daily), rivaroxaban (5 milligrams twice daily), or aspirin (100 milligrams once daily), found that those assigned to low dose rivaroxaban plus aspirin had better cardiovascular outcomes than those assigned to aspirin alone, although there were more major bleeding events [16]. In contrast, higher dose rivaroxaban did not result in better cardiovascular outcomes than aspirin alone and also resulted in more major bleeding events. A 2018 sub-analysis of 6391 patients with lower extremity PAD similarly demonstrated that patients assigned to low-dose rivaroxaban plus aspirin had reduced MACCE and MALE [17, 18]. Based on these data, among patients with symptomatic PAD, the use of low-dose rivaroxaban (2.5 milligrams twice daily) and low-dose aspirin is now a Class I recommendation by the 2024 AHA/ACC PAD guideline (Table 9.1).

Importantly, there is a lack of evidence supporting the use of dual antiplatelet therapy outside of a recent revascularization procedure (coronary or peripheral) in patients with symptomatic PAD (Class 2b recommendation by the 2024 AHA/ACC PAD guideline) (Table 9.1) [14]. Subgroup analyses of patients with PAD from larger trials, such as the Prevention of Cardiovascular Events in Patients with Prior Heart Attack Using Ticagrelor Compared to Placebo on a Background of Aspirin–Thrombolysis In Myocardial Infarction 54 (PEGASUS-TIMI 54) and the Clopidogrel for High Atherothrombotic Risk and Ischemic Stabilization, Management, and Avoidance (CHARISMA) trials, have been underpowered [19, 20]. The use of more potent antiplatelet therapies (e.g., vorapaxar) in patients with symptomatic PAD is also a Class 2b recommendation by the 2024 AHA/ACC PAD guideline (Table 9.1) [14]. The Thrombin Receptor Antagonist in Secondary Prevention of Atherothrombotic Ischemic Events–Thrombolysis In Myocardial Infarction 50 (TRA 2P–TIMI 50) trial randomized 26,449 patients with a history of MI, stroke, or symptomatic PAD to vorapaxar, an antagonist of the protease-activated receptor-1, or placebo [21]. While this study demonstrated a decreased risk of MALE in the cohort of 3787 patients with symptomatic PAD, there was an increased risk of bleeding. Finally, the use of full-intensity oral anticoagulation in the absence of another indication is not indicated in this population (Class 3 recommendation) (Table 9.1) [14]. This is supported by multiple RCTs and observational studies, such as Warfarin Antiplatelet Vascular Evaluation (WAVE), which demonstrated higher morbidity rates [22, 23]. However, this recommendation is distinct from recommendations regarding the addition of low-dose rivaroxaban to low-dose aspirin.

Antithrombotic Therapy After Endovascular or Surgical Revascularization

Among patients with symptomatic PAD who had recent lower extremity endovascular or surgical revascularization, there is an elevated residual risk of adverse cardiovascular and limb outcomes. To reduce the risk of MACCE and MALE in this population, the 2024 AHA/ACC PAD guideline recommends the use of low-dose rivaroxaban and low-dose aspirin (Class I recommendation) (Table 9.1) [14]. This is supported by the Vascular Outcomes Study of ASA [acetylsalicylic acid] Along with Rivaroxaban in Endovascular or Surgical Limb Revascularization for PAD (VOYAGER PAD) trial, which assessed the use of both low-dose rivaroxaban and low-dose aspirin in patients within 10 days of lower extremity revascularization who were not on anticoagulation for another indication or had planned P2Y12 inhibitor use [24]. The study found that this regimen reduced MACCE and MALE, compared with aspirin alone, mainly driven by a lower rate of acute limb ischemia. Smaller observational studies also support this recommendation in patients with CLTI after revascularization [25, 26].

Next, the 2024 AHA/ACC PAD guideline has a Class 2a recommendation for the use of dual antiplatelet therapy with low-dose aspirin and a P2Y12 antagonist for at least 1 to 6 months after endovascular revascularization (Table 9.1) [14]. This recommendation has been extrapolated from the use of dual antiplatelet therapy after percutaneous coronary intervention. Major contemporary trials on the use of different drug-coated devices support the use of dual antiplatelet therapy for a minimum for 2 to 6 months after revascularization [12, 13] However, the only trial that randomized patients to DAPT (daily dose of 100 milligrams of aspirin and 75 milligrams of clopidogrel for 6 months, or the same doses of aspirin plus placebo) after endovascular revascularization was underpowered and failed to demonstrate a long-term difference in outcomes compared to aspirin alone [27].

Despite limited evidence, the 2024 AHA/ACC PAD guideline also has a Class 2b recommendation for use of dual antiplatelet therapy with a P2Y12 antagonist and low-dose aspirin for at least 1 month after surgical revascularization with a prosthetic graft (Table 9.1) [14]. The 2000 Bypass Oral anticoagulants or Aspirin (Dutch BOA) trial, which randomized 2690 patients undergoing infrainguinal bypass to high intensity anticoagulation (international normalized ratio 3.0 to 4.5) with phenprocoumon or acenocoumarol or aspirin, found similar rates of graft occlusion between groups; a subgroup analysis also indicated that anticoagulation was associated with improved vein graft patency [28]. A later subanalysis from the Clopidogrel and Acetylsalicylic Acid in Bypass Surgery for Peripheral Arterial Disease (CASPAR) trial found that in 851 patients undergoing below-the-knee bypass grafting, the use of combination therapy with aspirin 81 milligrams daily and clopidogrel 75 milligrams daily was associated with a reduced risk of MALE or death compared to aspirin alone [29]. Importantly, there was no significant difference in rates of major bleeding between groups.

Current data and guidelines also support the benefit of single antiplatelet therapy after endovascular revascularization in patients on full-dose anticoagulation for another indication (e.g., atrial fibrillation or venous thromboembolism) and are not at elevated risk of bleeding (Class 2b recommendation) (Table 9.1) [14, 30]. However, the use of both dual antiplatelet therapy and full-intensity anticoagulation (i.e., triple therapy) is associated with a higher risk of bleeding.

Antithrombotic Therapy in Asymptomatic PAD

Finally, among patients with asymptomatic PAD, there is a lack of evidence supporting the use of aspirin [8, 31, 32]. In the Critical Leg Ischemia Prevention (CLIPS) trial, patients with asymptomatic PAD were randomized to treatment with aspirin or placebo; however, the study was stopped early and was found to be underpowered to assess the effect of aspirin in the subgroup of patients with asymptomatic PAD [8]. Other trials like Aspirin for Asymptomatic Atherosclerosis (AAA) and Prevention of Progression of Arterial Disease and Diabetes (POPADAD) had limited generalizability due to a higher ABI threshold for enrollment [31, 32]. Overall, despite the lack of supporting data, single antiplatelet therapy is still recommended in patients with asymptomatic PAD given the elevated risk of MACCE and mortality and high prevalence of CAD in this subgroup (Class 2b recommendation) (Table 9.1) [14, 33, 34]. Single antiplatelet therapy is also recommended in these patients with other clinical indications, such as CAD, cerebrovascular disease, and prior coronary revascularization.

Hyperlipidemia Management in PAD

Dyslipidemia is a significant predictor for adverse cardiovascular events and a modifiable risk factor in patients with PAD. The use of lipid-lowering therapies, such as statins, ezetimibe, proprotein convertase subtilisin/kexin type 9 (PCSK9) inhibitors, fibrates, icosapent ethyl, bempedoic acid, and inclisiran, has been associated with improved outcomes in this population.

The 2018 AHA/ACC cholesterol guideline and 2024 AHA/ACC PAD guideline have a Class 1 recommendation for treatment with high-intensity statin therapy to achieve a 50% or greater reduction in low-density lipoprotein cholesterol (LDL-C) levels in patients ≤75 years of age with atherosclerotic cardiovascular disease (CVD), including those with PAD [35]. Data based on subgroup analyses from randomized controlled trials (RCTs) further support the use of high-intensity statins to reduce the LDL-C level to less than 70 mg/dL [36–38]. High-intensity statins include atorvastatin 40–80 milligrams and rosuvastatin 20–40 milligrams [39].

The first subgroup analysis to analyze the use of statins to help lower the risk of MACCE in patients with PAD was from the 2007 Heart Protection Study [40]. In this RCT, 6748 patients with PAD were randomized to either simvastatin or placebo with a mean follow-up of 5 years. In the overall study population, simvastatin was associated with a 16% relative risk reduction in peripheral vascular events (4.7% versus 5.5%; $P = 0.002$), irrespective of the baseline LDL-C level. Numerous retrospective observational studies have also examined the role of statins in lowering adverse events in patients with PAD. For example, among 5861 patients with symptomatic PAD from the 2014 Reduction of Atherothrombosis for Continued Health registry, statin therapy was associated with a 14% relative risk reduction in the composite outcome of worsening claudication, critical limb ischemia, peripheral revascularization, and amputation at 4 years [41]. The largest study to date on the use of statins in this population involved 155,647 patients with PAD from the US Department of Veterans Affairs health care system between 2003 and 2014 [42]. This study found lower rates of amputation and death among patients treated with statins in both the unadjusted and adjusted analyses; interestingly, patients treated with high-intensity statin therapy were also found to have a 15% lower risk of mortality and a 22% lower risk of amputation compared to those treated with low-to-moderate–intensity statins. A more recent 2020 meta-analysis examining 138,060 patients with PAD similarly demonstrated that statins reduced the risk of MALE by 30%, amputation by 35%, and all-cause mortality by 39% [43]. Finally, a number of studies focused on patients with more severe manifestations of PAD, including those with chronic limb-threatening ischemia and those who had undergone revascularization or lower extremity amputation, reported positive associations between statin use and improvements in rates of amputation, revascularization, and all-cause mortality [44–50].

Next, the 2018 AHA/ACC cholesterol guideline and 2024 AHA/ACC PAD guideline have a Class 2a recommendation for initiating a PCSK9 inhibitor therapy in patients with PAD who are on maximally tolerated statin therapy and have an LDL-C level of ≥70 mg/dL [14, 35]. Data supporting this recommendation include a subanalysis of patients with symptomatic PAD from the Further Cardiovascular Outcomes Research with PCSK9 Inhibition in Subjects with Elevated Risk (FOURIER) RCT [36]. This analysis randomly assigned patients on statin therapy to a fixed dose of evolocumab or placebo. Use of a PCSK9 inhibitor therapy was associated with lower rates of MACCE (HR 0.79 [95% CI: 0.66–0.94]; $P = 0.0098$) and MALE (HR 0.63 [95% CI: 0.39–1.03]; $P = 0.063$) compared with the placebo group. Similarly, in a prespecified analysis from the 2018 Evaluation of Cardiovascular Outcomes After an Acute Coronary Syndrome During Treatment With Alirocumab (ODYSSEY OUTCOMES) trial, alirocumab was associated with a reduced risk of PAD events (HR 0.69 [95% CI: 0.54–0.89]; $P = 0.004$), particularly among those with high lipoprotein(a) levels [37]. Another prespecified analysis from this RCT demonstrated that although polyvascular disease (i.e., coronary, peripheral artery, and/or cerebrovascular disease) was associated with a higher risk of MACCE and death, alirocumab resulted in large absolute reductions.

The 2018 AHA/ACC cholesterol guideline and 2024 AHA/ACC PAD guideline also have a Class 2a recommendation for initiating ezetimibe in patients with PAD who are on maximally tolerated statin therapy and have an LDL-C level of ≥70 mg/dL [14, 35]. Data supporting this recommendation includes a subgroup analysis of the Improved Reduction of Outcomes: Vytorin Efficacy International Trial (IMPROVE-IT) trial, which examined over 1000 patients with extracoronary atherosclerotic arterial disease, including PAD [38]. This analysis found a lower rate of MACCE (45.2% versus 49.5%) among patients treated with ezetimibe over a follow-up period of 7 years. However, the use of ezetimibe to reduce the risk of MALE in patients with PAD has not yet been established.

Finally, lipid-lowering therapies, such as fibrates, icosapent ethyl, bempedoic acid, and inclisiran, are also utilized to help achieve target LDL-C goals, in particular among patients already on maximally tolerated statins or who are statin-intolerant. Large-scale studies like Fenofibrate Intervention and Event Lowering in Diabetes (FIELD), ACCORD, Reduction of Cardiovascular Events with Icosapent Ethyl-Intervention Trial (REDUCE-IT), CLEAR Outcomes, ORION 10, and ORION 11 support the use of these therapies to help lower lipid levels and reduce the risk of MACCE [51–55]. However, these medications have not been specifically studied in patients with PAD and most are not currently considered first-line therapies for secondary prevention.

Hypertension Management in PAD

Approximately 35% to 55% of patients with PAD have hypertension, the most common cardiovascular risk factor [56]. Current guidelines recommend aggressive treatment of hypertension in patients with PAD as the presence of both conditions can contribute to worse long-term outcomes, specifically MACCE [57]. Hypertension has also been associated with a decline in ankle-brachial index (ABI) in adults >65 years of age [58]. Although dedicated trials on the optimal antihypertensive therapies to use in patients with PAD are lacking, angiotensin-converting enzyme inhibitors (ACEi) or angiotensin-receptor blockers are considered first-line agents given their associated cardiovascular benefits in patients with PAD and hypertension, and have a Class I recommendation by the 2024 AHA/ACC PAD guideline [39]. β-blockers are also widely used, especially in patients with another indication like CAD, but are not included in the latest AHA/ACC recommendations (Table 9.1) [14, 35].

The 2017 ACC/AHA hypertension clinical practice guideline and 2024 AHA/ACC PAD guideline have a Class 1 recommendation for targeting a blood pressure of <130/80 mm Hg in patients with PAD and hypertension [14, 59]. Unfortunately, this recommendation is not supported by robust evidence as only a few studies have specifically included patients with PAD. Landmark trials like Systolic Blood Pressure Intervention Trial (SPRINT) demonstrated that in patients with known CVD, targeting a more aggressive systolic blood pressure goal of <120 mm Hg compared with the standard target of <140 mm Hg reduced rates of cardiovascular outcomes and associated mortality [60]. However, only 5.3% of the study population had PAD. Other studies, such as Appropriate Blood Pressure Control in Diabetes Study (ABCD), enrolled 950 patients (480 normotensive) and randomized them to either treatment with enalapril or nisoldipine (intensive blood pressure control) or placebo (moderate blood pressure control) and monitored them over 5 years. In a subset of 53 participants with PAD (defined as ABI <0.9), a more intensive blood pressure target (mean blood pressure of 128/75 mm Hg) was associated with a marked reduction in MACCE [61]. More recently, in a post-hoc analysis of 2699 hypertensive patients with concomitant PAD and CAD from the International Verapamil-SR/Trandolapril Study (INVEST), higher rates of MACCE were observed in patients with out-of-range high and low systolic blood pressures; this suggested that patients with PAD likely required a different target blood pressure goal compared to those without [62]. Similarly, Fudim et al. and Itoga et al. reported higher rates of MACCE in patients with PAD and concomitant high and low systolic blood pressures in the EUCLID trial and the Antihypertensive and Lipid-Lowering Treatment to Prevent Heart Attack Trial (ALLHAT) subanalysis, respectively [63, 64].

The benefits of ACEi therapy, in particular for PAD, were first demonstrated in the 2000 Heart Outcomes Prevention Evaluation (HOPE) trial, which randomized 9297 patients with vascular disease or diabetes to either ramipril 10 milligrams daily or placebo for 5 years. Within the study population, 44% of patients had PAD (defined as ABI ≤0.9) [65]. Overall, ramipril was associated with significantly lower risk of MACCE (14.0% versus 17.8%, RR 0.78 [95% CI: 0.70–0.86]; $P < 0.001$). In the subgroup analysis of patients with PAD, ramipril was associated with a similar reduction in risk of MI, stroke, or vascular death by 25%. Subsequently, the 2003 EUROPA trial randomized 12,218 patients, approximately 7% of which had PAD, to either perindopril or placebo and followed them over a mean period of 4.2 years [66]. Treatment with perindopril resulted in a 20% reduction in the primary endpoint of cardiovascular death, MI, or cardiac arrest compared with the placebo group ($P = 0.0003$). These findings persisted in the subgroup analysis of patients with PAD. In the following Ongoing Telmisartan Alone and in Combination with Ramipril Global Endpoint Trial (ONTARGET), ~25,000 patients with vascular disease or with risk factors, of which 13% had PAD, were randomized to receive either ramipril, telmisartan, or combination therapy [67]. This study found that ramipril and telmisartan had similar benefits on reducing the risk of MACCE; these findings were also similar in the PAD subgroup. Finally, these findings have also been demonstrated in the advanced PAD population. A 2015 observational analysis examining 464 patients with CLTI found that the use of ACEi or angiotensin-receptor blockers was associated with lower rates of MACCE (HR: 0.76 [95% CI: 0.58–0.99]; $P = 0.04$) and mortality (HR: 0.71 [95% CI: 0.53–0.95]; $P = 0.02$) [68]. No association was found with MALE.

Notably, the use of combination therapy has not been shown to provide additional benefit compared with either monotherapy in this population [68]. Instead, this is associated with a higher risk of adverse events like hyperkalemia and hypotension.

Although β-blockers are not considered a first-line therapy in patients with PAD and hypertension, they are commonly utilized in those with comorbid conditions like atrial fibrillation and CAD. Although there was initial concern about β-receptor antagonism causing compromised blood flow to the extremities via multiple proposed mechanisms (e.g., decreased cardiac output, increased reflex sympathetic activity, and imbalance of alpha and beta agonism in the peripheral vasculature), subsequent studies utilizing β-blockers did not demonstrate a signal of harm in terms of MALE; instead, a reduction in blood pressure was associated with improved claudication symptoms and overall functional status [69]. Studies supporting their use in this population include meta-analyses that found no impact of β-blockers on pain-free walking distance in patients with symptomatic PAD, as well as a more recent trial of 177 patients with PAD and claudication randomized to either nebivolol or hydrochlorothiazide that demonstrated similar limb outcomes between groups over a 24-week follow-up period [70–72]. While these results have been reassuring, larger prospective trials evaluating β-blockers and limb outcomes are still needed and no formal guideline recommendations currently exist supporting β-blockers in PAD management.

Diabetes Management in PAD

Diabetes is a major risk factor for PAD, as demonstrated by a two-fold increased prevalence of PAD in patients with diabetes relative to the general population [73]. In patients with established PAD, diabetes is associated with an increased risk of adverse outcomes, such as progression to CLTI, amputation, and death [74]. There are multiple proposed mechanisms for the association between diabetes and progressive PAD, including pathophysiological changes such as endothelial dysfunction, increased oxidative stress, and impaired arterial elastic properties [75, 76]. Observational studies also found that hyperglycemia is associated with lower rates of vessel patency and higher rates of adverse limb events in patients with diabetes undergoing peripheral angioplasty [77].

Multiple studies have demonstrated that improved glycemic control can reduce MACCE and MALE outcomes in patients with PAD [77–80]. This is in part due to a reduction in the risk of diabetic foot ulcers, which can lead to minor and major amputations. In a subgroup analysis of patients with diabetes from the EUCLID trial, there was an observed 14.2% increased relative risk of MACCE with every 1% increase in hemoglobin A1c [64]. Additionally, in the Strong Heart study examining 1974 patients with diabetes and no history of lower-extremity amputation, patients with PAD and an A1c of <6.5% had a lower age-adjusted odds ratio of major amputation during follow-up [81]. A meta-analysis of patients with diabetic foot ulcers also found a lower risk of amputation in patients with an A1c of <8% [78]. These findings have also been extended to the preprocedural setting [77, 79, 80]. Multiple observational studies have found that suboptimal glycemic control is associated with increased risk of MALE, including lower extremity amputation, among patients with PAD undergoing endovascular or surgical revascularization. Of note, these studies have included mixed PAD cohorts of both patients with claudication and those with CLTI, which can make interpretation of the findings more complex.

The 2024 AHA/ACC guideline has a Class I recommendation for the use of glucagon-like peptide-1 agonists (i.e., liraglutide and semaglutide) and sodium-glucose cotransporter-2 (SGLT-2 inhibitors) (i.e., canagliflozin, dapagliflozin, and empagliflozin) in patients with PAD and type 2 diabetes to reduce the risk of MACCE in patients with PAD [14]. Large-scale studies supporting the use of glucagon-like peptide-1 agonists in this population include Liraglutide Effect and Action in Diabetes: Evaluation of Cardiovascular Outcome Results (LEADER) and Trial to Evaluate Cardiovascular and Other Long-term Outcomes With Semaglutide in Subjects With Type 2 Diabetes (SUSTAIN-6) [82, 83]. In LEADER, the primary endpoint of MACCE occurred in 14.9% of patients in the placebo group compared with 13.0% of patients in the liraglutide group (HR: 0.87 [95% CI: 0.78–0.97]; $P < 0.001$) at a median follow-up of 3.8 years. Within the study population, 12.5% of patients had PAD. Similarly, in SUSTAIN-6, the primary endpoint of MACCE occurred in 6.6% of patients in the semaglutide group and 8.9% of patients in the placebo group (HR: 0.74 [95% CI: 0.58–0.95]; $P < 0.001$). In both trials, the presence of PAD was associated with an increased risk of MACCE. Additionally, there is an ongoing trial (SURPASS-CVOT) comparing tirzepatide, a glucagon-like peptide-1 agonist, to dulaglutide in patients with diabetes and CVD [84].

Prior RCTs have also established the benefit of SGLT-2 inhibitors in patients with type 2 diabetes and PAD. The Empagliflozin Cardiovascular Outcome Event Trial in Type 2 Diabetes Mellitus Patients (EMPA-REG OUTCOME) and CANagliflozin cardiovascular Assessment Study (CANVAS) trials demonstrated the role of SGLT-2 inhibitor in reducing the risk of MACCE [85, 86]. In EMPA-REG OUTCOME, 7020 patients, of which 21% had known PAD, were randomized to receive empagliflozin 10 milligrams or 25 milligrams or placebo once daily. Over a median follow-up period of 3.1 years, empagliflozin was shown to reduce the risk of MACCE (10.5% vs 12.1%; $P = 0.04$). Similarly, in CANVAS, 10,142 patients, of which 21% had known PAD, were randomized to receive either canagliflozin or placebo. Over a mean follow-up period of 3.6 years, canagliflozin was associated with a reduction in MACCE (HR: 0.86 [95% CI: 0.75–0.97]; $P < 0.01$).

However, this significant reduction in MACCE outcomes did not extend across all trials. In Dapagliflozin Effect on CardiovascuLAR Events-Thrombolysis In Myocardial Infarction 58 (DECLARE-TIMI 58), dapagliflozin was not associated with significant reduction in MACCE, though it did result in a reduction in cardiovascular death or hospitalization for heart failure (4.9% versus 5.8%; $P = 0.005$) [87]. Additionally, in Cardiovascular Outcomes Following Ertugliflozin Treatment in Type 2 Diabetes Mellitus Participants With Vascular Disease (VERTIS CV), ertugliflozin was found to be noninferior to placebo with respect to major adverse cardiovascular events [88]. It is also important to note that although the CANVAS trial demonstrated a reduced risk of MACCE with use of canagliflozin, there was also a higher risk of amputations in the treatment arm (6.3 versus 3.4 placebo per 1000 patient years; $P < 0.001$) [86]. Though the majority of these amputations were minor and occurred at the level of the toe or metatarsal bones, this raised questions about the safety of this medication in this patient population. Reassuringly, the subsequent data have been conflicting. Studies like Canagliflozin and Renal Events in Diabetes with Established Nephropathy Clinical Evaluation (CREDENCE) and a subgroup analysis of EMPA-REG OUTCOME did not demonstrate this finding, with the latter even showing improved limb survival in patients treated with empagliflozin [89–91]. Therefore, the FDA-issued black box warning associated with canagliflozin was removed in 2020 [91]. Additionally, it is now recommended that SGLT2 inhibitors be preferentially used in patients with PAD and comorbid heart failure to reduce MACCE [92].

Pharmacological Therapies for Improving Claudication Among Patients with Symptomatic PAD

Cilostazol, a phosphodiesterase III inhibitor that reduces platelet aggregation and enhances vasodilation, has been shown to improve walking distance and symptoms of claudication in patients with symptomatic stable PAD [93–96]. Cilostazol is the only FDA-approved medication with a Class I recommendation by the 2024 AHA/ACC PAD guideline for the treatment of intermittent claudication [14]. Multiple studies support its use in this patient population. A 2002 meta-analysis, which included 8 RCTs with 2702 patients with stable moderate to severe claudication, found that cilostazol significantly increased maximal and pain-free walking distances by 50% and 67%, respectively, and quality-of-life measures; these increases persisted across subgroups [97]. A subsequent 2010 meta-analysis examining 9 RCTs with 1258 patients treated with cilostazol 100 milligrams twice daily found that maximal walking distance improved by 50.7% compared with 24.3% in the placebo group, with an absolute increase of 42.1 meters ($P < 0.001$) [98]. A 2014 Cochrane review of 15 double-blind RCTs with 3718 participants also reported a positive association between cilostazol and improvement in claudication symptoms [94]. A 2021 network meta-analysis found that cilostazol improved maximal walking distance and ABI [95]. Finally, in a 2018 observational study performed in Hungary, 812 PAD patients who received cilostazol (50 or 100 milligrams twice daily) were found to have improved quality-of-life metrics and lower limb functional status when assessed by questionnaires [96].

Extending beyond patients with claudication symptoms, cilostazol has also been shown to reduce the risk of in-stent restenosis after endovascular treatment of femoropopliteal stenosis. In an RCT comparing cilostazol to a non-placebo control, cilostazol was found to improve primary patency at 3 years after bare-metal stent treatment of a femoropopliteal segment. In a sub-analysis of an RCT examining a paclitaxel-eluting stent, cilostazol reduced the rate of restenosis after stent treatment of femoropopliteal stenosis at 1 year [99]. In a meta-analysis of 8 studies with 3846 patients, cilostazol improved primary patency, target lesion revascularization, and MALE, including major amputation, when compared with placebo after femoropopliteal endovascular therapy at a median follow-up of 12.5 months [100].

Prior to cilostazol initiation, potential risks and side effects should also be considered. Notably, cilostazol is contraindicated in patients with heart failure of any severity [96, 101]. This is because of its pharmacologic similarity to oral milrinone, a phosphodiesterase inhibitor that has been associated with higher mortality rates in patients with advanced heart failure [102]. Other barriers to its use include potential side effects like diarrhea, headache, palpitations, and dizziness [103]. In a case series, 20% of patients who were prescribed cilostazol for claudication discontinued it by 3 months. This suggests that when prescribing cilostazol, assessing for patient tolerance early on (i.e., 2–4 weeks) may be beneficial.

Unfortunately, alternative therapies like pentoxifylline, a methylxanthine derivative, and chelation therapy (e.g., EDTA), are not recommended in current PAD guidelines. This is based on a lack of supporting evidence for their use in this population. A multicenter trial with 922 patients with moderate-to-severe claudication randomized to cilostazol 100 milligrams twice daily, pentoxifylline 400 milligrams three times daily, or placebo found that cilostazol resulted in a 54% increase in mean maximal walking distance compared with a 30% increase with pentoxifylline and a 34% increase with placebo at 24 weeks of follow up [103]. Additionally, there was no significant difference between pentoxifylline and placebo ($P = 0.82$). In a Cochrane review of chelation therapy that included 2 clinical trials with walking endpoints in patients with PAD, chelation therapy showed no significant improvement in claudication symptoms compared with placebo [104].

Conclusions

Current guidelines recommend a multimodal approach to the treatment of PAD, targeting broad risk factors for major cardiovascular events and adverse limb-related outcomes. This includes initiation of antiplatelets and/or anticoagulants, statins, antihypertensives, diabetes agents, and medications to reduce claudication symptoms. Although there is substantial data supporting the use of pharmacologic therapies in this high-risk population, there are still critical evidence gaps that must be addressed. This includes better elucidating the benefits of medical therapies among patients with asymptomatic PAD, determining the optimal antiplatelet and anticoagulant regimens for patients who have undergone revascularization, and developing effective novel therapies to improve functional status. Additionally, pharmacological therapy is highly underutilized in this population, with some data suggesting that as few as 19–27% of eligible patients even receive these therapies [3]. Future studies aimed at elucidating the underlying causes for these disparities will be critical. In the meantime, systems-wide changes will be necessary to improve uptake. This includes consideration for screening high-risk populations, improving patient awareness of PAD and the benefits of secondary prevention, ensuring physicians stay informed about the latest treatment guidelines and appropriate diagnostic methods, and addressing potential barriers to treatment access. Overall, given the significant social and economic burden of intermittent claudication, bridging these critical gaps with novel solutions will be paramount to reduce adverse outcomes and improve quality of life.

References

1. Kochar A, Mulder H, Rockhold FW, et al. Cause of death among patients with peripheral artery disease: insights from the EUCLID trial. Circ Cardiovasc Qual Outcomes. 2020;13(11):832–42.
2. Bonaca MP, Creager MA. Pharmacological treatment and current management of peripheral artery disease. Circ Res. 2015;116(9):1579–98.
3. Hua S, Isasi CR, Kizer JR, et al. Underuse of cardiovascular medications in individuals with known lower extremity peripheral artery disease: HCHS/SOL. J Am Heart Assoc. 2020;9(16):e015451.

4. Barnes JA, Eid MA, Creager MA, et al. Epidemiology and risk of amputation in patients with diabetes mellitus and peripheral artery disease. Arterioscler Thromb Vasc Biol. 2020;40:1808–17.
5. Mustapha JA, Fisher BT Sr, Rizzo JA, et al. Explaining racial disparities in amputation rates for the treatment of peripheral artery disease (PAD) using decomposition methods. J Racial Ethn Health Disparities. 2017;4:784–95.
6. Berger JS, Ladapo JA. Underuse of prevention and lifestyle counseling in patients with peripheral artery disease. JACC. 2017;69(18):2293–300.
7. Antithrombotic Trialists Collaboration. Collaborative meta-analysis of randomised trials of antiplatelet therapy for prevention of death, myocardial infarction, and stroke in high risk patients. BMJ. 2002;324:71–86.
8. Critical Leg Ischaemia Prevention Study (CLIPS) Group, Catalano M, Born G. Prevention of serious vascular events by aspirin amongst patients with peripheral arterial disease: randomized, double-blind trial. J Intern Med. 2007;261:276–84.
9. Berger JS, Krantz MJ, Kittelson JM, et al. Aspirin for the prevention of cardiovascular events in patients with peripheral artery disease: a meta-analysis of randomized trials. JAMA. 2009;301:1909–19.
10. CAPRIE Steering Committee. A randomised, blinded, trial of clopidogrel versus aspirin in patients at risk of ischaemic events (CAPRIE). Lancet. 1996;348:1329–39.
11. Chiarito M, Sanz-Sanchez J, Cannata F, et al. Monotherapy with a P2Y12 inhibitor or aspirin for secondary prevention in patients with established atherosclerosis: a systematic review and meta-analysis. Lancet. 2020;395:1487–95.
12. Gray WA, Keirse K, Soga Y, et al. A polymer-coated, paclitaxel-eluting stent (Eluvia) versus a polymer-free, paclitaxel-coated stent (Zilver PTX) for endovascular femoropopliteal intervention (IMPERIAL): a randomised, non-inferiority trial. Lancet. 2018;392:1541–51.
13. Dake MD, Ansel GM, Jaff MR, et al. Durable clinical effectiveness with paclitaxel-eluting stents in the femoropopliteal artery: 5-year results of the Zilver PTX randomized trial. Circulation. 2016;133:1472–83.
14. 2024 ACC/AHA/AACVPR/APMA/ABC/SCAI/SVM/SVN/SVS/SIR/VESS guideline for the Management of Lower Extremity Peripheral Artery Disease: a report of the American College of Cardiology/American Heart Association Joint Committee on Clinical Practice Guidelines. Circulation 2024;149(24):e1313–e1410.
15. Narula N, Dannenberg AJ, Olin JW, et al. Pathology of peripheral artery disease in patients with critical limb ischemia. J Am Coll Cardiol. 2018;72(18):2152–63.
16. Eikelboom JW, Connolly SJ, Bosch J, et al. Rivaroxaban with or without aspirin in stable cardiovascular disease. N Engl J Med. 2017;377:1319–30.
17. Anand SS, Bosch J, Eikelboom JW, et al. Rivaroxaban with or without aspirin in patients with stable peripheral or carotid artery disease: an international, randomised, double-blind, placebo-controlled trial. Lancet. 2018;391:219–29.
18. Anand SS, Caron F, Eikelboom JW, et al. Major adverse limb events and mortality in patients with peripheral artery disease: the COMPASS trial. J Am Coll Cardiol. 2018;71:2306–15.
19. Bonaca MP, Bhatt DL, Storey RF, et al. Ticagrelor for prevention of ischemic events after myocardial infarction in patients with peripheral artery disease. J Am Coll Cardiol. 2016;67:2719–28.
20. Cacoub PP, Bhatt DL, Steg PG, et al. Patients with peripheral arterial disease in the CHARISMA trial. Eur Heart J. 2009;30:192–201.
21. Bonaca MP, Scirica BM, Creager MA, et al. Vorapaxar in patients with peripheral artery disease: results from TRA2°P-TIMI 50. Circulation. 2013;127:1522–9.
22. Warfarin Antiplatelet Vascular Evaluation Trial Investigators, Anand S, Yusuf S, et al. Oral anticoagulant and antiplatelet therapy and peripheral arterial disease. N Engl J Med. 2007;357:217–27.
23. Johnson WC, Williford WO. Department of Veterans Affairs Cooperative Study #362. Benefits, morbidity, and mortality associated with long-term administration of oral

anticoagulant therapy to patients with peripheral arterial bypass procedures: a prospective randomized study. J Vasc Surg. 2002;35:413–21.
24. Bonaca MP, Bauersachs RM, Anand SS, et al. Rivaroxaban in peripheral artery disease after revascularization. N Engl J Med. 2020;382:1994–2004.
25. Soden PA, Zettervall SL, Ultee KH, et al. Dual antiplatelet therapy is associated with prolonged survival after lower extremity revascularization. J Vasc Surg. 2016;64:1633–1644 e1631.
26. Cho S, Lee YJ, Ko YG, et al. Optimal strategy for antiplatelet therapy after endovascular revascularization for lower extremity peripheral artery disease. J Am Coll Cardiol Intv. 2019;12:2359–70.
27. Tepe G, Bantleo R, Brechtel K, et al. Management of peripheral arterial interventions with mono or dual antiplatelet therapy--the MIRROR study: a randomised and double-blinded clinical trial. Eur Radiol. 2012;22(9):1998–2006.
28. Dutch Bypass Oral anticoagulants or Aspirin (BOA) Study Group. Efficacy of oral anticoagulants compared with aspirin after infrainguinal bypass surgery (The Dutch Bypass Oral Anticoagulants or Aspirin Study): a randomised trial. Lancet. 2000;355(9201):P346–51.
29. Belch JJ, Dormandy J, Committee CW, et al. Results of the randomized, placebo-controlled clopidogrel and acetylsalicylic acid in bypass surgery for peripheral arterial disease (CASPAR) trial. J Vasc Surg. 2010;52:825–833, 833 e821–822.
30. 2023 ACC/AHA/ACCP/HRS guideline for the diagnosis and management of atrial fibrillation. Circulation 2024;149:e1–e156.
31. Fowkes FG, Price JF, Stewart MC, et al. Aspirin for prevention of cardiovascular events in a general population screened for a low ankle brachial index: a randomized controlled trial. JAMA. 2010;303:841–8.
32. Belch J, MacCuish A, Campbell I, et al. The prevention of progression of arterial disease and diabetes (POPADAD) trial: factorial randomised placebo controlled trial of aspirin and antioxidants in patients with diabetes and asymptomatic peripheral arterial disease. BMJ. 2008;337:a1840.
33. Diehm C, Allenberg JR, Pittrow D, et al. Mortality and vascular morbidity in older adults with asymptomatic versus symptomatic peripheral artery disease. Circulation. 2009;120:2053–61.
34. Sartipy F, Sigvant B, Lundin F, et al. Ten year mortality in different peripheral arterial disease stages: a population based observational study on outcome. Eur J Vasc Endovasc Surg. 2018;55:529–36.
35. 2018 AHA/ACC/AACVPR/AAPA/ABC/ACPM/ADA/AGS/APhA/ASPC/NLA/PCNA guideline on the management of blood cholesterol: a report of the American College of Cardiology/American Heart Association task force on clinical practice guidelines. Circulation 2019;139:e1082–e1143.
36. Bonaca MP, Nault P, Giugliano RP, et al. Low-density lipoprotein cholesterol lowering with evolocumab and outcomes in patients with peripheral artery disease: insights from the FOURIER trial (further cardiovascular outcomes research with PCSK9 inhibition in subjects with elevated risk). Circulation. 2018;137:338–50.
37. Jukema JW, Szarek M, Zijlstra LE, et al. Alirocumab in patients with polyvascular disease and recent acute coronary syndrome: ODYSSEY OUTCOMES trial. J Am Coll Cardiol. 2019;74:1167–76.
38. Bonaca MP, Gutierrez JA, Cannon C, et al. Polyvascular disease, type 2 diabetes, and long-term vascular risk: a secondary analysis of the IMPROVE-IT trial. Lancet Diabetes Endocrinol. 2018;6:934–43.
39. 2024 ACC/AHA/AACVPR/APMA/ABC/SCAI/SVM/SVN/SVS/SIR/VESS Guideline for the Management of Lower Extremity Peripheral Artery Disease: a report of the American College of Cardiology/American Heart Association joint Committee on clinical practice guidelines. Circulation 2024;149(24):e1313–e1410.
40. Heart Protection Study Collaborative Group. Randomized trial of the effects of cholesterol-lowering with simvastatin on peripheral vascular and other major vascular outcomes in 20536 people with peripheral arterial disease and other high-risk conditions. J Vasc Surg. 2007;45:645–54.

41. Kumbhani DJ, Steg PG, Cannon CP, et al. REACH Registry Investigators. Statin therapy and long-term adverse limb outcomes in patients with peripheral artery disease: insights from the REACH registry. Eur Heart J. 2014;35:2864–72. https://doi.org/10.1093/eurheartj/ehu080.
42. Arya S, Khakharia A, Binney ZO, et al. Association of statin dose with amputation and survival in patients with peripheral artery disease. Circulation. 2018;137:1435–46.
43. Pastori D, Farcomeni A, Milanese A, et al. Statins and major adverse limb events in patients with peripheral artery disease: a systematic review and meta-analysis. Thromb Haemost. 2020;120:866–75.
44. Peters F, Kuchenbecker J, Kreutzburg T, et al. Long-term effectiveness and safety of initiating statin therapy after index revascularization in patients with peripheral arterial occlusive disease. J Am Heart Assoc. 2020;9:e018338.
45. Khariton Y, Patel KK, Chan PS, et al. Guideline-directed statin intensification in patients with new or worsening symptoms of peripheral artery disease. Clin Cardiol. 2018;41:1414–22.
46. Suckow BD, Kraiss LW, Schanzer A, et al. Statin therapy after infrainguinal bypass surgery for critical limb ischemia is associated with improved 5-year survival. J Vasc Surg. 2015;61:126–33.
47. Stavroulakis K, Borowski M, Torsello G, et al. Association between statin therapy and amputation-free survival in patients with critical limb ischemia in the CRITISCH registry. J Vasc Surg. 2017;66:1534–42.
48. Foley TR, Singh GD, Kokkinidis DG, et al. High-intensity statin therapy is associated with improved survival in patients with peripheral artery disease. J Am Heart Assoc. 2017;6:e005699.
49. DeCarlo C, Scher L, Shariff S, et al. Statin use and other factors associated with mortality after major lower extremity amputation. J Vasc Surg. 2017;66:216–25.
50. Schwartz GG, Steg PG, Szarek M, et al. Peripheral artery disease and venous thromboembolic events after acute coronary syndrome: role of lipoprotein(a) and modification by alirocumab: prespecified analysis of the ODYSSEY OUTCOMES randomized clinical trial. Circulation. 2020;141:1608–17.
51. Scott R, Best J, Forder P, et al. Fenofibrate intervention and event lowering in diabetes (FIELD) study: baseline characteristics and short-term effects of fenofibrate. Cardiovasc Diabetol. 2005;4:13.
52. The Action to Control Cardiovascular Risk in Diabetes Study Group. Effects of intensive glucose lowering in type 2 diabetes. N Engl J Med. 2008;358(24):2545–59.
53. Bhatt DL, Steg PG, Miller M, et al. Cardiovascular risk reduction with icosapent ethyl for hypertriglyceridemia. N Engl J Med. 2018;380:11–22.
54. Niseen SE, Lincoff AM, Brennan M, et al. Bempedoic acid and cardiovascular outcomes in statin-intolerant patients. N Engl J Med. 2023;388(15):1353–64.
55. Ray JJ, Wright RS, Kallend D, et al. Two phase 3 trials of inclisiran in patients with elevated LDL cholesterol. N Engl J Med. 2020;382:1507–19.
56. Clement DL, De Buyzere ML, Duprez DA. Hypertension in peripheral arterial disease. Curr Pharm Des. 2004;10:3615–20.
57. Piller LB, Simpson LM, Baraniuk S, et al. Characteristics and long-term follow-up of participants with peripheral arterial disease during ALLHAT. J Gen Intern Med. 2014;29:1475–83.
58. Kennedy M, Solomon C, Manolio TA, et al. Risk factors for declining ankle-brachial index in men and women 65 years or older: the Cardiovascular Health Study. Arch Intern Med. 2005;165:1896–902.
59. 2017 ACC/AHA/AAPA/ABC/ACPM/AGS/APhA/ASH/ASPC/NMA/PCNA guideline for the prevention, detection, evaluation, and management of high blood pressure in adults: a report of the American College of Cardiology/American Heart Association Task Force on Clinical Practice Guidelines. Hypertension 2018;71:e13–e115.
60. Sprint Research Group, Wright JT, Williamson JD, et al. A randomized trial of intensive versus standard blood-pressure control. N Engl J Med. 2015;373:2103–16.

61. Mehler PS, Coll JR, Estacio R, et al. Intensive blood pressure control reduces the risk of cardiovascular events in patients with peripheral arterial disease and type 2 diabetes. Circulation. 2003;107:753–6.
62. Bavry AA, Anderson RD, Gong Y, et al. Outcomes among hypertensive patients with concomitant peripheral and coronary artery disease: findings from the INternational VErapamil-SR/Trandolapril STudy. Hypertension. 2010;55:48–53.
63. Itoga NK, Tawfik DS, Lee CK, et al. Association of blood pressure measurements with peripheral artery disease events. Circulation. 2018;138:1805–14.
64. Low Wang CC, Blomster JI, Heizer G, et al. Cardiovascular and limb outcomes in patients with diabetes and peripheral artery disease: the EUCLID trial. J Am Coll Cardiol. 2018;72:3274–84.
65. Sleight P. The HOPE study (heart outcomes prevention evaluation). J Renin-Angiotensin-Aldosterone Syst. 2000;1:18–20.
66. Fox KM. EURopean trial on reduction of cardiac events with perindopril in stable coronary artery disease Investigators. Efficacy of perindopril in reduction of cardiovascular events among patients with stable coronary artery disease: randomised, double-blind, placebo-controlled, multicentre trial (the EUROPA study). Lancet. 2003;362(9386):782–8.
67. Investigators O, Yusuf S, Teo KK, et al. Telmisartan, ramipril, or both in patients at high risk for vascular events. N Engl J Med. 2008;358:1547–59.
68. Armstrong EJ, Chen DC, Singh GD, et al. Angiotensin-converting enzyme inhibitor or angiotensin receptor blocker use is associated with reduced major adverse cardiovascular events among patients with critical limb ischemia. Vasc Med. 2015;20:237–44.
69. Frohlich ED, Tarazi RC, Dustan HP. Peripheral arterial insufficiency. A complication of beta-adrenergic blocking therapy. JAMA. 1969;208:2471–2.
70. Radack K, Deck C. Beta-adrenergic blocker therapy does not worsen intermittent claudication in subjects with peripheral arterial disease. A meta-analysis of randomized controlled trials. Arch Intern Med. 1991;151:1769–76.
71. Paravastu SC, Mendonca D, Da Silva A. Beta blockers for peripheral arterial disease. Cochrane Database Syst Rev. 2008;(4):CD005508.
72. Diehm C, Pittrow D, Lawall H. Effect of nebivolol vs. hydrochlorothiazide on the walking capacity in hypertensive patients with intermittent claudication. J Hypertens. 2011;29:1448–56.
73. Soyoye DO, Abiodun OO, Ikem RT, et al. Diabetes and peripheral artery disease: a review. World J Diabetes. 2021;12(6):827–38.
74. Emerging Risk Factors Collaboration, Sarwar N, Gao P, Seshasai SR, et al. Diabetes mellitus, fasting blood glucose concentration, and risk of vascular disease: a collaborative metaanalysis of 102 prospective studies. Lancet. 2010;375:2215–22.
75. Makita S, Matsui H, Naganuma Y, et al. Diabetic state as a crucial factor for impaired arterial elastic properties in patients with peripheral arterial disease. Atherosclerosis. 2010;208:167–70.
76. Su Y, Liu XM, Sun YM, et al. Endothelial dysfunction in impaired fasting glycemia, impaired glucose tolerance, and type 2 diabetes mellitus. Am J Cardiol. 2008;102:497–8.
77. Singh S, Armstrong EJ, Sherif W, et al. Association of elevated fasting glucose with lower patency and increased major adverse limb events among patients with diabetes undergoing infrapopliteal balloon angioplasty. Vasc Med. 2014;19:307–14.
78. Lane KL, Abusamaan MS, Voss BF, et al. Glycemic control and diabetic foot ulcer outcomes: a systematic review and meta-analysis of observational studies. J Diabetes Complicat. 2020;34:107638.
79. Takahara M, Kaneto H, Iida O, et al. The influence of glycemic control on the prognosis of Japanese patients undergoing percutaneous transluminal angioplasty for critical limb ischemia. Diabetes Care. 2010;33:2538–42.
80. Arya S, Binney ZO, Khakharia A, et al. High hemoglobin A(1c) associated with increased adverse limb events in peripheral arterial disease patients undergoing revascularization. J Vasc Surg. 2018;67:217–228.e1.

81. Resnick HE, Carter EA, Sosenko JM, et al. Incidence of lower-extremity amputation in American Indians: the Strong Heart Study. Diabetes Care. 2004;27:1885–91.
82. Marso SP, Daniels GH, Brown-Frandsen K, et al. Liraglutide and cardiovascular outcomes in type 2 diabetes. N Engl J Med. 2016;375:311–22.
83. Cosmi F, Laini R, Nicolucci A. Semaglutide and cardiovascular outcomes in patients with type 2 diabetes. N Engl J Med. 2017;376:890.
84. Nicholls SJ, Bhatt DL, Buse JB, et al. Comparison of tirzepatide and dulaglutide on major adverse cardiovascular events in participants with type 2 diabetes and atherosclerotic cardiovascular disease: SURPASS-CVOT design and baseline characteristics. Am Heart J. 2024;267:1–11.
85. Zinman B, Wanner C, Lachin JM, et al. Empagliflozin, cardiovascular outcomes, and mortality in type 2 diabetes. N Engl J Med. 2015;373:2117–28.
86. Neal B, Perkovic V, Mahaffey KW, et al. Canagliflozin and cardiovascular and renal events in type 2 diabetes. N Engl J Med. 2017;377:644–57.
87. Wiviott SD, Raz I, Bonaca MP, et al. Dapagliflozin and cardiovascular outcomes in type 2 diabetes. N Engl J Med. 2019;380:347–57.
88. Cannon CP, Pratley R, Dagogo-Jack S, et al. Cardiovascular outcomes with ertugliflozin in type 2 diabetes. N Engl J Med. 2020;383:1425–35.
89. Perkovic V, Jardine MJ, Neal B, et al. Canagliflozin and renal outcomes in type 2 diabetes and nephropathy. N Engl J Med. 2019;380:2295–306.
90. Heyward J, Mansour O, Olson L, et al. Association between sodium-glucose cotransporter 2 (SGLT2) inhibitors and lower extremity amputation: a systematic review and meta-analysis. PLoS One. 2020;15:e0234065.
91. US Food and Drug Administration. FDA removes boxed warning about risk of leg and foot amputations for the diabetes medicine canagliflozin (Invokana, Invokamet, Invokamet XR). 2020. Accessed 1 Mar 2021. https://www.fda.gov/drugs/drug-safety-and-availability/fda-removes-boxed-warning-about-risk-leg-and-foot-amputations-diabetes-medicine-canagliflozin.
92. 2022 AHA/ACC/HFSA guideline for the management of heart failure: a report of the American College of Cardiology/American Heart Association Joint Committee on Clinical Practice Guidelines. Circulation 2022;145:e895–e1032.
93. Bedenis R, Stewart M, Cleanthis M, et al. Cilostazol for intermittent claudication. Cochrane Database Syst Rev. 2014:CD003748.
94. Mohammed M, Gosch K, Safley D, et al. Cilostazol and peripheral artery disease-specific health status in ambulatory patients with symptomatic PAD. Int J Cardiol. 2020;316:222–8.
95. Ma B, Fan X, Liu P. Therapeutic effects of medication use on intermittent claudication: a network meta-analysis. J Cardiovasc Pharmacol. 2021;77:253–62.
96. Farkas K, Kolossvary E, Jarai Z. Simple assessment of quality of life and lower limb functional capacity during cilostazol treatment – results of the SHort-tERm cIlostazol eFFicacy and quality of life (SHERIFF) study. Vasa. 2020;49:235–42.
97. Thompson PD, Zimet R, Forbes WP, Zhang P. Meta-analysis of results from eight randomized, placebo-controlled trials on the effect of cilostazol on patients with intermittent claudication. Am J Cardiol. 2002;90:1314–9.
98. Pande RL, Hiatt WR, Zhang P, et al. A pooled analysis of the durability and predictors of treatment response of cilostazol in patients with intermittent claudication. Vasc Med. 2010;15:181–8. https://doi.org/10.1177/1358863X10361545.
99. Soga Y, Hamasaki T, Edahiro R, et al. Sustained effectiveness of cilostazol after endovascular treatment of femoropopliteal lesions: midterm follow-up from the sufficient treatment of peripheral intervention by Cilostazol (STOP-IC) study. J Endovasc Ther. 2018;25:306–12.
100. Megaly M, Abraham B, Saad M, et al. Outcomes with cilostazol after endovascular therapy of peripheral artery disease. Vasc Med. 2019;24:313–23.
101. Otsuka Pharmaceutical Co. Pletal (cilostazol) [package insert]. Updated May 17, 2017. https://www.accessdata.fda.gov/drugsatfda_docs/label/2017/020863s024lbl.pdf.

102. Packer M, Carver JR, Rodeheffer RJ, et al. The PROMISE Study Research Group. Effect of oral milrinone on mortality in severe chronic heart failure. N Engl J Med. 1991;325:1468–75.
103. Dawson DL, Cutler BS, Hiatt WR, et al. A comparison of cilostazol and pentoxifylline for treating intermittent claudication. Am J Med. 2000;109:523–30.
104. Villarruz-Sulit MV, Forster R, Dans AL, et al. Chelation therapy for atherosclerotic cardiovascular disease. Cochrane Database Syst Rev. 2020;5:CD002785.
105. Hussain MA, et al. Antithrombotic therapy for peripheral artery disease: recent advances. J Am Coll Cardiol. 2018;71(21):2450–67.

Smoking Cessation in the Management of Claudication: Why and How

10

Kirthi S. Bellamkonda and Philip P. Goodney

Introduction

Smoking is a major risk factor in the development of peripheral arterial disease (PAD), a devastating condition that affects more than 12 million adults; smoking causes 500,000 deaths in the United States each year [1–5]. Because it is strongly associated with smoking, PAD is most prevalent among populations deemed "vulnerable," including low-income patients, those with significant mental illness, racial/ethnic groups such as African Americans and Hispanic patients, and Veterans [1, 6, 7]. Given that more deaths are attributable every year to cigarette smoking than any other cause, quitting smoking gives patients on average up to 10 years of additional survival [3, 5].

Smoking Over Time

History of Smoking

The first use of tobacco is documented via the discovery of charred tobacco seeds in the Wishbone site in northern Utah, at a settlement over 10,000 years old [8]. In 1528, Europeans returning from the Americas brought tobacco with them, and by the end of the sixteenth century, use and production was growing throughout Europe. Royalty, religious leadership, and normal people alike touted the health benefits. Monastic communities in Italy and elsewhere farmed tobacco. Ultimately, however, tobacco use likely had modest health effects until the post-industrial revolution explosion in manufactured cigarettes [9].

K. S. Bellamkonda (✉) · P. P. Goodney
Section of Vascular Surgery, Heart and Vascular Center, Dartmouth Hitchcock Medical Center, Lebanon, NH, USA
e-mail: kirthi.s.bellamkonda@hitchcock.org; Philip.P.Goodney@hitchcock.org

W. P. Robinson III, J. P. Simons (eds.), *The Patient-Centered Approach to Claudication*, https://doi.org/10.1007/978-3-032-02460-2_10

The Start of Cessation Efforts

Since the early days of its introduction to Europe, there have been critics of tobacco. Pope Urban VIII banned its use in churches in a 1642 publication "Cum Ecclesiae," due to the sneezing which snuff consumption caused, and King James I/VI of England and Scotland was an avid smoking cessationist, describing it as a "custome … dangerous to the lungs." However, no clear pathophysiological explanation was derived until the modern era. A medical argument for limiting tobacco exposure was made at the end of the nineteenth century, when it was observed that those with occupational exposure to tobacco had a proclivity for lung cancer [9].

The statistical association between smoking and lung cancer was elucidated in a series of reports in the first half of the twentieth century, culminating in a landmark 1964 Surgeon General's Report on Smoking and Health, which drove a 1966 labelling requirement on cigarette packaging [10]. Since then, a number of public health programs, advertising regulations, and treatment strategies have been developed, resulting in a decline in smoking from 52% in 1965 to 15% in 2017 among American men [10]. Some of these gains have been offset by losses due to a sharp uptick in the use of electronic cigarettes ("vaping") in recent years [11–14].

Quality and Quantity of Nicotine Consumption

Cigarette smoking is the most frequently encountered type of tobacco use. E-cigarettes are now the second most commonly used form of nicotine, and are the top choice among younger smokers [15]. Due to the relative recency of their popularity, it is not commonly known how to estimate the intensity of nicotine use. A popular brand on the market advertises 5% nicotine capsules, with approximately 40 mg per pod and an absorption equivalence of 1 pack [16]. However, it is important to note that unlike cigarettes, which are highly regulated, there is more variability in the nicotine refill industry, and many do-it-yourself refills, which may result in dramatically higher dosages.

Electronic cigarette use has increased dramatically, especially in younger patients. In many cases, years, even decades of declines in smoking have dramatically reversed with the adoption of electronic cigarettes.

PAD, Smoking, and Disparities

Rates of PAD are much higher among certain vulnerable patient populations due in large part to the high rates of smoking. While great progress has been made in reducing rates of smoking in the United States overall, this progress has been uneven. Smoking rates among patients with PAD remain high among demographic groups representing low-income and low-education segments of the population [17, 18]. For example, the gradient in smoking ranges from 31% for those with an income<$15,000 to 12.8% for those with an income >$50,000 [17, 18]. Even greater disparities in rates of smoking are evident for education levels. Smoking rates are nearly 50% for those with a GED diploma compared with 5.6% for those with a graduate degree. These trends are evident in large longitudinal studies as well. A study based on data from the National Health and Nutrition Examination Survey found that PAD was nearly 3 times higher among those in the lowest income and education level categories compared with those in the highest [19].

Harms of Smoking in PAD

Despite the importance of smoking cessation for persons with PAD and the existence of evidence-based clinical practice guidelines for smoking cessation (which include physician advice, nicotine replacement therapy, and longitudinal counseling) [20–23], fewer than one in five PAD patients receives evidence-based help with quitting smoking around the time of invasive treatments [24–26].

Smoking Increases Risk of Development of PAD

A number of studies have confirmed a link with smoking and the development of PAD. Active smoking, a history of smoking without current smoking, and even secondhand smoke exposure are all associated with an increased risk of developing PAD [27–29]. Ingolfsson et al., along with a large volume of other literature, demonstrate a strongly linear dose-dependent relationship with the incidence of PAD and smoking, with a relative risk of 2.3 for former smokers, 2.6 for 1–14 cigarette/day smokers, 7.7 for 15–24 cigarette/day smokers, and 10.2 for 25+ cigarette/day smokers [28, 30]. When comparing PAD, coronary heart disease, and stroke, cigarette smoking and dose is most strongly associated with PAD [31]. In a study of 5686 never smokers, it was found that exposure to >40 hours per week of secondhand tobacco smoke was associated with a 5.5× increase in the incidence of symptomatic or asymptomatic PAD [32]. There is extremely limited epidemiological data on the use of electronic cigarettes and the development of any atherosclerotic disease.

Smoking is associated with worse outcomes in every category of PAD progression—ABI measurements over time, severity of claudication, development of rest pain, and development of tissue loss [33]. In a study of interval ABI changes in patients with PAD, smoking was a significant independent predictor of large-vessel PAD progression [34]. Among 138 patients with intermittent claudication, the active smokers had a shorter time to onset of claudication pain and a longer recovery from claudication pain [35]. Progression to critical limb threatening ischemia (CLTI) was also worse in smokers—in a study of 224 claudicants, smoking was associated with an increased risk of developing rest pain [36, 37].

Smoking Worsens Outcomes After Revascularization

Among smokers, outcomes for both open and endovascular surgery demonstrate worse vascular patency and increased amputation rates. In a study of the Vascular Study Group of New England, smokers were found to have inferior primary and assisted primary patency of lower extremity bypass grafts [38]. Patients who smoked had a three-fold increase in graft failure, independent of type of conduit [39]. Compared with non-smokers, respiratory complications were more common among smokers undergoing any type of lower extremity revascularization [40].

Benefits of Cessation

Several meta-analyses (Table 10.1) have shown that quitting smoking offers benefits in nearly all cardiovascular outcomes, including overall mortality [21, 41, 42]. These benefits are especially evident in the perioperative period for patients treated for PAD with invasive procedures and are more pronounced for vulnerable groups, given their higher underlying risks of smoking [21–23, 42–50].

Despite the importance of smoking cessation for persons with PAD and the existence of evidence-based clinical practice guidelines for smoking cessation (which include physician advice, nicotine replacement therapy, and longitudinal counseling) [20–23], fewer than one in five PAD patients receives evidence-based help with quitting smoking around the time of invasive treatments [24–26]. PAD patients with lower socioeconomic status (SES) are more likely to smoke and less likely to receive smoking cessation advice than those with higher SES [24].

Smoking Cessation Strategies

Smoking cessation is a long, complex process rife with setback and failure—although the majority of adults who smoke wanted to quit in the preceding year, only 1 in 20 were able to do so without medical assistance. With assistance, 1 in 10 are successful, but an increase in the number of quit attempts increases the

Table 10.1 Meta-analyses of benefits of smoking cessation

Study	Outcome measure	Key findings
Critchley et al., JAMA 2003 [41]	All-cause mortality	Smoking cessation has an independent effect on mortality across all age groups
Stead et al., Cochrane Review 2013 [42]	Mortality at 20 years	Physician advice had a small but measurable effect on quit rates
Rigotti et al., Cochrane Review 2012 [21]	Mortality at 2 years	Interventions for hospitalized smokers increase smoking cessation
Jha et al., NEJM 2013 [51]	Hazard ratios for death	Hazard ratio for death for smokers is 2.7–3.3x greater than non-smokers
Selvin et al., Circulation 2004 [6]	Cardiovascular disease	PAD increases with age; disproportionately affects African Americans

likelihood of ultimate lasting cessation [1]. Most patients who sustain cessation will go through multiple attempts. Thus, multiple frameworks have arisen for broaching the topic of smoking cessation.

The VAPOR Study

Our group, with support from the Society for Vascular Surgery, designed and conducted a pilot study of a smoking cessation program designed for patients with PAD, called the Physician Offer and Report (VAPOR) Trial [52–58]. This study determined the feasibility and potential efficacy of an evidence-based standardized smoking cessation intervention delivered by vascular surgeons to smokers with peripheral arterial disease.

Across 8 vascular practices in the United States, we performed a cluster-randomized trial of current adult smokers referred for vascular care from September 1, 2014, to July 31, 2015. A three-component smoking cessation intervention (physician advice, nicotine replacement therapy, and telephone-based quitline referral) was compared with usual care. The primary outcome was smoking cessation for 7 days, assessed 3 months after the intervention. Secondary outcomes were patients' nicotine dependence and health expectancies of smoking assessed using Patient Reported Outcomes Measurement Information System (PROMIS; RAND Corporation, Santa Monica, Calif).

There were 156 patients enrolled (65 in four intervention practices, 91 in four control practices), and 141 (90.3%) completed follow-up. Patients in the intervention and control practices were similar in age (mean, 61 years), sex (68% male), cigarettes per day (mean, 14), and prior quit attempts (77%). All three components of the intervention were delivered to 75% of patients in intervention practices vs to 7% of patients at control practices ($P < 0.001$) (Fig. 10.1). At 3 months, 23 of 57 patients (40.3%) in the intervention group quit smoking (23 of 56 patients quit who completed follow-up, plus 1 death included in the analysis in the denominator as a smoker), and 26 of 84 patients (30.9%) in the control group quit smoking (26 patients of 84 who completed follow-up, including 2 deaths included in the denominator as smokers). This difference (40.3% quit rate in intervention, 31% quit rate in control; $P = 0.250$) was not statistically significant in crude analyses ($P = 0.250$) or analyses adjusted for clustering ($P = 0.470$) (Fig. 10.2). Multivariable analysis showed factors associated with smoking cessation were receipt of physician advice (odds ratio for cessation, 1.96; 95% confidence interval, 1.28–3.02; $P < 0.002$) and nicotine replacement therapy (odds ratio, 1.92; 95% confidence interval, 1.43–2.56; $P < 0.001$).

Overall, our study found that implementation of a brief, surgeon-delivered smoking cessation intervention is feasible for patients with peripheral arterial disease. A larger trial will be necessary to determine whether this is effective for smoking cessation.

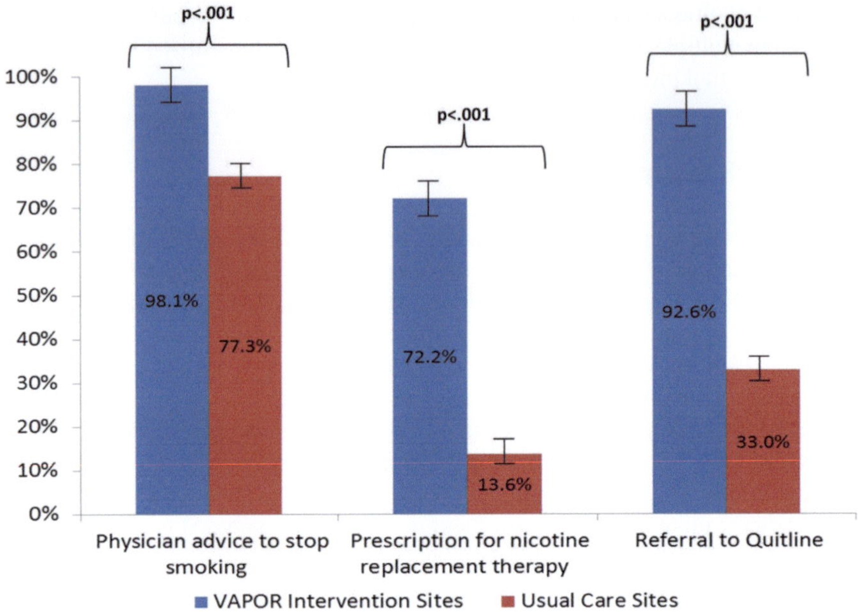

Fig. 10.1 Effects of various interventions in the VAPOR trial

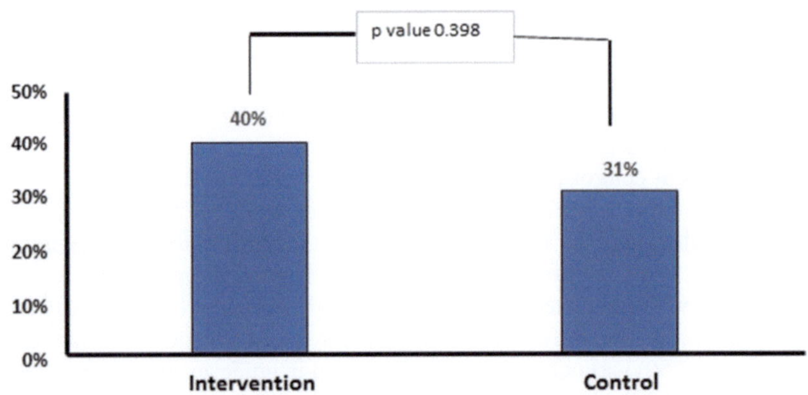

Fig. 10.2 Smoking cessation rate in intervention and control group of VAPOR trial

Other Society-Based Advice on Smoking Cessation

The US Public Health Service promulgates the now widely adopted "5 A's framework" for tobacco cessation, which is elaborated in the American Association of Family Physicians (AAFP) guidelines and the 2018 American College of Cardiology (ACC) decision pathway. The World Health Organization (WHO) endorses this intervention for patients ready to quit, and also further elaborates on this [59–61].

Of note, the ACC switches the "Assess" and "Advise" steps in their decision tool compared to other organizations.

1. *Ask*—Ask patients about their tobacco use at every clinical encounter and categorize patients into "current," "former," and "never" smokers. As discussed above, patients who are younger or less educated may be unaware of the nicotine content of non-cigarette products. It is thus important to ask about use patterns in thorough, but easily understood terms.
2. *Advise*—Encourage patients to quit. Only about half of the patients are motivated to quit, so it is important to present information to patients about the many benefits of cessation. For PAD patients, this can be focused on amputation and adverse limb events, which are typically of central focus for patients. In addition, patients may consider the economic benefits of cessation, or may be motivated by insurance coverage for prescription cessation products, whereas they may not have chosen to purchase over-the-counter products which are costly.
3. *Assess*—There are two interpretations of the assessment step. The ACC recommends an assessment of nicotine dependence, including number of cigarettes per day and time to first cigarette after waking, as well as prior quit attempts for active smokers. For former smokers, assessment may include risk of relapse, while for never smokers, this may include secondhand exposure. The WHO recommends asking "would you like to be a non-tobacco user?" and "do you think you have a chance of quitting successfully?" while the AAFP recommends a combination of these two assessment tactics.
4. *Assist*—For patients willing to quit, two modalities of therapy should be offered, pharmacologic and behavioral, which are both discussed below. A key component of the assist and arrange stages is setting a quit date, ideally within 2 weeks. The WHO provides a helpful acronym, the STAR method: set a quit date, tell loved ones, anticipate challenges, and remove tobacco products from the patient.
5. *Arrange*—Continuous engagement is important for cessation. The ACC recommends a follow-up call or visit at 2–4 weeks, ongoing monitoring of treatment and adherence, reinforcement at each visit, and for non-smokers, ongoing monitoring of non-smoking status.

A list of systematic reviews of various smoking cessation strategies is given in Table 10.2.

Pharmacologic Treatment

Pharmacologic treatment is an important tool in controlling the addiction and withdrawal symptoms of smoking, and almost all smokers should be considered. For some smokers who smoke <1/2 pack per day or non-daily, dosages may be reduced.

There are three agents approved by the FDA for the treatment of nicotine use—varenicline, bupropion, and nicotine replacement products [59, 64]. Some of these products are used to prevent cravings before they happen (bupropion, varenicline,

Table 10.2 Meta-analyses of different smoking cessation treatment strategies

Study	Key exposure	Summary of effect
Thomsen et al., Cochrane database systematic Review [50]	Peri-op interventions	Even brief interventions increase cessation by 41%
Stead et al., Cochrane database systematic Review [42]	Physician advice	Intensive interv. 37% more effective than brief
Lancaster et al., Cochrane database systematic Review [62]	Behavioral counseling	56% increase in quit rate with counseling
Hartmann et al., Cochrane database systematic Review [46]	Interventions for cessation	Up to 57% increase in cessation with multimodality
Civljak et al., Cochrane database systematic Review [63]	Web-based interventions	Variable, but up to 2.05 RR increase in quit rate

and the nicotine patch) while other products are used to treat cravings when they arise (lozenges, gum, inhaler, and nasal spray). Varenicline is the most effective of these options, but the *ACC recommends that a first-line treatment in PAD may include either varenicline or combination-NRT* (both patch and short-acting agent). Bupropion and single-agent NRT are less effective, including in depressed smokers, as the nicotine-use effects of bupropion are separate from the antidepressant effects [65]. If one agent produces partial remission, then two agents may be used. If none of the FDA approved agents produce an effect, then non-FDA-approved uses of nortriptyline or clonidine have been described. A full description of the order in which to attempt treatment may be found in the ACC 2018 consensus statement [59].

In the VAPOR trial, a simple treatment card was created to guide clinicians in providing advice as well as patches, nicotine therapy, and pharmacologic agents (Fig. 10.3).

Non-pharmacological Treatment

Patients ready to quit smoking should be offered *both* pharmacologic *and* non-pharmacologic treatment, which is more effective than either alone. Compared to the seven FDA-approved pharmacologic agents, there are a myriad of non-pharmacological interventions for smoking cessation. It is very important to note here that of all the non-pharmacological interventions, only a subset of behavioral interventions is demonstrated to have efficacy. There is little evidence for the use of acupuncture, electrostimulation, hypnotherapy, laser therapy, or any type of bio-medical feedback in the treatment of smoking cessation [66]. There is some controversy about the use of motivational interviewing, which the ACC recommends but the AAFP does not. However, behavioral interventions with consensus efficacy include phone/text-based support, web/print-based resources, group or individual counselling, psychotherapy, and ongoing clinical advice [67–69]. Smoking cessation support exists through government organizations at the national and local level, as well as through insurance and hospital systems. Refer to your organization's resource guidelines, as well as your state's public health web page for further information.

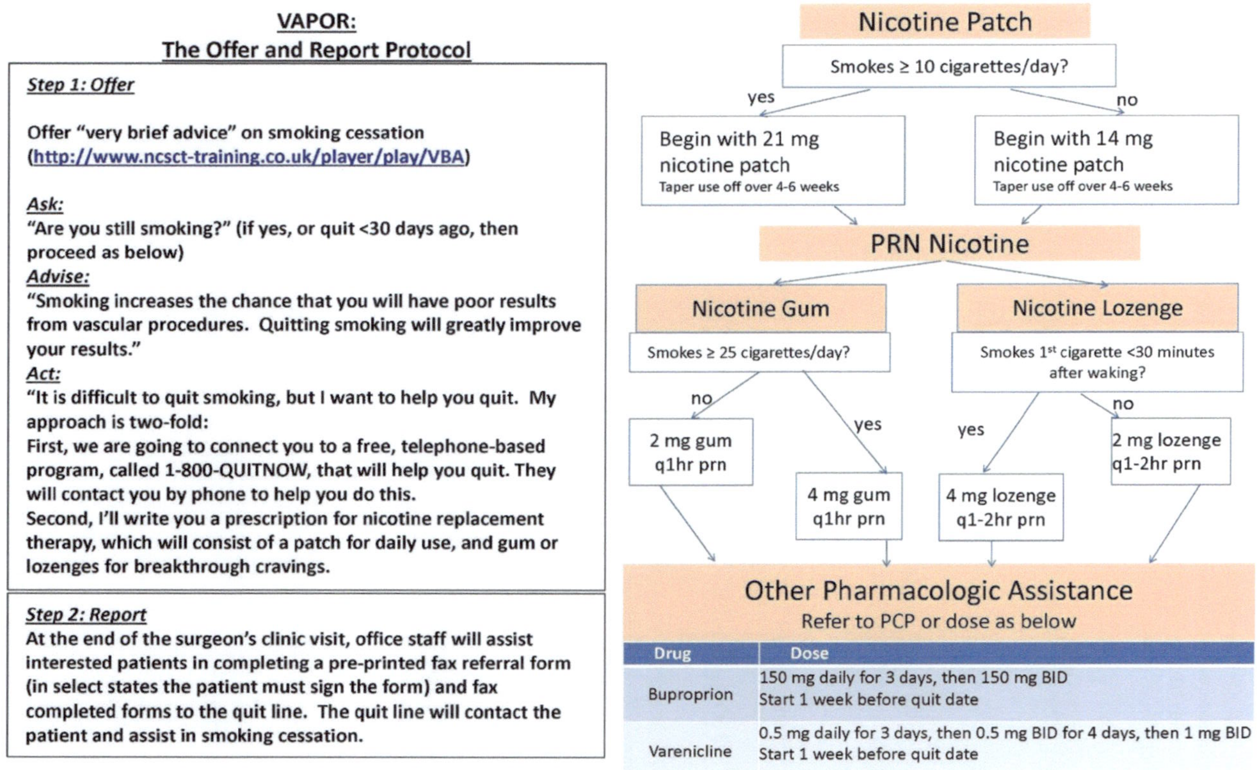

Fig. 10.3 VAPOR trial's intervention protocol on a simple treatment card to guide clinicians

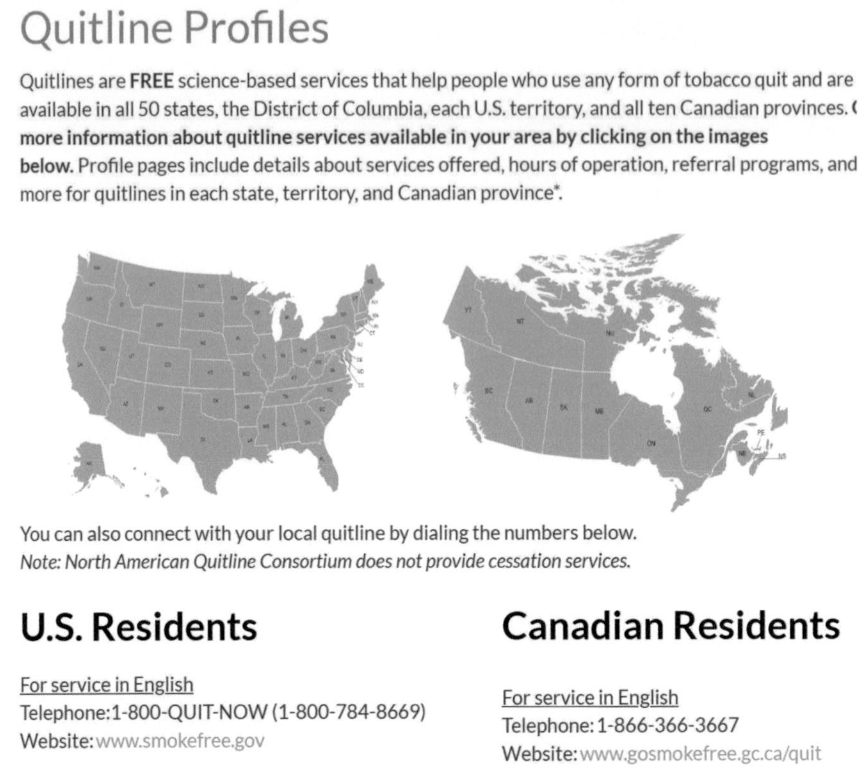
Quitline Profiles
Quitlines are FREE science-based services that help people who use any form of tobacco quit and are available in all 50 states, the District of Columbia, each U.S. territory, and all ten Canadian provinces. more information about quitline services available in your area by clicking on the images below. Profile pages include details about services offered, hours of operation, referral programs, and more for quitlines in each state, territory, and Canadian province*.
You can also connect with your local quitline by dialing the numbers below.
Note: North American Quitline Consortium does not provide cessation services.
U.S. Residents
For service in English
Telephone:1-800-QUIT-NOW (1-800-784-8669)
Website: www.smokefree.gov
Canadian Residents
For service in English
Telephone: 1-866-366-3667
Website: www.gosmokefree.gc.ca/quit

Fig. 10.4 Quitlines in the United States and Canada, available regionally

1-800-QUIT NOW

Quitlines are phone-based resources that provide free, evidence-based smoking cessation advice (https://www.naquitline.org/page/quitlineprofiles). An example of these resources is shown in Fig. 10.4.

Conclusions

Smoking is a key risk factor for the development and progression of PAD, and smoking cessation successfully mitigates this risk. First-line pharmacologic treatment should be varenicline or combination nicotine replacement therapy, and behavioral therapy may be accessed through local institutional or governmental programs, especially 1-800-QUIT-NOW. At every visit, cessation should be addressed with active smokers, while relapse should be addressed with former smokers, and secondhand smoke exposure should be addressed with never smokers.

References

1. VanFrank B. Adult smoking cessation—United States, 2022. MMWR Morb Mortal Wkly Rep. 2024;73:633.
2. Harris E. Systematic review finds the Most effective smoking cessation aids. JAMA. 2023;330(15):1421–2. https://doi.org/10.1001/jama.2023.18742.
3. Rigotti NA, Kruse GR, Livingstone-Banks J, et al. Treatment of tobacco smoking: a review. JAMA. 2022;327(6):566–77. https://doi.org/10.1001/jama.2022.0395.
4. Force USPST, Krist AH, Davidson KW, et al. Interventions for tobacco smoking cessation in adults, including pregnant persons: US preventive services task force recommendation statement. JAMA. 2021;325(3):265–79. https://doi.org/10.1001/jama.2020.25019.
5. Prod'homme C, Jacquemin D, Touzet L, et al. Barriers to end-of-life discussions among hematologists: a qualitative study. Palliat Med. 2018;32(5):1021–9. https://doi.org/10.1177/0269216318759862. [published Online First: 2018/05/15].
6. Selvin E, Erlinger TP. Prevalence of and risk factors for peripheral arterial disease in the United States: results from the National Health and Nutrition Examination Survey, 1999–2000. Circulation. 2004;110(6):738–43. https://doi.org/10.1161/01.cir.0000137913.26087.f0.
7. The L. Nicotine addiction, reduction, and smoking cessation. Lancet. 2017;390(10096):716. https://doi.org/10.1016/S0140-6736(17)32240-7.
8. Duke D, Wohlgemuth E, Adams KR, et al. Earliest evidence for human use of tobacco in the Pleistocene Americas. Nat Hum Behav. 2022;6(2):183–92.
9. Proctor RN. The global smoking epidemic: a history and status report. Clin Lung Cancer. 2004;5(6):371–6.
10. Office USPHS. Introduction, conclusions, and the evolving landscape of smoking cessation. Smoking cessation: a report of the surgeon general [Internet]: US Department of Health and Human Services 2020.
11. Eissenberg T, Shihadeh A. Electronic nicotine-delivery systems for smoking cessation. N Engl J Med. 2024;390(19):1830–1. https://doi.org/10.1056/NEJMc2403709.
12. Hartmann-Boyce J, Lindson N, Butler AR, et al. Electronic cigarettes for smoking cessation. Cochrane Database Syst Rev. 2022;11(11):CD010216. https://doi.org/10.1002/14651858.CD010216.pub7. [published Online First: 20221117].
13. Rigotti NA. Electronic nicotine-delivery systems for smoking cessation. Reply. N Engl J Med. 2024;390(19):1832. https://doi.org/10.1056/NEJMc2403709.
14. Rigotti NA. Electronic cigarettes for smoking cessation – have we reached a tipping point? N Engl J Med. 2024;390(7):664–5. https://doi.org/10.1056/NEJMe2314977.
15. Jamal A. Tobacco use among middle and high school students—United States, 2011–2016. MMWR Morb Mortal Wkly Rep. 2017;66:47.
16. Prochaska JJ, Vogel EA, Benowitz N. Nicotine delivery and cigarette equivalents from vaping a JUULpod. Tob Control. 2022;31(e1):e88–93.
17. Subherwal S, Patel MR, Chiswell K, et al. Clinical trials in peripheral vascular disease: pipeline and trial designs: an evaluation of the ClinicalTrials.gov database. Circulation. 2014;130(20):1812–9. https://doi.org/10.1161/CIRCULATIONAHA.114.011021.
18. Subherwal S, Patel MR, Tang F, et al. Socioeconomic disparities in the use of cardioprotective medications among patients with peripheral artery disease: an analysis of the American College of Cardiology's NCDR PINNACLE Registry. J Am Coll Cardiol. 2013;62(1):51–7. https://doi.org/10.1016/j.jacc.2013.04.018.
19. Pande RL, Creager MA. Socioeconomic inequality and peripheral artery disease prevalence in US adults. Circ Cardiovasc Qual Outcomes. 2014;7(4):532–9. https://doi.org/10.1161/CIRCOUTCOMES.113.000618.
20. Fiore MC, Bailey WC, Cohen SJ, et al. Smoking cessation clinical practice guideline, vol. 276. Rockville: Agency for Health Care Policy and Research,Public Health Service, US Dept of Health and Human Services; 1996.

21. Rigotti NA, Clair C, Munafo MR, et al. Interventions for smoking cessation in hospitalised patients. Cochrane Database Syst Rev. 2012;5:CD001837. https://doi.org/10.1002/14651858.CD001837.pub3.
22. Stead LF, Perera R, Bullen C, et al. Nicotine replacement therapy for smoking cessation. Cochrane Database Syst Rev. 2012;11:CD000146. https://doi.org/10.1002/14651858.CD000146.pub4. [doi] [published Online First: 2012/11/16].
23. Thomsen T, Villebro N, Moller AM. Interventions for preoperative smoking cessation. Cochrane Database Syst Rev. 2014;3:CD002294. https://doi.org/10.1002/14651858.CD002294.pub4.
24. Spangler EL, Farber A, Rigotti N, et al. Characteristics of patients enrolling in VAPOR: a SVS-sponsored trial of a smoking cessation intervention. J Vasc Surg. 2015;61:151S.
25. Black JH 3rd. Evidence base and strategies for successful smoking cessation. J Vasc Surg. 2010;51(6):1529–37. https://doi.org/10.1016/j.jvs.2009.10.124.
26. Thorndike AN, Rigotti NA, Stafford RS, et al. National patterns in the treatment of smokers by physicians. JAMA. 1998;279(8):604–8.
27. Wang W, Zhao T, Geng K, et al. Smoking and the pathophysiology of peripheral artery disease. Front Cardiovasc Med. 2021;8:704106.
28. Willigendael EM, Teijink JA, Bartelink M-L, et al. Influence of smoking on incidence and prevalence of peripheral arterial disease. J Vasc Surg. 2004;40(6):1158–65.
29. Aday AW, Matsushita K. Epidemiology of peripheral artery disease and polyvascular disease. Circ Res. 2021;128(12):1818–32.
30. Ingolfsson IÖ, Sigurdsson G, Sigvaldason H, et al. A marked decline in the prevalence and incidence of intermittent claudication in Icelandic men 1968–1986: a strong relationship to smoking and serum cholesterol—the Reykjavik Study. J Clin Epidemiol. 1994;47(11):1237–43.
31. Ding N, Sang Y, Chen J, et al. Cigarette smoking, smoking cessation, and long-term risk of 3 major atherosclerotic diseases. J Am Coll Cardiol. 2019;74(4):498–507.
32. Lu L, Mackay DF, Pell JP. Association between level of exposure to secondhand smoke and peripheral arterial disease: cross-sectional study of 5686 never smokers. Atherosclerosis. 2013;229(2):273–6.
33. Lu L, Mackay D, Pell J. Meta-analysis of the association between cigarette smoking and peripheral arterial disease. Heart. 2014;100(5):414–23.
34. Aboyans V, Criqui MH, Denenberg JO, et al. Risk factors for progression of peripheral arterial disease in large and small vessels. Circulation. 2006;113(22):2623–9.
35. Gardner AW. The effect of cigarette smoking on exercise capacity in patients with intermittent claudication. Vasc Med. 1996;1(3):181–6.
36. Jonason T, Ringqvist I. Factors of prognostic importance for subsequent rest pain in patients with intermittent claudication. Acta Med Scand. 1985;218(1):27–33.
37. Cronenwett JL, Warner KG, Zelenock GB, et al. Intermittent claudication: current results of nonoperative management. Arch Surg. 1984;119(4):430–6.
38. Jones DW, Goodney PP, Eldrup-Jorgensen J, et al. Active smoking in claudicants undergoing lower extremity bypass predicts decreased graft patency and worse overall survival. J Vasc Surg. 2018;68(3):796–806. e1
39. Willigendael EM, Teijink JA, Bartelink M-L, et al. Smoking and the patency of lower extremity bypass grafts: a meta-analysis. J Vasc Surg. 2005;42(1):67–74.
40. Reitz KM, Althouse AD, Meyer J, et al. Association of smoking with postprocedural complications following open and endovascular interventions for intermittent claudication. JAMA Cardiol. 2022;7(1):45–54.
41. Critchley JA, Capewell S. Mortality risk reduction associated with smoking cessation in patients with coronary heart disease: a systematic review. JAMA. 2003;290(1):86–97. https://doi.org/10.1001/jama.290.1.86.
42. Stead LF, Buitrago D, Preciado N, et al. Physician advice for smoking cessation. Cochrane Database Syst Rev. 2013;5:CD000165. https://doi.org/10.1002/14651858.CD000165.pub4. [published Online First: 2013/06/04].

43. Aveyard P, Begh R, Parsons A, et al. Brief opportunistic smoking cessation interventions: a systematic review and meta-analysis to compare advice to quit and offer of assistance. Addiction. 2012;107(6):1066–73. https://doi.org/10.1111/j.1360-0443.2011.03770.x.
44. Bryant J, Passey ME, Hall AE, et al. A systematic review of the quality of reporting in published smoking cessation trials for pregnant women: an explanation for the evidence-practice gap? Implement Sci. 2014;9:94. https://doi.org/10.1186/s13012-014-0094-z.
45. Hartmann-Boyce J, Stead LF, Cahill K, et al. Efficacy of interventions to combat tobacco addiction: Cochrane update of 2012 reviews. Addiction. 2013;108(10):1711–21. https://doi.org/10.1111/add.12291.
46. Hartmann-Boyce J, Stead LF, Cahill K, et al. Efficacy of interventions to combat tobacco addiction: Cochrane update of 2013 reviews. Addiction. 2014;109(9):1414–25. https://doi.org/10.1111/add.12633.
47. Munafo M, Rigotti N, Lancaster T, et al. Interventions for smoking cessation in hospitalised patients: a systematic review. Thorax. 2001;56(8):656–63.
48. Stead LF, Hartmann-Boyce J, Perera R, et al. Telephone counselling for smoking cessation. Cochrane Database Syst Rev. 2013;8:CD002850. https://doi.org/10.1002/14651858.CD002850.pub3. [doi] [published Online First: 2013/08/13].
49. Stead LF, Perera R, Lancaster T. A systematic review of interventions for smokers who contact quitlines. Tob Control. 2007;16(Suppl 1):i3–8. 16/Suppl_1/i3 [pii]. https://doi.org/10.1136/tc.2006.019737. [doi] [published Online First: 2007/12/01].
50. Thomsen T, Villebro N, Moller AM. Interventions for preoperative smoking cessation. Cochrane Database Syst Rev. 2010;(7):CD002294. https://doi.org/10.1002/14651858.CD002294.pub3.
51. Jha P, Ramasundarahettige C, Landsman V, et al. 21st-century hazards of smoking and benefits of cessation in the United States. N Engl J Med. 2013;368(4):341–50. https://doi.org/10.1056/NEJMsa1211128.
52. Goodney PP, Spangler EL, Newhall K, et al. Feasibility and pilot efficacy of a brief smoking cessation intervention delivered by vascular surgeons in the vascular physician offer and report (VAPOR) trial. J Vasc Surg. 2017;65(4):1152–60 e2. https://doi.org/10.1016/j.jvs.2016.10.121. [published Online First: 20170209]
53. Hoel AW, Nolan BW, Goodney PP, et al. Variation in smoking cessation after vascular operations. J Vasc Surg. 2013;57(5):1338–44; quiz 44 e1–4. https://doi.org/10.1016/j.jvs.2012.10.130. [published Online First: 20130130].
54. Howard R, Albright J, Osborne N, et al. Impact of a regional smoking cessation intervention for vascular surgery patients. J Vasc Surg. 2022;75(1):262–9. https://doi.org/10.1016/j.jvs.2021.07.103. [published Online First: 20210721]
55. Jones DW, Goodney PP, Eldrup-Jorgensen J, et al. Active smoking in claudicants undergoing lower extremity bypass predicts decreased graft patency and worse overall survival. J Vasc Surg. 2018;68(3):796–806 e1. https://doi.org/10.1016/j.jvs.2017.12.044. [published Online First: 20180306].
56. Newhall K, Burnette M, Brooke BS, et al. Smoking cessation counseling in vascular surgical practice using the results of interviews and focus groups in the vascular surgeon offer and report smoking cessation pilot trial. J Vasc Surg. 2016;63(4):1011–7 e2. https://doi.org/10.1016/j.jvs.2015.10.086. [published Online First: 20151230].
57. Newhall K, Suckow B, Spangler E, et al. Impact and duration of brief surgeon-delivered smoking cessation advice on attitudes regarding nicotine dependence and tobacco harms for patients with peripheral arterial disease. Ann Vasc Surg. 2017;38:113–21. https://doi.org/10.1016/j.avsg.2016.06.005. [published Online First: 20160810].
58. Spangler EL, Goodney PP. Smoking cessation strategies in vascular surgery. Semin Vasc Surg. 2015;28(2):80–5. https://doi.org/10.1053/j.semvascsurg.2015.10.001. [published Online First: 20151008].
59. Barua RS, Rigotti NA, Benowitz NL, et al. 2018 ACC expert consensus decision pathway on tobacco cessation treatment: a report of the American College of Cardiology Task Force on Clinical Expert Consensus Documents. J Am Coll Cardiol. 2018;72(25):3332–65.

60. Okuyemi KS, Nollen NL, Ahluwalia JS. Interventions to facilitate smoking cessation. Am Fam Physician. 2006;74(2):262–71.
61. World Health Organization. Toolkit for delivering the 5A's and 5R's brief tobacco interventions to TB patients in primary care. 2014.
62. Lancaster T, Stead LF. Individual behavioural counselling for smoking cessation. Cochrane Database Syst Rev. 2005;(2):CD001292. https://doi.org/10.1002/14651858.CD001292.pub2.
63. Civljak M, Sheikh A, Stead LF, et al. Internet-based interventions for smoking cessation. Cochrane Database Syst Rev. 2010;(9):CD007078. https://doi.org/10.1002/14651858.CD007078.pub3.
64. Ratchford E, Khoury S. Smoking cessation in peripheral artery disease. American College; 2020. p. 367.
65. Cinciripini PM, Kypriotakis G, Green C, et al. The effects of varenicline, bupropion, nicotine patch, and placebo on smoking cessation among smokers with major depression: a randomized clinical trial. Depress Anxiety. 2022;39(5):429–40.
66. White AR, Rampes H, Liu JP, et al. Acupuncture and related interventions for smoking cessation. Cochrane Database Syst Rev. 2014;2014(1):CD000009.
67. Whittaker R, McRobbie H, Bullen C, et al. Mobile phone-based interventions for smoking cessation. Cochrane Database Syst Rev. 2016;4:CD006611.
68. Vinci C. Cognitive behavioral and mindfulness-based interventions for smoking cessation: a review of the recent literature. Curr Oncol Rep. 2020;22:1–8.
69. Ford P, Clifford A, Gussy K, et al. A systematic review of peer-support programs for smoking cessation in disadvantaged groups. Int J Environ Res Public Health. 2013;10(11):5507–22.

Behavioral and Mental Health Considerations for Patients Experiencing Vasculogenic Claudication

11

Santiago Callegari, Carlos Mena-Hurtado, and Kim G. Smolderen

Introduction

Health and disease are multidimensional constructs. With the rise of chronic diseases over the past century, especially cardiovascular diseases, the need to address the multifaceted nature of disease and its treatment was again underscored by clinician scholars such as George Engel in the late 1970s. Engel referenced the importance of understanding and treating disease from the perspective of a biopsychosocial model. More recent examples of this call are the increased recognition of the role of social determinants of health play, and we might even go further as to include economic or commercial determinants of health if we were to extend the different impacts of macro-economic and geopolitical forces on how health, disease, and treatment is being constructed and contribute to the contemporary global chronic disease burden [1]. Other examples of theories that speak to the multidimensional nature of health is the socio-ecological theory [2], which emphasizes that in addition to individual (intrapsychic) factors, individuals experience health and disease in the larger context of family, their friends and neighborhood where they spend time, and the broader community and social settings they participate in (Fig. 11.1) [2]. This multidimensional view of health and illness is recognized in multiple societies, including the World Health Organization, recognizing health as an optimal state of physical, mental, and social health [3].

S. Callegari · C. Mena-Hurtado
Vascular Medicine Outcomes Program, Section of Cardiovascular Medicine, Department of Internal Medicine & Department of Psychiatry, Yale University, New Haven, CT, USA
e-mail: santiago.callegari@yale.edu; carlos.mena-hurtado@yale.edu

K. G. Smolderen (✉)
Vascular Medicine Outcomes Program, Section of Cardiovascular Medicine, Department of Internal Medicine & Department of Psychiatry, Yale University, New Haven, CT, USA

Department of Psychiatry, Yale School of Medicine, New Haven, CT, USA
e-mail: kim.smolderen@yale.edu

W. P. Robinson III, J. P. Simons (eds.), *The Patient-Centered Approach to Claudication*, https://doi.org/10.1007/978-3-032-02460-2_11

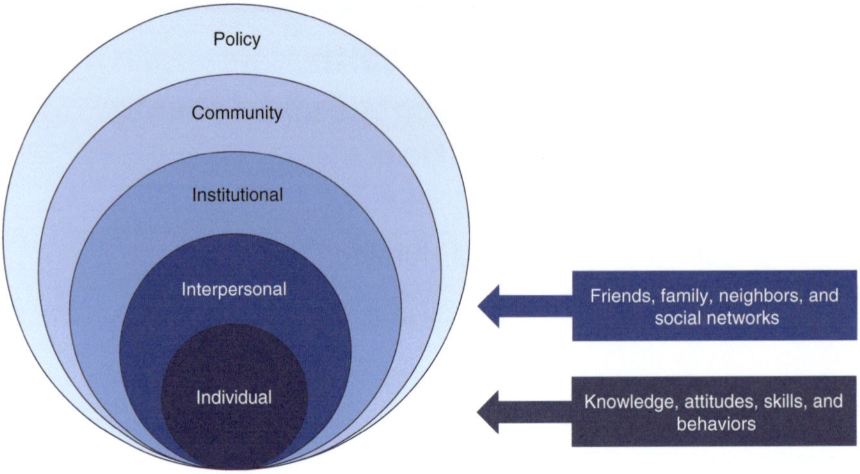

Fig. 11.1 The socioecological model explains how a person's health is dictated by multiple factors beyond the individual (intrapsychic) to include interpersonal, institutional, community, and policy level factors. In this chapter, we focus on the individual (intrapsychic) and interpersonal (interpsychic) factors that influence a person's claudication experience, focusing on the psychological risk perspective specifically. (Adapted from the book Ecological systems theory by Urie Bronfenbrenner [2])

As the chronic disease burden for cardiovascular diseases such as peripheral artery disease (PAD) (Table 11.1) is expected to grow globally [4, 5], addressing factors that influence and impact the occurrence and progression of disease in its totality are essential to make a meaningful impact on the health of individuals, their families, and the health of a society at large. PAD includes three distinct manifestations: asymptomatic disease, intermittent claudication, and chronic limb-threatening ischemia. PAD is estimated to impact over 230 million individuals worldwide, and cardiovascular risk factors contributing to its risk are expected to exponentially grow, especially among minorities [6, 7]. For PAD patients manifesting with claudication, care is focused on addressing atherosclerotic risk factors and improving physical function and health-related quality of life [8].

Claudication was initially described by a French veterinarian in a horse affected by progressive limping and lameness consequent to a fibrous clot that occluded the femoral arteries of the posterior limbs [9–11]. Later on, it was Charcot in 1846 who clearly defined and described the syndrome (and used the term "intermittent claudication") in humans [9–11]. He described it as a pain reproducibly elicited by walking-induced muscle ischemia and consistently relieved by rest that allows reperfusion of the affected limb [9–11]. This biological basis for the claudication, initially described in an animal model, set the foundations of the current view of PAD that we still have to this day. In 1898, it was Erb who in his description of 13 case reports suggested that PAD occurred earlier in life than previously thought and that it seemed that smoking was one of the primary risk factors for claudication [12]. The Framingham risk studies later confirmed that the predominant risk factors

Table 11.1 Summary of the factors that have been associated with peripheral artery disease incidence or outcomes

Domain	Category	Factors	Associations	References
Intrapsychic	Personality	Anger proneness	Higher incidence of PAD	[27]
		Acts of hostility	Severity of PAD	[28]
		Type D personality	Higher mortality	[29]
			Lower quality of life	
			More depressive symptoms	
		Neuroticism	Higher PAD prevalence	[30]
	Mood disorders	Depression	Bilateral relationship with PAD	[31–34, 36]
			Mortality	
			Longer hospital stay	
			Periprocedural complications of revascularization	
			Higher costs during admissions	
			Health status	
	Substance use disorder	Smoking	PAD prevalence	[37, 39]
			Mortality	
			Major amputation	
		Methamphetamines and cocaine use	PAD admissions among users	[40]
		Cannabis users	PAD prevalence	[42]
			Decrease in bypass patency	
			Amputations after bypass	
		Alcohol use	Prevalence of PAD	[43, 44]
		Opioid use	PAD readmissions	[47]
			Longer hospital length of stay	[48]
			Higher risk of postoperative complication	
			Major amputation	
	Chronic pain		Severe pain related to PAD	[53, 54]
	PTSD		PAD prevalence	[64]
	ADHD		PAD incidence	[65]
	Perceived stress		Higher PAD mortality	[66, 67]
			Lower health status	
	Health behaviors	Motivational therapy	Improved symptom relief	[57, 60–63]
			Adherence to exercise therapy	
Interpsychic factors	Social support	Perceived social support	PAD incidence	[71, 72]
			Lower health status	
	Social deprivation		Delayed disease presentation	[74, 75]
			Worse outcomes after revascularization	
	Family and caregivers		Qualitative work	{Egberg, 2013 #634}

for developing PAD were diabetes and smoking [13]. Claudication, as a central symptom of the condition, remained the main diagnostic element for PAD until the ankle-brachial index (ABI) was introduced in the mid twentieth century, which demonstrated that claudication vastly underestimates the actual prevalence of PAD [14, 15], and since then, an abnormal ankle-brachial index, defined as ABI ≤ 0.9, is used as a supportive diagnostic element in contemporary medicine [8]. As with all the other atherosclerotic conditions, clinical trials demonstrated benefit for treating its risk factors through lipid-lowering therapies, antihypertensive therapy, exercise therapy, antithrombotic therapy, and smoking cessation, among other lifestyle modifications in patients with PAD [8, 15–20].

PAD is conceptualized as an arterial obstruction problem as well as a systemic atherosclerotic disorder. Therefore, improving local perfusion alone does not address the systemic factors that are the root causes of atherosclerotic diseases such as PAD. Most of the risk factors for PAD are related to lifestyle, such as smoking, a sedentary lifestyle, metabolic risk factors, e.g., diabetes, hyperlipidemia, and unhealthy dietary patterns. Exposure to psychological stress has been added to the list of risk factors for atherosclerotic diseases such as PAD, and forms either a direct or indirect relationship with disease incidence, and progression, as well as the management of risk factors. Decades worth of mechanistic evidence supporting the association between psychological stress and cardiovascular disease across the spectrum of arterial beds has been documented, and evidence-based behavioral/psychological interventions based on these insights have become available to improve the quality of life and outcomes in patients with atherosclerotic diseases [21].

This chapter will discuss the different ways in which psychological stress may affect atherosclerosis, and next, focus on the intra- and interpsychic risk factors for which there has been evidence found for either the incidence or the disease progression and experience and impacts on PAD treatments. It will conclude with considerations for psychological assessment and interventions in PAD and will describe future areas for development. It will focus on Rutherford categories 1–3 (mild to severe claudication). The management of more advanced stages of disease, characterized by ischemic rest pain, non-healing wounds, ulceration, and gangrene/amputation are beyond the scope of the current chapter.

A Model of Psychological Stress for Atherosclerotic Diseases

Many underlying mechanisms for the relationship between psychological stress and atherosclerosis have been studied, with the following resulting comprehensive model explaining the multitude of ways in which underlying stress can promote atherosclerosis throughout the system [21]. Chronic stress and stress due to affective disorders and other psychiatric conditions lead to activation of the hypothalamic-pituitary-adrenal (HPA) axis and the sympathetic nervous system, which can further affect behaviors (e.g., disturbed sleep, reduced physical activity, change in appetite and diet, substance use). Due to the prolonged activation and the release of stress

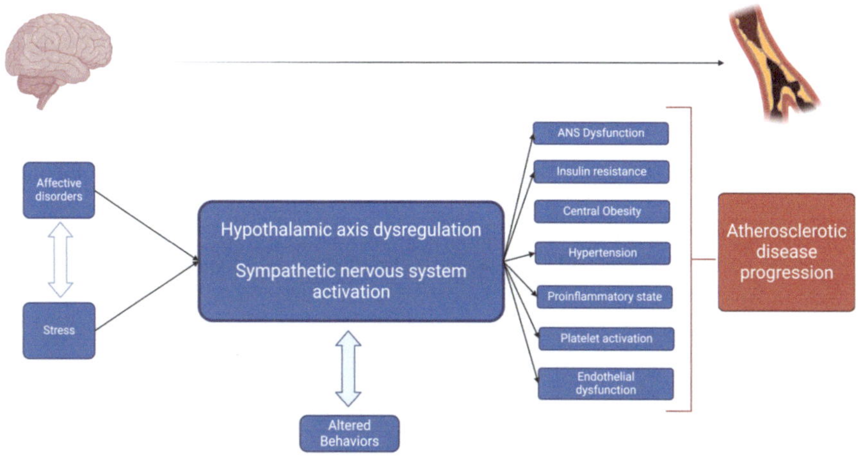

Fig. 11.2 Adapted from the original Rozanski et al. which attempts to explain the underlying mechanisms that link psychological stress to atherosclerotic disease progression

hormones (adrenaline and cortisol), the system is in a "fight or flight" mode, and this is associated with an imbalance of the autonomic nervous system. This imbalance further results in heightened physiologic responsiveness to acute stress, which can also interact with chronic stressors that cause more downstream neuroendocrine, sympathetic, and behavioral effects, such as insulin resistance, obesity, hypertension, increased inflammation, platelet reactivity, and endothelial dysfunction, among others. All of these mechanisms can contribute to the increased risk of atherosclerotic disease progression (Fig. 11.2). There are no specific conceptual models for the impact of chronic stress on peripheral vasculature specifically, except for some incidental mechanistic evidence stemming from animal studies and sympathectomy procedures in humans. In animal studies, TRPV and TRPA channels, nerve growth factor (NGF), collateral arteries' response, among others, are all biological mediators that link the sympathetic nervous system response as a direct mediator of peripheral vascular perfusion [22–25]. In humans, sympathectomy procedures in end-stage PAD were able to demonstrate relief from rest pain and increase skin blood flow and warmth, with over 70% of patients experiencing improvement in their symptoms [26].

Intra-psychic Factors of Relevance for PAD

Personality

In atherosclerotic diseases, the role of personality traits that are prone to developing disease has been the subject of study for many decades. For PAD specifically, the role of anger proneness, as measured by the Spielberger Anger Expression Scale, has been associated with an increased risk of developing PAD in a dose-response fashion, over the course of a mean follow-up time of 9.7 years as documented in the Atherosclerosis Risk in Communities Study [27].

In cross-sectional work, the role of hostility has been investigated in PAD. Through the use of the Bedford Foulds personality deviance questionnaire, information on extrapunitiveness, intropunitiveness, and dominance was derived, and an independent association was found between more acts of hostility and severity of PAD in the Edinburgh Artery Study [28].

Furthermore, the role of a distressed personality, or Type D personality, as assessed by the Type D Scale–14, and which consists of a combination of social inhibition and negative affectivity, has been associated with an increased risk of mortality in those with intermittent claudication, an impaired quality of life, and increased risk of experiencing depressive symptoms [29].

Finally, neuroticism, has also been associated with PAD, as compared with control groups in a smaller sample in the primary care setting [30].

Mood Disorders

Patients with PAD are at increased risk of experiencing depressive symptoms, with estimates ranging from 16% to 35% [31]. Depression has been associated with a 24% increased risk of mortality [31]. Furthermore, depressive symptoms have been associated with an increased risk of post-procedural complications, longer hospital stays, and more costly admissions characterized by major amputation [32, 33]. Individuals under 65 years old are more at risk of having a diagnosed depressive disorder, and depressive symptoms go hand in hand with reduced physical activity patterns in PAD, as illustrated in a cohort of patients with intermittent claudication [34, 35]. The more patients reduce their physical activity, the higher the risk of developing subsequent depressive symptoms [34]. Lastly, there are also differences by sex, in which women with PAD present with the double the depression burden compared to men, which results also in more compromised health status states for women vs. men with intermittent claudication [36].

Substance Use Disorders

One of the primary risk factors for PAD has traditionally been smoking. When compared to never-smokers, individuals who are current smokers have a 2.3-fold increase in the prevalence of PAD, and the prevalence continues to be higher even in former-smokers [37]. At a national level, in countries with heavy tobacco use (i.e., 30% of the population are smokers), 50% of PAD could be attributed to smoking alone [37]. Around 30–40% of individuals with new or worsening claudication presenting at a vascular specialty clinic will have an active smoking status [38]. While smoking cessation is one of the key recommendations that clinicians treating PAD will provide, few patients receive tobacco cessation counseling for cessation support. This is despite smoking cessation being associated with a 60% reduction in all-cause mortality at 5 years and improved amputation-free survival [39]. Moreover, relapse rates for smoking are high with more than 1/3 of initial quitters relapsing with 72% of all individuals who smoke, having an active smoking status at 12 months following diagnosis. These findings were noted in the longitudinal PORTRAIT study, following an international cohort of individuals with intermittent claudication [38].

A few studies have explored the association of other substance use (disorders) and PAD. Among individuals using methamphetamine in the National Inpatient Sample database, PAD-related admissions among methamphetamine users have been on the rise annually, with an almost six-fold change between 2008 and 2020 [40]. An increase in PAD-related admissions among cocaine users has also been noted [40]. For cannabis abuse disorder, and risk of a PAD diagnosis in the NIS database it was demonstrated that the disorder was associated with more than three times the odds of having PAD, but without a significant association with in-hospital mortality or requiring endovascular revascularization [41]. Cannabis use has also been associated with worse outcomes after lower extremity bypass with a decreased bypass patency at 30 days and 1 year, as well as a higher risk of amputations at 1 year after lower extremity bypass compared to non-cannabis users [42].

Alcohol consumption studies have demonstrated a nonlinear association with PAD, similar to other cardiovascular disorders. A recent meta-analysis of cohort studies identifying more than 70,000 patients with alcohol use and among which 2544 cases of PAD over a median follow-up period of 21.9 years found a U-shaped association with the prevalence of PAD. The risk of PAD was significantly reduced among those who drank <2 drinks a day, but heavy alcohol use (>10 drinks/day) was associated with an increasing risk of developing PAD [43]. Another study evaluating moderate alcohol consumption in US male physicians found similar results [44].

Lastly, and importantly, another frequently used substance among patients with PAD is opioids. In a national database, individuals with PAD were deemed as "high opioid users" (defined as ≥2 opioid prescriptions within a 1-year period) occurred in 1 in 4 patients [45]. A new diagnosis of PAD carried a significantly higher likelihood of having high-opioid use, with 21.7% of individuals having high opioid use before diagnosis compared to 27.3% after diagnosis [45]. Importantly, even after revascularization, the high opioid use was not reduced. After revascularization (and excluding periprocedural opioid use), the percentage of high opioid users went from 25.8% before treatment to 29.6% after revascularization [45]. Chronic opioid use, defined as consistent opioid prescription filling in the 3 months prior to the procedure, is also common in PAD. In a single-center study in North Carolina, of patients with PAD undergoing revascularization, 34% of patients undergoing either endovascular or bypass revascularization had preoperative chronic opioid use (defined as consistent opioid prescription filling in the 3 months prior to the procedure) [46]. Female sex, chronic musculoskeletal pain, benzodiazepine use, and self-reported illicit drug use were significantly associated with preoperative chronic opioid use. After revascularization, more than 85% with preoperative chronic opioid use continued to have chronic opioid use, and 10% of patients who were not chronically taking opioids before the procedure developed chronic opioid use [46].

Furthermore, a diagnosed opioid use disorder (OUD) has been known to be associated with worse outcomes in PAD. A study using the national inpatient sample (NIS) identified hospitalizations with PAD using ICD10 codes, and further classified them according to OUD or major depressive disorder (MDD) codes [47]. A total of 13 million admissions were included, in which individuals with OUD and MDD had higher odds of being readmitted at 30 and 90 days as well as having the longest hospital stay over those without these comorbidities. Moreover, patients with OUD and no MDD had the highest median cost of admission compared to patients without OUD [47]. A comparable study evaluating the outcomes of patients with OUD undergoing bypass in the NIS database found similar results, with OUD being associated with a higher risk of postoperative respiratory complications, sepsis, infections, acute kidney injury, major amputations, higher costs, and longer length of stay [48].

Chronic Pain

Related to the issue of opioid use is the experience of chronic pain. Pain is one of the main symptoms in PAD and the characteristic pain associated with intermittent claudication is one of its defining features. Typical symptoms of claudication originally defined by Dr. Rose, i.e., ischemic pain that is triggered by exercise that is resolved within 10 min of resting, are present in a minority of individuals. The prevalence of claudication among individuals with PAD is frequently less than 10% in study cohorts [49]. Most (~60%) individuals with PAD in the community are asymptomatic [49–51]. Individuals with leg pain on exertion and rest have almost double the prevalence of diabetes compared to patients with the classic intermittent claudication (48.9% vs 26.7%), as well as worse sensory neuropathy when assessed with a monofilament test [52].

Negative health beliefs and other chronic pain conditions (pain conditions lasting longer than 3–6 months) [53, 54] are more likely to be associated with more severe pain in individuals with claudication. The description of the phenomenology of pain experiences in PAD is still in its early stages. As pain too is subject to biopsychosocial factors, and the complexity of the origin of pain in PAD may be multi-factorial, we have yet to understand how tailored biopsychosocial pain treatment programs may look in PAD. The complexity of pain arises from multiple regional factors that can be the cause of the pain (inflammatory, neuropathic, nociceptive, ischemic), as well as also central regulators by cortical pathways that influence pain that can also be affected by psychological factors and behaviors. The pain experience might also differ by sex, and rest pain and atypical leg symptoms are more prevalent in women, while intermittent claudication is more frequently seen in men [55]. Lastly, the pain experience also evolves depending on disease progression. While pain in claudication is more ischemic in nature, at later stages of the disease (CLTI), pain tends to be more neuropathic in nature [56].

Claudication treatments are focused on improving functioning. Exercise therapy is designed to increase the pain-free and maximum walking distance through repeated sessions of walking where one gradually tries to walk through the pain and increase the distance at which one can walk without pain [57]. Mechanisms are not entirely clear, but if compliant, patients tend to improve their walking ability and quality of life [58]. Invasive treatment, either through endovascular or surgical revascularization, is an option if patients are not responsive to medical management and exercise therapy alone, and have significant detriment to their daily lifestyle as a result of their symptoms [8, 59].

In both strategies, concerns related to intrapsychic factors are of relevance to the chances of success. Adherence and motivational issues play a major role in whether patients will experience relief with exercise therapy, and programs combining exercise therapy with motivational interviewing and cognitive behavioral therapy interventions tend to improve success rates [57, 60–63]. For revascularization, having anxiety, depression, or OUD has been associated with an increased risk of multiple complications, and with this risk, also prolonged episodes of pain.

No multimodal pain management protocols exist for PAD-related pain, in contrast to conditions like chronic back pain, or migraine; further mechanistic study and implementation research and program design around pain management in PAD is needed to understand the complexity of the phenomenon. Especially due to the risks associated with opioids, including dependence, overdose, and mortality, developing alternative pain management approaches in PAD is crucial.

Other Psychiatric Conditions and Psychological Factors

Increased risk of PAD has also been associated with other mental health conditions aside from mood and addiction disorders, including posttraumatic stress disorders and attention-deficit hyperactivity disorders. In a population-based study cohort in Germany, almost 1500 elderly individuals were evaluated for diagnostic criteria for PTSD and scores on the Posttraumatic Diagnostic Scale (PTSD) [64]. Trauma exposure was present in 29.1%, and PTSD diagnosis was made on 4.6% of the cohort. When compared to individuals without trauma, trauma exposure was associated with multiple cardiovascular disorders (coronary artery disease, heart failure, PAD) as well as hypertension and dyslipidemia. PTSD vs. no PTSD was significantly associated with an almost two-fold increased odds of PAD [64]. In another population-based cohort study performed in Sweden, which identified 5 million individuals among which 37,027 were identified as having ADHD, the association between ADHD and incident cardiovascular disease was examined for a mean follow-up of 11.80 ± 2.85 years [65]. The association between ADHD and PAD was among the strongest associations after adjusting for sociodemographics and medical comorbidities (nearly twice the risk of those without ADHD); after adjusting for psychiatric comorbidities the association was still significant.

Levels of perceived stress, not tied to a mental health disorder, have also been associated with worse outcomes among patients with PAD. In a multicenter national study, patients experiencing higher chronic stress over the first 6 months after diagnosis demonstrated poorer recovery in disease-specific health status outcomes at 1 year. After adjustment for biopsychosocial comorbidities, the association was still statistically significant. Similarly, high levels of perceived stress were also associated with a greater long-term mortality risk [66, 67].

Health Behaviors

Lifestyle recommendations consist of modifiable health behavior changes that patients are encouraged to make to manage their disease, including smoking cessation, increases in their exercise and walking regimens, dietary modifications, diabetes management, etc. To maximize success, factors such as self-efficacy, adaptive illness representations, and coping skills will need to be in place per the Common Sense model of health developed by Leventhal, a widely used model for understanding predictors of health behavior changes (Fig. 11.3) [68]. Furthermore,

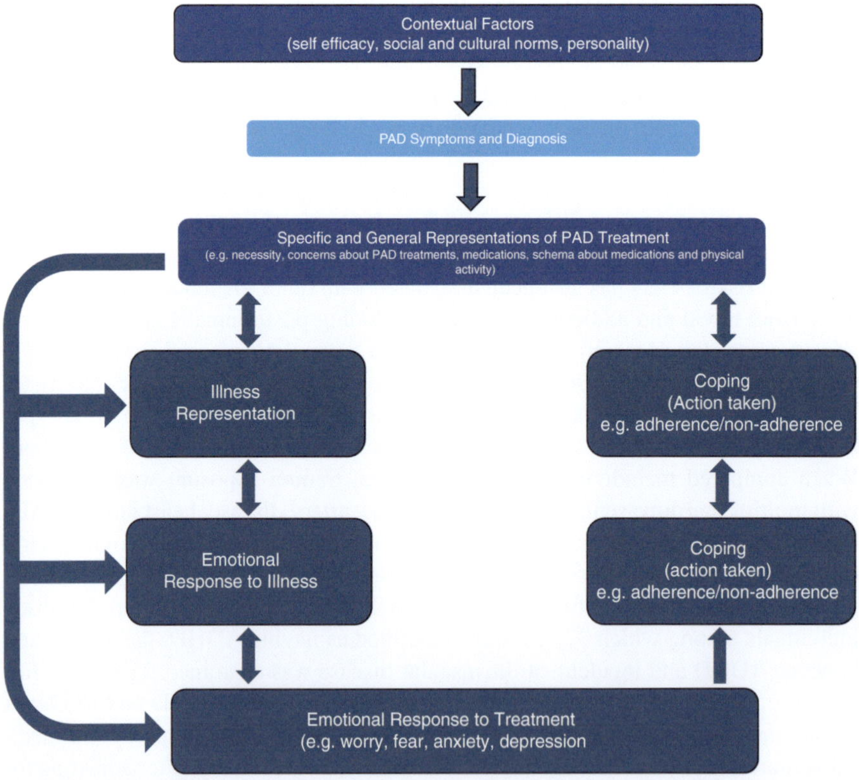

Fig. 11.3 Model adapted from the commonsense model of health developed by Leventhal to understand predictors of health behavior changes in peripheral artery disease (PAD). (Adapted from Leventhal et al. [68] in European Psychologist)

understanding adherence to making lifestyle changes and improving daily habits is also crucial in maximizing chances for success.

A multitude of factors go into whether a patient can adhere to recommended lifestyle changes. Aspects of motivation, abilities and skills, cues in people's environment, and whether patients can execute the changes (e.g., safety in neighborhoods may prevent patients from being able to comply with a home-based walking regimen) are all factors to consider. As for the motivational aspects, not every patient may be in the same stage of readiness to make changes. The stages-of-change model as developed by Prochaska and DiClemente divides individuals into 5 stages of readiness in which, while originally thought to be linear, is now described as a cyclical or "spiral" pattern. This is believed to be the more accurate depiction of change for most individuals [69]. The 5 stages are: (1) Precontemplation, in which there is no intention to change the behavior in the foreseeable future and individuals are often unaware of their problems; (2) Preparation, in which they are intending to enact change, and may demonstrate small behavioral changes but not yet an effective action; (3) Action, in which individuals modify their behavior, experience, or environment to overcome their problems; (4) Maintenance, in which individuals concentrate in preventing relapse and consolidating gains from previous stage; and (5) Termination, in which individuals have completed the change process and no longer need to work on relapse [69]. The different stages of change need to be evaluated and it is important to evaluate the patient's stage of change; tailored motivational language (motivational interviewing) would work best to support them in their claudication management journey [70].

Several trials have shown improved results in symptom relief and treatment success for exercise programs when adding these insights to the intervention protocol [57, 60–63]. Similar approaches would be beneficial for any health behavior change that the patient is recommended to make, for example, smoking cessation or dietary changes.

Interpsychic Factors of Relevance for PAD

Interpsychic factors (psychological factors that influence interactions with others) in PAD have been shown to be important as well, and should be considered in evaluating an individual's disease risk, and the management of their PAD.

Social Support and Social Isolation

Claudication is a diagnosis that has an impact on patients' daily functioning in different domains of life, not only the physical impairment, but also their mental and social functioning. They may need to rely on others for help. Social roles and dynamics may be impacted by the condition. Engagement in social activities may also be impacted. Less social support has been associated with PAD risk, which was partially explained by the level of depressive and fatigue symptoms in the

Atherosclerosis Risk in Communities (ARIC) study [71]. Furthermore, in an international cohort of individuals with intermittent claudication, a total of 18.2% indicated they had low social support as measured by the Enhancing Recovery in Coronary Heart Disease Patients (ENRICHD) Social Support Inventory (ESSI), and it was found that low social support was independently associated with a lower PAD-specific health status a year following the start of their initial treatment for PAD [72]. A promising group-based home-based exercise intervention where support group meetings were facilitated with a coach was able to demonstrate an improvement in social functioning at 6 month follow up [73].

Social Deprivation

In a larger context of social determinants of health, patients who are the most at risk of experiencing PAD often live in neighborhoods where several forms of deprivation exist in terms of access to education, health care, healthy food options, clean air and walkable spaces, among other disadvantages. Different metrics have been used to measure the effects of deprivation, and consistently, a relationship has been shown with delayed disease presentation [74], and worse disease outcomes following revascularization [75]. Awareness of patients' socio-economic background is crucial to consider, as additional resources may be needed to be able to allow for them to benefit equally from therapeutic options that are available, and a larger framework for continuous advocacy and community-based approaches are needed to address these factors in more systemic ways [76].

Family, Caregivers

As chronic disease not only impacts the individual patient, but also the social systems around them, it is important to consider the potential for realization of health behavior changes in the context of the family system and their environment. Additionally, it is important to consider the burden that caring for an individual with chronic disease may involve. Besides some initial qualitative work {Egberg, 2013 #634}, the impact of PAD on the family and caregivers has not been fully elucidated, especially for the early stages of disease. By extrapolating from other cardiovascular chronic conditions, we have learned that involving the caregiver and family in interventions for disease management is an impactful strategy to promote the rehabilitation process and improve outcomes [77].

Assessment and Treatment Considerations

Management of cardiovascular risk factors in patients with PAD requires a consideration of the total biopsychosocial context, and incorporating these insights in the work-up and treatment plan is important. Integrated behavioral care pathways have been described before [78], and could form important strategies for enhancing day-to-day disease management. This entails having a heightened awareness for their risk of mood disorders and other mental health conditions that may simultaneously need to be treated in the context of PAD management to optimize outcomes. Encouraging evidence has been emerging in the context of exercise therapy options that, when enhanced with evidence based behavioral interventions such as cognitive behavioral therapy, or motivational interviewing, better outcomes (completion rates, daily physical activity) are achieved as compared with interventions without those enhancements [79–81].

Future Directions

Despite the origins of the biological model that initially explained the condition of PAD, in recent decades, the paradigm of PAD has increasingly shifted to also recognize and include psychological factors that play a role in PAD for disease risk, disease management, and treatment outcomes. To effectively improve outcomes in PAD, a multidimensional approach is needed to effectively address the mental health burden of the disease, support patients to make lifestyle changes, and help improve their symptoms and quality of life. Program design and implementation for integrated care options for PAD are still in their infancy; additional evidence is needed to demonstrate the impact these care pathways can have on improving clinical and patient-centered outcomes for PAD. In addition, larger advocacy efforts regarding awareness, training, and reimbursement are required for full maturation of these multidisciplinary pathways. Furthermore, thorough understanding of how psychological factors impact and interact with PAD management and outcomes is still unfolding; more evidence is needed particularly for high-risk groups such as minorities, and women who may have a higher risk of distress, exposure to trauma, and lack of support. Chronic pain and substance use disorders in PAD are additional topics that need more dedicated research efforts, both from a mechanistic and intervention/prevention standpoints. Team-based approaches are becoming more and more common for cardiovascular disease management [82], given their complex risk profile, and associated needs for their disease management; their application to PAD care specifically is a promising development [78, 82].

Conclusion

Effective management of patients with claudication requires a holistic and team-based approach to the disease. Despite the origins of the biological model to explain PAD, in recent decades, the understanding of the patient experience with claudication has evolved to also include mental health considerations and psychological factors that play a role in terms of risk for developing PAD, barriers to modifying them, and the impact of PAD and its treatment on precipitating or exacerbating mental health problems. To effectively improve outcomes in patients with claudication, a multidimensional and multidisciplinary approach is warranted. Understanding the intrapsychic and interpsychic factors, in the larger context of social determinants of health, that explain how a disease develops and how it affects the disease history (pain, functional status, cardiovascular risk), is instrumental for holistic care. It broadens the framework of risk assessment, the interventions we offer, and the outcomes measure to evaluate treatment success. It is imperative that treatment success for patients with claudication includes the wider patient experience and their psychological functioning across the different stages of disease.

Acknowledgments N/A

Disclosures Dr. Mena-Hurtado reports unrestricted research grants from Philips and Shockwave and is a consultant for Abbott Vascular, Cook, Medtronic, and Terumo; Dr. Smolderen reports unrestricted research grants from Philips, Merck, Shockwave, and Johnson & Johnson; she is a consultant for Terumo, Cook, and Twill Inc. The other authors report no competing interests.

Sources of Funding N/A

References

1. Gilmore AB, Fabbri A, Baum F, Bertscher A, Bondy K, Chang HJ, et al. Defining and conceptualising the commercial determinants of health. Lancet. 2023;401(10383):1194–213.
2. Bronfenbrenner U. Ecological systems theory (1992). Making human beings human: bioecological perspectives on human development. Thousand Oaks: Sage; 2005. p. 106–73.
3. International Health C. Summary report on proceedings, minutes and final acts of the International Health Conference held in New York from 19 June to 22 July 1946. New York/Geneva: United Nations, World Health Organization, Interim Commission; 1948.
4. Pearson-Stuttard J, Guzman-Castillo M, Penalvo JL, Rehm CD, Afshin A, Danaei G, et al. Modeling future cardiovascular disease mortality in the United States: national trends and racial and ethnic disparities. Circulation. 2016;133(10):967–78.
5. Mensah GA, Fuster V, Murray CJL, Roth GA, Global Burden of Cardiovascular D, Risks C. Global burden of cardiovascular diseases and risks, 1990-2022. J Am Coll Cardiol. 2023;82(25):2350–473.
6. Song P, Rudan D, Zhu Y, Fowkes FJI, Rahimi K, Fowkes FGR, et al. Global, regional, and national prevalence and risk factors for peripheral artery disease in 2015: an updated systematic review and analysis. Lancet Glob Health. 2019;7(8):e1020–e30.
7. Peri-Okonny PA, Romain G, Callegari S, Cleman J, Vashist A, Smolderen KG, et al. Prediction of health status in patients undergoing lower extremity intervention for claudication. Ann Vasc Surg. 2025;110(Pt A):314–22.
8. Gornik HL, Aronow HD, Goodney PP, Arya S, Brewster LP, Byrd L, et al. 2024 ACC/AHA/AACVPR/APMA/ABC/SCAI/SVM/SVN/SVS/SIR/VESS Guideline for the Management of Lower Extremity Peripheral Artery Disease: a report of the American College of Cardiology/American Heart Association Joint Committee on Clinical Practice Guidelines. Circulation. 2024;149(24):e1313–e410.
9. Bollinger A, Eckert J, Rüttimann B, Becker F. Die «galoppierende» Geschichte der Claudicatio intermittens. Vasa. 2000;29(4):295–9.
10. Charcot J-M. Sur la claudication intermittente observée dans un cas d'oblitération complète de l'une des artères iliaques primitives. CR Soc Biol (Paris). 1858;5:225.

11. Bronas UG, Regensteiner JG. Connecting the past to the present: a historical review of exercise training for peripheral artery disease. Vasc Med. 2022;27(2):174–85.
12. Erb W. Ueber das „intermittirende Hinken“ und andere nervöse Störungen in Folge von Gefässerkrankungen. Deutsche Zeitschrift für Nervenheilkunde. 1898;13(1):1–76.
13. Murabito JM, D'Agostino RB, Silbershatz H, Wilson WF. Intermittent claudication. A risk profile from the Framingham heart study. Circulation. 1997;96(1):44–9.
14. McDermott MM. Peripheral artery disease: past and future. Circulation. 2024;149(15):1151–3.
15. Campia U, Gerhard-Herman M, Piazza G, Goldhaber SZ. Peripheral artery disease: past, present, and future. Am J Med. 2019;132(10):1133–41.
16. Bhatt DL, Flather MD, Hacke W, Berger PB, Black HR, Boden WE, et al. Patients with prior myocardial infarction, stroke, or symptomatic peripheral arterial disease in the CHARISMA trial. J Am Coll Cardiol. 2007;49(19):1982–8.
17. Bonaca MP, Bauersachs RM, Anand SS, Debus ES, Nehler MR, Patel MR, et al. Rivaroxaban in peripheral artery disease after revascularization. N Engl J Med. 2020;382(21):1994–2004.
18. Ostergren J, Sleight P, Dagenais G, Danisa K, Bosch J, Qilong Y, et al. Impact of ramipril in patients with evidence of clinical or subclinical peripheral arterial disease. Eur Heart J. 2004;25(1):17–24.
19. Heart Protection Study Collaborative G. Randomized trial of the effects of cholesterol-lowering with simvastatin on peripheral vascular and other major vascular outcomes in 20,536 people with peripheral arterial disease and other high-risk conditions. J Vasc Surg. 2007;45(4):645–54; discussion 53–4.
20. CAPRIE Steering Committee. A randomised, blinded, trial of clopidogrel versus aspirin in patients at risk of ischaemic events (CAPRIE). Lancet. 1996;348(9038):1329–39.
21. Rozanski A, Blumenthal JA, Davidson KW, Saab PG, Kubzansky L. The epidemiology, pathophysiology, and management of psychosocial risk factors in cardiac practice: the emerging field of behavioral cardiology. J Am Coll Cardiol. 2005;45(5):637–51.
22. Xing J, Gao Z, Lu J, Sinoway LI, Li J. Femoral artery occlusion augments TRPV1-mediated sympathetic responsiveness. Am J Physiol Heart Circ Physiol. 2008;295(3):H1262–H9.
23. Xing J, Li J. Proteinase-activated receptor-2 sensitivity of amplified TRPA1 activity in skeletal muscle afferent nerves and exercise pressor reflex in rats with femoral artery occlusion. Cell Physiol Biochem. 2017;44(1):163–71.
24. Lu J, Xing J, Li J. Role for NGF in augmented sympathetic nerve response to activation of mechanically and metabolically sensitive muscle afferents in rats with femoral artery occlusion. J Appl Physiol (1985). 2012;113(8):1311–22.
25. Taylor JC, Li Z, Yang HT, Laughlin MH, Terjung RL. Alpha-adrenergic inhibition increases collateral circuit conductance in rats following acute occlusion of the femoral artery. J Physiol. 2008;586(6):1649–67.
26. Alexander JP. Chemical lumbar sympathectomy in patients with severe lower limb ischaemia. Ulster Med J. 1994;63(2):137–43.
27. Wattanakit K, Williams JE, Schreiner PJ, Hirsch AT, Folsom AR. Association of anger proneness, depression and low social support with peripheral arterial disease: the atherosclerosis risk in communities study. Vasc Med. 2005;10(3):199–206.
28. Whiteman MC, Deary IJ, Fowkes FGR. Personality and social predictors of atherosclerotic progression: Edinburgh artery study. Psychosom Med. 2000;62(5):703–14.
29. Aquarius AE, Smolderen KG, Hamming JF, De Vries J, Vriens PW, Denollet J. Type D personality and mortality in peripheral arterial disease: a pilot study. Arch Surg. 2009;144(8):728–33.
30. Toth-Vajna G, Toth-Vajna Z, Balog P, Konkoly Thege B. Depressive symptomatology and personality traits in patients with symptomatic and asymptomatic peripheral arterial disease. BMC Cardiovasc Disord. 2020;20(1):304.
31. Scierka LE, Mena-Hurtado C, Ahmed ZV, Yousef S, Arham A, Grimshaw AA, et al. The association of depression with mortality and major adverse limb event outcomes in patients with peripheral artery disease: a systematic review and meta-analysis. J Affect Disord. 2023;320:169–77.

32. Harris KM, Mena-Hurtado C, Burg MM, Vriens PW, Heyligers J, Smolderen KG. Association of depression and anxiety disorders with outcomes after revascularization in chronic limb-threatening ischemia hospitalizations nationwide. J Vasc Surg. 2023;77(2):480–9.
33. Arya S, Lee S, Zahner GJ, Cohen BE, Hiramoto J, Wolkowitz OM, et al. The association of comorbid depression with mortality and amputation in veterans with peripheral artery disease. J Vasc Surg. 2018;68(2):536–45 e2.
34. Yazgan I, Bartlett V, Romain G, Cleman J, Petersen-Crair P, Spertus JA, et al. Longitudinal pathways between physical activity, depression, and perceived stress in peripheral artery disease. Circ Cardiovasc Qual Outcomes. 2023;16(8):544–53.
35. Harris KM, Mena-Hurtado C, Arham A, Burg MM, Freedland KE, Sinha R, et al. Increasing prevalence of critical limb ischemia hospitalizations with distinct mental health burden among younger adults. J Am Coll Cardiol. 2021;78(21):2126–8.
36. Smolderen KG, Spertus JA, Vriens PW, Kranendonk S, Nooren M, Denollet J. Younger women with symptomatic peripheral arterial disease are at increased risk of depressive symptoms. J Vasc Surg. 2010;52(3):637–44.
37. Willigendael EM, Teijink JA, Bartelink ML, Kuiken BW, Boiten J, Moll FL, et al. Influence of smoking on incidence and prevalence of peripheral arterial disease. J Vasc Surg. 2004;40(6):1158–65.
38. Patel KK, Jones PG, Ellerbeck EF, Buchanan DM, Chan PS, Spertus JA, et al. Abstract 19534: change in smoking behavior in actively smoking patients with symptomatic peripheral artery disease-insights from the international PORTRAIT registry. Circulation. 2017;136(suppl_1):A19534-A.
39. Armstrong EJ, Wu J, Singh GD, Dawson DL, Pevec WC, Amsterdam EA, et al. Smoking cessation is associated with decreased mortality and improved amputation-free survival among patients with symptomatic peripheral artery disease. J Vasc Surg. 2014;60(6):1565–71.
40. Ali S, Al-Yafeai Z, Hossain MI, Bhuiyan MS, Duhan S, Aishwarya R, et al. Trends in peripheral artery disease and critical limb ischemia hospitalizations among cocaine and methamphetamine users in the United States: a nationwide study. Front Cardiovasc Med. 2024;11:1412867.
41. Vyas H, Jain H, Benz M. C-31 | Impact of marijuana use on prevalence and interventions in peripheral artery disease. J Soc Cardiovasc Angiogr Interv. 2023;2(3):100817.
42. Braet DJ, Albright J, Brown C, Osborne NH, Henke PK. Impact of cannabis use on outcomes after lower extremity bypass. Ann Vasc Surg. 2023;89:43–51.
43. Yuan S, Wu J, Chen J, Sun Y, Burgess S, Li X, et al. Association between alcohol consumption and peripheral artery disease: two de novo prospective cohorts and a systematic review with meta-analysis. Eur J Prev Cardiol. 2024;32(2):149–55.
44. Camargo CA, Stampfer MJ, Glynn RJ, Gaziano JM, Manson JE, Goldhaber SZ, et al. Prospective study of moderate alcohol consumption and risk of peripheral arterial disease in US male physicians. Circulation. 1997;95(3):577–80.
45. Itoga NK, Sceats LA, Stern JR, Mell MW. Association of opioid use and peripheral artery disease. J Vasc Surg. 2019;70(4):1271–9 e1.
46. Velazquez-Ramirez G, Krebs J, Stafford JM, Ur R, Craven TE, Stutsrim AE, et al. Prevalence of chronic opioid use in patients with peripheral arterial disease undergoing revascularization. J Vasc Surg. 2022;75(1):186–94.
47. Amenyedor K, Lee M, Algara M, Siddiqui WT, Hardt M, Romain G, et al. Impact of comorbid opioid use disorder and major depressive disorder on healthcare utilization outcomes in patients with peripheral artery disease: a National Readmission Database analysis. Vasc Med. 2024;29(2):163–71.
48. Narayanan M, Alnahhal KI, Lingutla R, Irshad A, Iafrati M, Suarez L, et al. Outcomes of infrainguinal bypass in patients with cannabis vs opioid use disorder. Ann Vasc Surg. 2022;82:144–55.
49. McDermott MM. Lower extremity manifestations of peripheral artery disease: the pathophysiologic and functional implications of leg ischemia. Circ Res. 2015;116(9):1540–50.

50. Fowkes FG, Housley E, Cawood EH, Macintyre CC, Ruckley CV, Prescott RJ. Edinburgh Artery Study: prevalence of asymptomatic and symptomatic peripheral arterial disease in the general population. Int J Epidemiol. 1991;20(2):384–92.
51. Criqui MH, Fronek A, Klauber MR, Barrett-Connor E, Gabriel S. The sensitivity, specificity, and predictive value of traditional clinical evaluation of peripheral arterial disease: results from noninvasive testing in a defined population. Circulation. 1985;71(3):516–22.
52. McDermott MM, Greenland P, Liu K, Guralnik JM, Criqui MH, Dolan NC, et al. Leg symptoms in peripheral arterial disease: associated clinical characteristics and functional impairment. JAMA. 2001;286(13):1599–606.
53. Merskey HE. Classification of chronic pain: descriptions of chronic pain syndromes and definitions of pain terms. Pain. 1986;3:S1–S226.
54. Treede RD, Rief W, Barke A, Aziz Q, Bennett MI, Benoliel R, et al. A classification of chronic pain for ICD-11. Pain. 2015;156(6):1003–7.
55. Porras CP, Bots ML, Teraa M, van Doorn S, Vernooij RWM. Differences in symptom presentation in women and men with confirmed lower limb peripheral artery disease: a systematic review and meta-analysis. Eur J Vasc Endovasc Surg. 2022;63(4):602–12.
56. Ruger LJ, Irnich D, Abahji TN, Crispin A, Hoffmann U, Lang PM. Characteristics of chronic ischemic pain in patients with peripheral arterial disease. Pain. 2008;139(1):201–8.
57. Treat-Jacobson D, McDermott MM, Bronas UG, Campia U, Collins TC, Criqui MH, et al. Optimal exercise programs for patients with peripheral artery disease: a scientific statement from the American Heart Association. Circulation. 2019;139(4):e10–33.
58. Murphy TP, Cutlip DE, Regensteiner JG, Mohler ER 3rd, Cohen DJ, Reynolds MR, et al. Supervised exercise, stent revascularization, or medical therapy for claudication due to aortoiliac peripheral artery disease: the CLEVER study. J Am Coll Cardiol. 2015;65(10):999–1009.
59. Woo K, Siracuse JJ, Klingbeil K, Kraiss LW, Osborne NH, Singh N, et al. Society for Vascular Surgery appropriate use criteria for management of intermittent claudication. J Vasc Surg. 2022;76(1):3–22 e1.
60. Elgersma KM, Brown RJL, Salisbury DL, Stigen L, Gildea L, Larson K, et al. Adherence and exercise mode in supervised exercise therapy for peripheral artery disease. J Vasc Nurs. 2020;38(3):108–17.
61. Quirk F, Dickinson C, Baune B, Leicht A, Golledge J. Pilot trial of motivational interviewing in patients with peripheral artery disease. Int Angiol. 2012;31(5):468–73.
62. McDermott MM, Liu K, Guralnik JM, Criqui MH, Spring B, Tian L, et al. Home-based walking exercise intervention in peripheral artery disease: a randomized clinical trial. JAMA. 2013;310(1):57–65.
63. Treat-Jacobson D, McDermott MM, Beckman JA, Burt MA, Creager MA, Ehrman JK, et al. Implementation of supervised exercise therapy for patients with symptomatic peripheral artery disease: a science advisory from the American Heart Association. Circulation. 2019;140(13):e700–e10.
64. Glaesmer H, Brahler E, Gundel H, Riedel-Heller SG. The association of traumatic experiences and posttraumatic stress disorder with physical morbidity in old age: a German population-based study. Psychosom Med. 2011;73(5):401–6.
65. Li L, Chang Z, Sun J, Garcia-Argibay M, Du Rietz E, Dobrosavljevic M, et al. Attention-deficit/hyperactivity disorder as a risk factor for cardiovascular diseases: a nationwide population-based cohort study. World Psychiatry. 2022;21(3):452–9.
66. Malik AO, Peri-Okonny P, Gosch K, Thomas M, Mena C, Hiatt WR, et al. Association of perceived stress levels with long-term mortality in patients with peripheral artery disease. JAMA Netw Open. 2020;3(6):e208741.
67. Malik AO, Poghni P-O, Gosch K, Thomas MB, Mena-Hurtado C, Hiatt W, et al. Association of perceived stress with health status outcomes in patients with peripheral artery disease. J Psychosom Res. 2021;140:110313.
68. Leventhal H, Phillips LA, Burns E. The common-sense model of self-regulation (CSM): a dynamic framework for understanding illness self-management. J Behav Med. 2016;39(6):935–46.

69. Prochaska JO, Velicer WF. The transtheoretical model of health behavior change. Am J Health Promot. 1997;12(1):38–48.
70. Quirk F, Dickinson C, Baune B, Leicht A, Golledge J. Improving health behaviour outcomes through motivational interviewing in patients with chronic disease. J Sci Med Sport. 2010;1:e61.
71. Honda Y, Mok Y, Mathews L, Hof JRV, Daumit G, Kucharska-Newton A, et al. Psychosocial factors and subsequent risk of hospitalizations with peripheral artery disease: the atherosclerosis risk in communities (ARIC) study. Atherosclerosis. 2021;329:36–43.
72. Callegari S, Romain G, Cleman J, Scierka L, Peri-Okonny PA, Spertus J, et al. Association of social support and health status outcomes in peripheral artery disease. J Vasc Surg. 2024;80(6):1824–35 e7.
73. Rejeski WJ, Spring B, Domanchuk K, Tao H, Tian L, Zhao L, et al. A group-mediated, home-based physical activity intervention for patients with peripheral artery disease: effects on social and psychological function. J Transl Med. 2014;12:29.
74. Mota L, Marcaccio CL, Zhu M, Moreira CC, Rowe VL, Hughes K, et al. Impact of neighborhood social disadvantage on the presentation and management of peripheral artery disease. J Vasc Surg. 2023;77(5):1477–85.
75. Gwilym B, Chandy T, Edwards C, Hampton C, Lewis DR. Deprivation and supervised exercise for intermittent claudication. J Vasc Soc G B Irel. 2022;1(4):130–6.
76. Allison MA, Armstrong DG, Goodney PP, Hamburg NM, Kirksey L, Lancaster KJ, et al. Health disparities in peripheral artery disease: a scientific statement from the American Heart Association. Circulation. 2023;148(3):286–96.
77. Bakas T, McCarthy MJ, Miller EL. Systematic review of the evidence for stroke family caregiver and dyad interventions. Stroke. 2022;53(6):2093–102.
78. Gaffey AE, Harris KM, Mena-Hurtado C, Sinha R, Jacoby DL, Smolderen KG. The Yale roadmap for health psychology and integrated cardiovascular care. Health Psychol. 2022;41(10):779–91.
79. Cleary CM, Adajian A, Gifford ED, Orosco E, Li YH, Healy L, et al. Incentives and individualized coaching improve completion rates of supervised exercise therapy for claudication. J Vasc Surg. 2024;80(3):821–30 e3.
80. Aalami OO, Lin J, Savage D, Ho V, Bertges D, Corriere M. Use of an app-based exercise therapy program including cognitive-behavioral techniques for the management of intermittent claudication. J Vasc Surg. 2022;76(6):1651–6 e1.
81. Abaraogu UO, Dall P, Seenan C, Rhodes S, Gorely T, McParland J, et al. Effect of behavior-change interventions on daily physical activity in patients with intermittent claudication: the OPTIMA systematic review with meta-analysis. Eur J Prev Cardiol. 2024;32(2):156–68.
82. Collins T, Lunos S. Home-based walking therapy improves walking ability and quality of life in persons with diabetes mellitus and peripheral arterial disease. Vasc Med. 2010;15(2):155.

Exercise Therapy for Peripheral Artery Disease: Mechanisms, Outcomes, and Optimal Methods

12

Mary M. McDermott

Walking exercise is first-line therapy for intermittent claudication due to lower extremity peripheral artery disease (PAD) [1–3]. PAD is defined by atherosclerotic blockages of the arteries supplying the legs and affects approximately 10–15% of people aged 65 and older [4, 5]. The number of people living with PAD is likely increasing, as older people live longer with chronic disease [3]. PAD is characterized by lower extremity ischemia during walking activity, when demand for oxygen in lower extremity muscles exceeds oxygen supply. Lower extremity ischemia during walking activity typically results in leg tightness, pain, cramping, or weakness. These symptoms typically resolve within 10 min of rest, when oxygen supply meets demand.

People with PAD have greater functional impairment, more rapid functional decline, and faster mobility loss than those without PAD [6–12]. Among 666 people (412 with PAD) in the Walking and Leg Circulation Study (WALCS), those with severe PAD were 4.2 times more likely and those with mild PAD were 3.2 times more likely to become unable to walk ¼ mile or climb a flight of stairs without assistance at 5-year follow-up, compared to age-matched controls without PAD, adjusting for comorbidities and other confounders [10]. Even people with PAD who report no exertional leg symptoms have greater walking impairment and faster rates of walking decline, compared to age-matched people without PAD [6, 7, 9].

Few medications have been identified that improve walking performance in people with intermittent claudication due to PAD [2]. Cilostazol, a phosphodiesterase 3 inhibitor, is the only drug that is both FDA approved and recommended by clinical practice guidelines [1, 2]. Cilostazol has a modest effect on walking performance and is frequently discontinued due to adverse effects, such as palpitations, headache, and diarrhea [1, 2, 13–16]. Walking exercise is the most effective non-invasive therapy for improving walking impairment in people with intermittent claudication

M. M. McDermott (✉)
Feinberg School of Medicine, Northwestern University, Chicago, IL, USA
e-mail: mdm608@northwestern.edu

W. P. Robinson III, J. P. Simons (eds.), *The Patient-Centered Approach to Claudication*, https://doi.org/10.1007/978-3-032-02460-2_12

[1, 2]. Supervised treadmill walking exercise has been considered the most effective medical therapy for claudication, based on multiple randomized clinical trials demonstrating benefits of supervised exercise for claudication [17–24]. Based on evidence of benefit in multiple clinical trials, in 2017 the Center for Medicare Services (CMS) agreed to cover supervised exercise for people with intermittent claudication due to PAD [25]. However, few people participate in CMS covered supervised exercise [26–29]. Furthermore, while CMS covers up to 24 weeks of exercise, supervised exercise does not have a persistent benefit on walking performance in PAD [30]. While advising people with claudication to walk for exercise at home in an unsupervised setting has not demonstrated significant benefit, multiple randomized clinical trials that incorporate behavioral methods to help people adhere to consistent home-based exercise have demonstrated significant benefit on walking performance for people with PAD [23, 24, 31–34]. This review summarizes current evidence regarding optimal exercise interventions to improve walking performance in people with intermittent claudication due to PAD. Mechanisms of walking exercise are also reviewed.

Supervised Exercise for Intermittent Claudication Due to PAD

Overview

Supervised exercise for claudication typically consists of walking for exercise on a treadmill for up to 60 min per session, three times a week, at an exercise center or rehabilitation facility under the supervision of a physician, advanced practice clinician, exercise physiologist or a Registered Nurse [35–37]. Results of more than 30 randomized clinical trials have tested the effects of supervised walking exercise on walking performance in people with claudication. In a meta-analysis of 25 randomized clinical trials of supervised walking exercise that included 1054 people with PAD, compared to a non-exercise control group, supervised walking exercise was associated with significantly improved maximum treadmill walking distance [+180 m (95% CI: +130, +230 m)] and with significantly improved pain-free treadmill walking distance [+128 m (95% CI: +92, +165 m)] [17]. Supervised treadmill exercise is particularly effective for improving treadmill walking performance and some of the effects of supervised treadmill exercise on treadmill walking performance are due to a learning effect on the treadmill walking outcome, since supervised treadmill exercise is performed on a treadmill [38, 39]. However, relatively few clinical trials of supervised exercise have included the 6-min walk test as an outcome measure [17, 18]. Of the clinical trials that included the 6-min walk test as an outcome measure, the typical effect of supervised treadmill exercise on improved 6-min walk has been approximately 30–35 m, consistent with a large clinically important effect [20–22, 39]. Effects of supervised treadmill exercise on patient-reported outcomes or quality of life measures have been less consistent, with variable effects of supervised walking exercise on patient-reported outcome measures in people with claudication [20–24, 40]. Effects of supervised treadmill exercise on physical activity levels in people with claudication remain unclear. In a network meta-analysis of eight randomized clinical trials that included 656 patients with claudication, supervised exercise therapy increased daily physical activity by 803 steps/day, measured by a pedometer, compared to control [41]. However, the included randomized clinical trials were of moderate quality [41]. A randomized clinical trial of 156 participants with PAD demonstrated significant effects of supervised treadmill exercise on 6-min walk distance and treadmill walking distance, but had no effect on daily physical activity, compared to a control group that did not exercise [20]. Overall, supervised treadmill exercise significantly improves treadmill walking performance in people with symptomatic PAD, compared to a non-exercise control group, but effects on quality of life and physical activity are less consistent and less clear [20–24, 36]. In addition, some of the large effects of supervised treadmill walking on the treadmill walking outcome are due to a learning effect associated with a "training to the outcome measure" for the treadmill walking outcome [38, 39].

CMS Coverage of Supervised Exercise for People with Intermittent Claudication Due to PAD

Based on clinical trial evidence showing significant benefits of supervised treadmill exercise for people with claudication, the Center for Medicare and Medicaid Services (CMS) published a decision memorandum in 2017, describing their intention to cover supervised exercise therapy for symptomatic PAD [24]. Medicare currently covers three supervised exercise sessions per week lasting 30–60 min per session for a duration of 12 weeks (i.e., a total of 36 exercise sessions) [25, 35]. In order to cover exercise rehabilitation for PAD, CMS requires that patients have a face-to-face meeting with a physician to obtain the referral. CMS also requires that the exercise facility be located in a hospital or outpatient hospital setting, that the exercise intervention be delivered by qualified personnel (such as an exercise physiologist or nurse) with training in exercise therapy for patients with PAD, and that the exercise program must be carried out under direct physician supervision [25, 35]. Exercise covered by Medicare can consist of any supervised exercise activity, so long as the exercise is supervised and takes place at a physician office or medical center or hospital. If a patient with claudication completes the 12 weeks of Medicare-covered exercise and continues to report ischemic leg symptoms with walking, a second referral can be provided by a physician [25, 35]. Medicare will pay for a second set of 36 sessions of supervised walking exercise. In contrast to the first referral, the second set of 36 sessions are not required to take place over a 12-week period, but can occur over a longer time period. Medicare will not authorize additional referrals beyond these two referrals. The Medicare-covered supervised exercise includes a co-pay of approximately $11 per session, which can be difficult for many patients to afford [27]. For patients who take part in all 36 sessions, the total co-payment is $396.

Despite Medicare coverage for supervised treadmill exercise, few people with claudication participate in supervised treadmill exercise. In a Medicare Claims Database study of 129,699 people with PAD-related intermittent claudication treated between June 1, 2017 and December 31, 2018, only 1735 (1.3%) enrolled in supervised treadmill exercise covered by CMS [26]. Of the 1735 who began CMS covered supervised exercise, only 89 (5.1%) completed all 36 sessions covered by Medicare [26].

Optimal Methods for Supervised Treadmill Exercise in Intermittent Claudication Due to PAD

Relatively few clinical trials have studied optimal methods of supervised treadmill exercise in people with PAD. However, effective supervised exercise programs have typically instructed patients to walk for exercise at a pace that induces ischemic leg symptoms within 10 min of each "bout" or "episode" of exercise and advised patients to walk to maximal ischemic leg symptoms during each exercise "bout" or episode [20–24]. Patients should be instructed to rest when ischemic leg symptoms reach a 4 or 5 on a 1–5 Likert scale, where 5 is the worst possible pain. Once leg symptoms abate during rest, the participant should be advised to begin a new bout of walking exercise. The treadmill walking speed and the treadmill incline should be increased gradually, as the patient improves, in order to attain near-maximal ischemic leg symptoms within 10 min of onset of each bout of walking. Supervised treadmill exercise interventions should be tailored to each patient's walking ability. Patients may need to begin at a walking speed as low as 0.50 miles per hour, depending on their ability, and may be able to begin with only about 20 min of walking exercise, depending on their ability. In a 12-week walking exercise program, the treadmill speed or treadmill incline should be increased at least once weekly to ensure that the patient is walking at a sufficient intensity to experience moderate to severe ischemic leg symptoms within 10 min of each bout of exercise. If the participant is able to walk for more than 10 min without significant ischemic leg symptoms, the walking speed or treadmill incline should be increased for the next bout of exercise [37].

Helping Patients with Claudication Attain Realistic Expectations About Benefits of Exercise

In contrast to lower extremity revascularization, a walking exercise intervention has gradual effects on improvement in walking ability in people with intermittent claudication due to PAD [42]. Prior work showed that approximately 8 weeks of supervised treadmill exercise were required before large and statistically significant improvement in treadmill walking distances were observed [43]. Many patients with claudication are not aware that the benefits of walking exercise can require weeks before they have noticeable effects on walking ability. The gradual effect of walking exercise on improvement in walking distance should be discussed with patients, so that their expectations align with their likely trajectory of improvement in walking ability. Furthermore, the benefits of walking exercise are not durable, after the walking exercise is discontinued. Patients should be advised to continue walking exercise, once coverage of supervised exercise ends.

Barriers to Participation in Supervised Treadmill Exercise

Even among the small number of patients with PAD who obtain a referral for supervised exercise, adherence rates to supervised exercise are low, with fewer than 5% of patients completing all 36 walking exercise sessions covered by Medicare [26]. Potential barriers explaining the low participation rates in supervised exercise programs by these patients include: lack of physician referrals, inadequate availability of supervised exercise programs, cost and burden associated with travel to an exercise facility, and the $11 copay per exercise session for supervised exercise covered by CMS [27–29].

In an online questionnaire completed by 135 US vascular surgeons, cardiologists, and vascular medicine physicians that included at least one physician from all 50 states, 54% of physicians reported that they did not have a supervised exercise program at their institution, and 5% were uncertain whether their institution had a supervised exercise program available for PAD [28]. Forty-nine percent of physicians had never referred a patient with claudication to supervised exercise, and 26% were not aware that CMS covered supervised treadmill exercise [28]. While this study demonstrated poor availability of supervised exercise programs and poor physician awareness of CMS supervised exercise coverage for claudication in the United States, the study was limited by a questionnaire response rate of 15%. In a questionnaire of 489 people with PAD from the Chicago area, 357 (73.2%) people reported willingness to travel to an exercise facility three times per week for supervised exercise but of these 357, only 214 (59.9%) reported that they would be willing and able to pay the $11 CMS copay required by Medicare for each exercise session [27]. Additional study documented that people with claudication were unwilling or unable to participate in supervised exercise even when there were no monetary costs for exercise participation [29]. Many people with claudication find that participating in supervised exercise is burdensome and difficult, in part because of lack of interest in traveling for exercise or presence of comorbid illnesses that made exercise difficult [20]. Post-hoc results from 2 randomized clinical trials of supervised treadmill exercise that included 366 participants with PAD reported a mean attendance rate of 75% over a 6-month period of supervised exercise, even though transportation to the exercise facility was provided and exercise costs were paid by the research study [44].

Home-Based Walking Exercise

Home-based exercise is typically defined as walking exercise that takes place outside of a medical center, often in, around, or near a patient's home, without the physical presence of a coach. Compared to supervised exercise, advantages of home-based walking exercise include the greater convenience of exercise that takes place in or near home, flexibility associated with the ability to walk for exercise at a time and location most convenient for the patient, and absence of expenses associated with the insurance co-pay, rehabilitation facility, or an in-person coach.

In 2024, the AHA/ACC clinical practice guidelines designated home-based (termed "community-based") exercise as a Class I recommendation, determining for the first time that home-based (i.e., community-based) exercise is a first-line therapy for intermittent claudication due to PAD, based on evidence from multiple randomized clinical trials demonstrating significant benefit of home-based exercise to improve walking performance in people with PAD. In the 2024 AHA/ACC practice guidelines, supervised and home-based walking exercise were each recommended as a first-line therapy for PAD-related walking impairment [2]. Even though supervised exercise and home-based exercise are each designated first-line therapy for PAD, home-based exercise has traditionally been considered less effective than supervised exercise to improve walking performance in people with claudication. This bias favoring supervised exercise may have started with the 2006 AHA/ACC clinical practice guidelines which stated that there was "no evidence" for advising patients with PAD to "go home and walk" [45]. Since the 2006 practice guidelines were published, multiple randomized clinical trials have been completed that tested the hypothesis that home-based exercise improves walking performance in people with claudication. The home-based exercise interventions in these clinical trials have typically featured a coach who meets once weekly or less frequently with the participants or contacts them by telephone to encourage regular walking exercise at home [31–34, 46–48]. However, randomized clinical trials of home-based exercise interventions for patients with claudication have yielded mixed results, with several randomized clinical trials demonstrating significant and meaningful benefit, while others showed no beneficial effect of home-based exercise for claudication [31–34, 46–48]. The mixed results of these randomized clinical trials are likely due to the fact that home-based exercise interventions for PAD have varied between clinical trials, differing with regard to frequency and type of intervention, coach interactions, the degree to which behavioral change methods are incorporated, and the use of devices, such as step counters or other activity devices, to monitor walking exercise activity [31–34, 46–48]. In contrast, supervised treadmill exercise interventions for claudication have been consistent with regard to the nature of the intervention and consistent regarding their benefits. The homogeneity of the typical supervised treadmill exercise intervention has likely contributed to the inconsistency of observed benefits of supervised treadmill exercise for claudication [49]. Additionally, the use of maximal treadmill walking distance as the primary outcome for most clinical trials of supervised exercise has also likely accentuated the benefits of supervised treadmill exercise for claudication, due to a "training to the outcome

Table 12.1 Characteristics of supervised and home-based exercise for intermittent claudication due to peripheral artery disease

	Supervised walking exercise	Home-based walking exercise
Definition	Walking exercise that takes place at a medical center in the presence of a coach	Walking exercise in or outside of the home that takes place without the physical presence of a coach. Also referred to as community-based exercise
2024 AHA/ACC clinical practice guideline recommendation	Class I, Level of Evidence A	Class I, Level of Evidence A
Typical efficacy	Preferentially improves treadmill walking distance. Improves treadmill walking distance by about 180 m and 6-min walk by about 30–35 m, compared to control	Preferentially improves overground walking. The most effective home-based exercise interventions improve 6-min walk by 45 to approximately 54 m. Home-based exercise improves treadmill walking distance, but to a lesser degree than supervised exercise
Insurance coverage	Covered by many insurance companies, including Medicare	Not covered by insurance typically
Proposed optimal methods	Three times weekly exercise, conducted at an intensity that induces ischemic leg symptoms within 10 min of the start of exercise. Treadmill speed and grade should be increased as needed to ensure ischemic leg symptoms during exercise	Five times weekly exercise should be conducted, working up to 50 min of exercise per session. Walking exercise should be conducted at a pace inducing ischemic leg symptoms within 10 min of each bout of exercise

measure" effect [49]. Growing evidence suggests that home-based exercise has the potential to be highly potent for improving walking performance (Table 12.1).

Effective Home-Based Exercise Interventions for People with Intermittent Claudication Due to PAD

Since 2011, at least eight randomized clinical trials of home-based exercise with sample sizes of more than 100 people with PAD have been published [22, 23, 31, 32, 34, 46–48]. Results of these trials were mixed, with some showing no benefit of home-based exercise on walking impairment in claudication and others demonstrating large gains of up to 41–53 m improvement in 6-min walk distance, compared to a non-exercise control group [22, 23, 31, 32, 34, 46–48]. Four clinical trials that demonstrated meaningful effects of home-based walking exercise on walking performance are summarized below.

Gardner et al. published results from two randomized clinical trials that demonstrated significant and meaningful benefits of home-based walking exercise on walking performance in patients with claudication due to PAD. In the first clinical trial, 119 people with intermittent claudication were randomized to either supervised treadmill exercise, home-based walking exercise, or attention control for 12 weeks. The supervised treadmill exercise group attended treadmill exercise sessions 3 times weekly and walked for exercise on the treadmill for up to 40 min per session. The home-based exercise group was asked to walk for exercise around their home three times per week at a self-guided pace, working up to 45 min of walking exercise per exercise session. Participants randomized to home-based walking exercise received a step counter to objectively monitor their exercise activity and met with a coach every 2–4 weeks to receive feedback about their exercise activity recorded on their activity monitor. At 12-week follow-up, peak treadmill walking time significantly improved by 215 s in the supervised exercise group and by 124 s in the home-based exercise group, but declined by 10 s in the control group. At 12-week follow-up, pain-free treadmill walking time significantly improved by 165 s in the supervised exercise group and by 134 s in the home-based exercise group, but declined by 16 s in the control group. Supervised treadmill exercise and home-based walking exercise each improved peak treadmill walking time and pain-free treadmill walking time significantly more than the control group, and effects of supervised treadmill exercise did not significantly differ from the effects of home-based exercise on walking performance. In a second clinical trial, Gardner et al. randomized 180 patients with claudication due to PAD to home-based walking exercise, supervised treadmill exercise, or a control group for 12 weeks [24]. At 12-week follow-up, the supervised treadmill exercise and home-based exercise groups each significantly improved pain-free treadmill walking time and maximal treadmill walking time, compared to the control group. At 12-week follow-up, the home-based exercise group significantly improved 6-min walk distance by 45 m, while the supervised treadmill exercise group improved 6-min walk by 15 m, and the control group improved 6-min walk by 4 m. The home-based walking exercise group significantly improved the 6-min walk more than both the control group and the supervised treadmill exercise group, respectively [24]. The supervised treadmill exercise group did not significantly improve 6-min walk distance, compared to the control group. This clinical trial suggested, for the first time, that home-based exercise may be better than supervised exercise for improving 6-min walk distance. This finding was surprising because of prior work suggesting that supervised treadmill exercise significantly and consistently improved treadmill walking performance more than home-based exercise [50]. This result was likely in part due to a "training to the outcome measure" phenomenon, in which patients who walk for exercise on the treadmill specifically improve their treadmill walking ability [38, 39].

McDermott et al. also published results from two separate randomized clinical trials of home-based walking exercise, demonstrating large effects of the home-based walking exercise intervention on 6-min walk distance. In the GOALS Trial, 194 people with claudication due to PAD were randomized into one of two parallel groups: a Group Mediated Cognitive Behavioral (GMCB) intervention or an attention control group [31]. The GMCB intervention consisted of weekly in-person meetings with other PAD participants and a coach, during which group support and behavioral change methods were discussed, to help participants adhere to home-based exercise [31]. Participants in the GMCB group were advised to walk for exercise in or around their home five times weekly, working up to 50 min of exercise per session, when possible. Participants in the attention control group met weekly with other PAD participants for a lecture about a health topic not related to exercise. At 6-month follow-up, the GMCB intervention improved 6-min walk by 53.5 m (95% CI: 33.2, 73.8, $P < 0.001$), compared to the attention control group. The GMCB intervention also significantly improved accelerometer-measured physical activity over 7 days, treadmill walking time, and patient-reported outcomes, including the Walking Impairment Questionnaire distance score and the Walking Impairment Questionnaire speed score. A second clinical trial by McDermott MM et al. that included 305 participants with claudication due to PAD demonstrated that walking for exercise at a pace inducing ischemic leg symptoms was necessary to improve 6-min walk and treadmill walking distance. In this clinical trial, the 305 participants from four cities in the United States were randomized to home-based walking exercise at a pace inducing ischemic leg symptoms (high-intensity exercise), home-based walking exercise at a comfortable pace without ischemic leg symptoms (low-intensity exercise), or an attention control group for 12 months [34]. The two exercise groups received weekly telephone calls from the same coach who provided support and advice, using behavioral methods, to help participants walk for exercise five times weekly for up to 50 min per session if possible. The high-intensity group was advised to walk for exercise at a pace inducing ischemic leg symptoms, while the low-intensity group was advised to walk for exercise at a comfortable pace without ischemic leg symptoms. The attention control group received weekly telephone calls with information about health topics not related to exercise. The median intensity of exercise, measured by accelerometer, was 728 activity units in the low-intensity exercise group vs. 1584 activity units in the high-intensity exercise group ($P < 0.001$). Over the 12-month intervention, although both exercise groups were advised to walk for exercise five times weekly, working up to 50 min of exercise per session, the low-intensity group exercised more days per week (3.5 vs. 2.8) and for more minutes per week (145 vs. 77 min), compared to the high-intensity exercise group. At 12-month follow-up, the high-intensity exercise group significantly improved 6-min walk distance more than the low-intensity group (difference: +40.9 m) and more than the control group (+49.6 m) [34]. The LITE clinical trial demonstrated the importance of walking for exercise at a high-intensity pace that induces ischemic leg symptoms, in order to attain benefit from a home-based exercise walking intervention.

While Gardner et al. and McDermott et al. each reported that home-based exercise improved 6-min walk by 41–53.5 m, compared to a control group that did not exercise, in interventions ranging from 12-week to 12-month durations, several other randomized clinical trials demonstrated either smaller effects of home-based exercise on 6-min walk or no effect of home-based exercise on 6-min walk [32, 46–48]. For example, Bearne et al. reported that a 12-week home-based exercise intervention improved 6-min walk by a relatively modest and statistically significant 16.7 m, while other trials have failed to demonstrate significant beneficial effects of home-based exercise on 6-min walk distance [32, 46–48]. These heterogeneous effects likely have contributed to confusion about whether home-based exercise is effective and also about the most optimal home-based exercise program to improve walking distance in claudication [49].

A recent meta-analysis of 23 studies with 1907 participants with PAD reported that home-based walking exercise interventions that incorporated more frequent monitoring of exercise activity by a coach, that emphasized walking exercise at least three times weekly, and that were designed to encourage walking for exercise at moderate or maximum ischemic pain were associated with greater benefit than home-based walking exercise interventions without these characteristics [51]. However, further studies are needed to define the optimal home-based exercise intervention for improving walking performance. Further study is also needed to evaluate whether some individuals benefit more from supervised, compared to home-based exercise and vice versa.

Relative Effects of Home-Based Walking Exercise, Compared to Supervised Exercise for Intermittent Claudication Due to PAD

Based on the 2024 AHA/ACC guidelines, either home-based or supervised exercise could be recommended as first-line for people with claudication. Few data are available regarding direct comparisons of highly potent home-based exercise interventions with supervised exercise interventions. Gardner et al. reported that home-based exercise improved the 6-min walk significantly more than supervised exercise in people with claudication [24]. An individual participant data meta-analysis of 719 participants from 3 clinical trials of supervised treadmill exercise and 2 clinical trials of home-based walking exercise reported that supervised treadmill exercise and home-based walking exercise were each associated with significantly improved 6-min walk distance, maximum treadmill walking distance, and pain-free treadmill walking distance, compared to attention control [40]. In this meta-analysis, the magnitude of effect of supervised treadmill exercise, compared to control, was less than the magnitude of effect of home-based exercise compared to control for the outcome of improvement in 6-min walk distance [−23.1 m (95% CI: −43.9, −3.6)] [40]. In comparison, supervised treadmill exercise, compared to control, was associated with a greater magnitude of benefit for the outcome of maximal treadmill walking distance [+132.5 m (95% CI: 72.1, 192.9)] [40]. These results suggest that home-based walking exercise preferentially has greater effects on improving 6-min walk distance, compared to supervised treadmill exercise, while supervised treadmill exercise preferentially improves treadmill walking performance, compared to home-based walking exercise [40]. Compared to control, effects of home-based exercise on patient-reported outcomes were greater than effects of supervised exercise, but further study is needed that directly compares supervised and home-based exercise on patient-reported outcomes in patients with claudication.

Biologic Pathway by Which Walking Exercise Improves Walking Performance in Intermittent Claudication Due to PAD

Despite the fact that walking exercise is the most effective non-invasive therapy for claudication, the biologic pathways responsible for the benefits of exercise remain largely unknown. Identifying the biologic pathways by which walking exercise improves walking performance is likely to help identify targets for future drug therapies for PAD-related walking impairment. Walking exercise does not alter atherosclerotic plaque or change the ankle brachial index. While multiple hypothesized biologic mechanisms by which exercise improves walking performance in claudication have been proposed, there is no definitive evidence for any proposed mechanism [52, 53]. Potential biologic pathways by which walking exercise may improve walking performance include effects of exercise to increase capillary density, improve lower extremity perfusion, favorably alter walking mechanics via a more efficient gait, improve mitochondrial activity and biogenesis, reduce blood viscosity, and increase eNOS activity and plasma nitrite abundance [52, 53, 54, 55]. Exercise may also increase lower extremity myofiber quality and quantity.

Lower Extremity Exercise and Mitochondrial Activity in Intermittent Claudication Due to PAD

Preliminary evidence suggests that exercise may increase citrate synthase, a measure of mitochondrial abundance and activity, in lower extremity skeletal muscle of people with intermittent claudication due to PAD. For example, Van Schaardenburgh et al. randomized 29 PAD patients to either home-based calf raise exercise with ischemic pain ($N = 14$) or home-based walking exercise conducted 3× weekly for 30 min per session ($N = 15$) [54]. At 8-week follow-up, both exercise groups improved pain-free and maximal treadmill walking time, but improvement in treadmill walking time was statistically significant only in those randomized to calf raises [54]. Results of lower extremity muscle biopsies showed that citrate synthase, a measure of mitochondrial abundance and activity, significantly increased in the calf raise group ($P = 0.02$), but not in the group randomized to walking exercise ($P = 0.10$) [54]. The small sample size may have limited statistical power to detect a significant improvement in the group randomized to walking exercise. However, other measures of improved mitochondrial activity, such as measures of mitochondrial Complex I and Complex I + II, did not improve in either exercise group [54].

Walking Exercise and Capillary Density

Currently, there is no high-quality evidence from clinical trials that walking exercise improves capillary density in lower extremity muscle, compared to a non-exercise control group. In one randomized clinical trial of 35 PAD participants randomized to either supervised treadmill exercise or simply advice to walk for exercise at home for 12 weeks, supervised exercise significantly increased gastrocnemius muscle biopsy capillary density from 216 to 286 capillaries/mm^2 and also improved treadmill walking distance among those randomized to supervised treadmill exercise [55]. In contrast, the advice to walk for exercise at home did not improve capillary density or treadmill walking distance. However, there were no statistically significant differences in change in capillary density between those randomized to supervised treadmill exercise vs. advice to walk for exercise at home. Vascular endothelial growth factor (VEGF-A), which stimulates angiogenesis, did not significantly increase in the gastrocnemius muscle biopsy lysates [56]. In contrast, vascular endothelial growth factor $(VEGF)_{165}b$, an antiangiogenic factor, increased in the gastrocnemius muscle biopsy lysates [56]. A randomized clinical trial of lower extremity resistance training for 24 weeks in 20 participants with claudication significantly improved 6-min walk distance, gastrocnemius muscle Type I fiber area, gastrocnemius muscle Type II fiber area, and capillary density, compared to a control group that did not exercise [57]. Given that strength training is less effective than walking exercise for claudication, the significance of these findings is unclear.

Walking Exercise, eNOS Activity, and Plasma Nitrite

Walking exercise may stimulate endothelial nitric oxide synthase (eNOS) production of nitric oxide through increased arterial shear stress and muscle contraction during exercise. The nitric oxide produced by eNOS during exercise is partially oxidized to nitrite, a biomarker for eNOS-dependent nitric oxide bioavailability. Change in plasma nitrite levels between the beginning and end of a maximal exercise test, Δ nitrite, measures the net bioavailability of nitric oxide during exercise, reflecting both eNOS production of nitric oxide during exercise and consumption of nitric oxide by oxidative stress. The biomarker Δ nitrite is significantly reduced in untrained people with PAD, compared to untrained people without PAD, and preliminary evidence suggests that exercise training increases nitric oxide bioavailability, most likely through adaptations that increase nitric oxide production by eNOS and reduce nitric oxide consumption by oxidative stress [58]. In 21 untrained people without cardiovascular disease, plasma nitrite levels between the beginning and end of a maximal exercise stress test (i.e., Δ nitrite) increased by 39.3%, but declined by 44.2% in 28 untrained people with PAD [59]. In 14 people with PAD who engaged in 12 weeks of supervised exercise, Δ nitrite increased by 33% (from −28% to +6.6%) between baseline and 12-week follow-up, indicating improved nitric oxide bioavailability during exercise activity after 12 weeks of a supervised exercise intervention [58]. Greater increases in Δ nitrite were associated with greater improvement in pain-free treadmill walking time in response to exercise (R squared: +0.59, $P < 0.001$) [58]. Despite these promising findings, overall, the biologic pathway by which exercise improves walking performance in claudication remains unclear.

Exercise Interventions Other Than Walking for People with Intermittent Claudication Due to PAD

Randomized clinical trials of modest size have consistently reported that upper and lower extremity ergometry, consisting of cycling with the arms and legs, respectively, can improve walking performance in people with intermittent claudication due to PAD [60–62]. For example, in a clinical trial of 104 people randomized to either upper extremity ergometry, lower extremity ergometry, or a non-exercise control for 6 months, the upper extremity ergometry group improved pain-free walking distance by 51% and the lower extremity ergometry group improved pain-free walking distance by 57%, compared to the non-exercise control group [60]. Exercise interventions occurred twice weekly and consisted of ten cycles of 2-min bouts of arm or leg cycling ergometry alternating with 2-min rest periods. The upper extremity ergometry group increased maximal treadmill walking distance by 29% and the lower extremity ergometry group increased maximal treadmill walking distance by 31%, compared to the control group ($P < 0.001$ for each comparison). These results were consistent with other randomized clinical trials of upper and lower extremity ergometry for improving walking performance in people with PAD [62–63].

Resistance Training for Intermittent Claudication Due to PAD

People with PAD have reduced lower extremity muscle area and abnormalities in mitochondrial activity and structure in lower extremity skeletal muscle. Lower extremity resistance training may improve walking performance in people with claudication, but randomized clinical trial evidence shows a smaller effect of resistance training on walking performance, compared to walking exercise [20, 63]. In a clinical trial of 156 people with claudication who were randomized to supervised treadmill exercise, supervised lower extremity resistance training, or attention control for 6-months, supervised treadmill exercise increased 6-min walk by 35.9 m (95% CI: +15.3, +56.5, $P < 0.001$), compared to control, and resistance training improved 6-min walk by 12.4 m (95% CI: −8.4, +33.3, $P = 0.24$), compared to control [20]. In this trial, lower extremity resistance training consisted of three sessions per week with a trainer and included 3 sets of 8 repetitions of leg curls, leg press, and knee extension exercises, with weights increased as tolerated during the clinical trial [20]. In a systematic review and meta-analysis that studied the effect of resistance training on improvements in treadmill walking and 6-min walk distance in claudication and included 17 randomized clinical trials with 826 participants, resistance training significantly improved treadmill walking distance [standard mean difference 0.45 (95% CI: 0.23, 0.79)] but did not significantly improve 6-min walk distance [mean difference +25.6 m, (95% CI: −3.1, +54.2)] compared to control [63]. In this meta-analysis, the two largest studies, including the clinical trial by McDermott et al. with 156 participants, showed no effect of resistance training on 6-min walk distance, compared to control [20, 63]. Overall, clinical trial evidence suggests that walking exercise is a more effective exercise intervention in claudication than resistance training (Table 12.2).

Table 12.2 Summary of clinical trials of effective home-based exercise interventions for intermittent claudication due to peripheral artery disease

	Sample size	Duration	Intervention	Result
Gardner et al. [23]	119	12 weeks	Participants were randomized to supervised treadmill exercise, home-based walking exercise, or a non-exercise control. The home-based walking exercise group was asked to walk three sessions/week for up to 45 min/session. A step counter monitored the home-based walking exercise activity, and participants randomized to home-based exercise received feedback from an in-person coach every 2–4 weeks	Peak treadmill walking time improved by 215 s in the supervised exercise group, by 124 s in the home-based exercise group, and declined by 10 s in the control group. Improvements in the supervised and home-based exercise were significantly greater than the control
McDermott et al. [31]	194	Six months	Participants were randomized to a home-based walking exercise intervention, consisting of a group mediated cognitive behavioral (GMCB) intervention, consisting of weekly in-person meetings with other PAD participants and a coach. Participants were asked to walk for exercise at home 5 days/week working up to 50 min/session. Behavioral change principles, such as group support, goal-setting, self-efficacy building, and self-monitoring were used in the intervention group	At 6-month follow-up, the GMCB intervention improved 6-min walk by 53.5 m (95% CI: 33.2, 73.8, $P < 0.001$), compared to the attention control group. The exercise intervention also significantly improved patient-reported outcomes and treadmill walking and physical activity, compared to the control group

(continued)

Table 12.2 (continued)

	Sample size	Duration	Intervention	Result
Gardner et al. [24]	180	12 weeks	Participants were randomized to supervised treadmill exercise, home-based walking exercise, or a non-exercise control. The home-based walking exercise group was asked to walk three sessions/week for up to 45 min/session. A step counter monitored the home-based walking exercise activity, and participants randomized to home-based exercise received feedback from an in-person coach every 2–4 weeks	Supervised exercise improved 6-min walk by 15 m; home-based exercise improved 6-min walk by 45 m, and the control group improved 6-min walk by 4 m. Home-based exercise improved 6-min walk significantly more than the supervised exercise group and significantly more than the control group
McDermott et al. [34]	305	12 months	Participants were randomized to walking exercise at a pace inducing ischemic leg symptoms (high intensity), walking exercise at a comfortable pace without ischemic leg symptoms (low intensity) or a control group that did not exercise. Participants received weekly telephone calls from a coach and wore an ActiGraph accelerometer to monitor exercise intensity. Behavioral change principles, such as goal-setting, self-efficacy building, and self-monitoring, were used in the intervention group	The high-intensity exercise group significantly improved 6-min walk distance more than the low-intensity group (difference: +40.9 m) and more than the control group (+49.6 m). The high-intensity exercise group improved treadmill walking time significantly more than both the low-intensity and the control group. Both the high-intensity and the low-intensity exercise group improved patient-reported outcomes more than control

(continued)

Table 12.2 (continued)

	Sample size	Duration	Intervention	Result
Bearne et al. [32]	190	3-months	Participants were randomized to either the home-based walking exercise intervention or control. The exercise intervention consisted of four in-person intervention sessions with a physical therapist, who used motivational interviewing to encourage home-based walking exercise. Behavioral principles were applied in the intervention to help participants set goals and monitor progress	At 3-month follow-up, 6-min walk increased by 16.7 m, compared to the control group

Conclusions

Walking exercise is the most effective medical intervention for improving walking impairment in people with intermittent claudication due to PAD. Both supervised walking exercise and home-based walking exercise are highly effective therapies, and both are now recommended as first-line therapy to improve walking distance in people with claudication. While CMS covers supervised exercise therapy for claudication, medical insurance currently does not cover home-based exercise and future investigation should develop an accessible infrastructure for delivering home-based exercise. Home-based walking exercise has been shown to have greater effects on improving 6-min walk distance, compared to supervised treadmill exercise, while supervised treadmill exercise preferentially improves treadmill walking performance, compared to home-based walking exercise. Biologic pathways by which exercise improves walking performance in PAD remain unclear.

References

1. Polonsky TS, McDermott MM. Lower extremity peripheral artery disease without chronic limb-threatening ischemia: a review. JAMA. 2021;325(21):2188–98.
2. Writing Committee Members: Gornik HL, Aronow HD, Goodney PP, Arya S, Brewster LP, Byrd L, Chandra V, Drachman DE, Eaves JM, Ehrman JK, Evans JN, Getchius TSD, Gutierrez JA, Hawkins BM, Hess CN, Ho KJ, Schuyler Jones W, Kim ESH, Kinlay S, Kirksey L, Kohlman-Trigoboff D, Long CA, Pollak AW, Sabri SS, Sadwin LB, Secemsky EA, Serhal M, Shishenhbor MH, Treat-Jacobson D, Wilkins LR. 2024 ACC/AHA/AACVPR/APMA/ABC/SCAI/SVM/SVN/SVS/SIR/VESS Guideline for the management of lower extremity peripheral artery disease: a report of the American College of Cardiology/American Heart Association

Joint Committee on Clinical Practice Guidelines. Circulation. 2024;149:e1313–410. https://doi.org/10.1016/jacc.2024.02.013.

3. Criqui MH, Matsushita K, Aboyans V, Hess CN, Hicks CW, et al. Lower extremity peripheral artery disease: contemporary epidemiology, management gaps, and future directions: a scientific statement from the American Heart Association. Circulation. 2021;144(9):e171–91.
4. Newman AB, Siscovick DS, Manolio TA, Polak J, Fried LP, Borhani NO, Wolfson SK. Ankle-arm index as a marker of atherosclerosis in the cardiovascular health study. Cardiovascular Heart Study (CHS) Collaborative Research Group. Circulation. 1993;88:837–45. PMID: 8353913.
5. Criqui MH, Aboyans V. Epidemiology of peripheral artery disease. Circ Res. 2015;116:1509–26.
6. McDermott MM, Fried L, Simonsick E, Ling S, Guralnik JM. Asymptomatic peripheral arterial disease is independently associated with impaired lower extremity functioning: the women's health and aging study. Circulation. 2000;101:1007–12. PMID: 10704168.
7. McDermott MM, Greenland P, Liu K, Guralnik JM, Criqui MH, Dolan NC, Chan C, Celic L, Pearce WH, Schneider JR, Sharma L, Clark E, Gibson D, Martin GJ. Leg symptoms in peripheral arterial disease: associated clinical characteristics and functional impairment. JAMA. 2001;286:1599–606. PMID: 11585483.
8. McDermott MM, Greenland P, Liu K, Guralnik JM, Celic L, Criqui MH, Chan C, Martin GJ, Schneider J, Pearce WH, Taylor LM, Clark E. The ankle brachial index is associated with leg function and physical activity: the walking and leg circulation study. Ann Intern Med. 2002;136:873–83. PMID: 12069561.
9. McDermott MM, Liu K, Greenland P, Guralnik JM, Criqui MH, Chan C, Pearce WH, Schneider JR, Ferrucci L, Celic L, Taylor LM, Vonesh E, Martin GJ, Clark E. Functional decline in peripheral arterial disease: associations with the ankle brachial index and leg symptoms. JAMA. 2004;292:453–61.
10. McDermott MM, Guralnik JM, Tian L, Liu K, Ferrucci L, Liao Y, Sharma L, Criqui MH. Associations of borderline and low normal ankle-brachial index values with functional decline at 5-year follow-up: the WALCS (walking and leg circulation study). J Am Coll Cardiol. 2009;53:1056–62. PMID: 19298919. PMCID: PMC3215766.
11. McDermott MM, Guralnik JM, Tian L, Ferrucci L, Liu K, Liao Y, Criqui MH. Baseline functional performance predicts the rate of mobility loss in persons with peripheral arterial disease. J Am Coll Cardiol. 2007;50:974–82. PMID: 17765125. PMCID: PMC2645658.
12. Gardner AW, Montgomery PS, Killewich LA. Natural history of physical function in older men with intermittent claudication. J Vasc Surg. 2004;40:73–8. PMID: 15218465.
13. Stevens JW, Simpson E, Harnan S, Squires H, Meng Y, Thomas S, Michaels J, Stansby G. Systematic review of the efficacy of cilostazol, naftidrofuryl oxalate and pentoxifylline for the treatment of intermittent claudication. Br J Surg. 2012;99:1630–8. PMID: 23034699.
14. Dawson DL, Cutler BS, Meissner MH, Strandness DE Jr. Cilostazol has beneficial effects in treatment of intermittent claudication: results from a multicenter, randomized, prospective, double-blind trial. Circulation. 1998;98:678–86. PMID: 9715861.
15. Money SR, Herd JA, Isaacsohn JL, Davidson M, Cutler B, Heckman J, Forbes WP. Effect of cilostazol on walking distances in patients with intermittent claudication caused by peripheral vascular disease. J Vasc Surg. 1998;27:267–74; discussion 274-275. PMID: 9510281.
16. Beebe HG, Dawson DL, Cutler BS, Herd JA, Strandness DE Jr, Bortey EB, Forbes WP. A new pharmacological treatment for intermittent claudication: results of a randomized, multicenter trial. Arch Intern Med. 1999;159:2041–50. PMID: 10510990.
17. Fakhry F, van de Luijtgaarden KM, Bax L, den Hoed PT, Hunink MG, Rouwet EV, et al. Supervised walking therapy in patients with intermittent claudication. J Vasc Surg. 2012;56(4):1132–42.
18. Gommans LN, Saarloos R, Scheltinga MR, Houterman S, de Bie RA, Fokkenrood HJ, et al. Editor's choice—the effect of supervision on walking distance in patients with intermittent claudication: a meta-analysis. Eur J Vasc Endovasc Surg. 2014;48(2):169–84.
19. Lane R, Harwood A, Watson L, Leng GC. Exercise for intermittent claudication. Cochrane Database Syst Rev. 2017;12(12):CD000990.

20. McDermott MM, Ades P, Guralnik JM, Dyer A, Ferrucci L, Liu K, et al. Treadmill exercise and resistance training in patients with peripheral arterial disease with and without intermittent claudication: a randomized controlled trial. JAMA. 2009;301(2):165–74.
21. McDermott MM, Ferrucci L, Tian L, Guralnik JM, Lloyd-Jones D, Kibbe MR, et al. Effect of granulocyte-macrophage colony-stimulating factor with or without supervised exercise on walking performance in patients with peripheral artery disease: the PROPEL randomized clinical trial. JAMA. 2017;318(21):2089–98.
22. McDermott MM, Bazzano L, Peterson CA, Sufit R, Ferrucci L, Domanchuk K, et al. Effect of telmisartan on walking performance in patients with lower extremity peripheral artery disease: the TELEX randomized clinical trial. JAMA. 2022;328(13):1315–25.
23. Gardner AW, Parker DE, Montgomery PS, Scott KJ, Blevins SM. Efficacy of quantified home-based exercise and supervised exercise in patients with intermittent claudication: a randomized controlled trial. Circulation. 2011;123(5):491–8.
24. Gardner AW, Parker DE, Montgomery PS, Blevins SM. Step-monitored home exercise improves ambulation, vascular function, and inflammation in symptomatic patients with peripheral artery disease: a randomized controlled trial. J Am Heart Assoc. 2014;3(5):e001107.
25. Jensen TS, Chin J, Ashby L, Schafer J, Dolan D. Proposed national coverage determination for supervised exercise therapy (SET) for symptomatic peripheral artery disease (PAD). Available from: https://www.cms.gov/medicare-coverage-database/details/nca-proposed-decision-memo.aspx?NCAId=287. Accessed 1 Jan 2025.
26. Divakaran S, Carroll BJ, Chen S, Shen C, Bonaca MP, Secemsky EA. Supervised exercise therapy for symptomatic peripheral artery disease among medicare beneficiaries between 2017 and 2018: participation rates and outcomes. Circ Cardiovasc Qual Outcomes. 2021;14(8):e007953. https://doi.org/10.1161/CIRCOUTCOMES.121.007953. Epub 2021 Jul 23. PMID: 34293930; PMCID: PMC8373731.
27. Cetlin MD, Polonsky T, Ho K, Zhang D, Tian L, Zhao L, et al. Barriers to participation in supervised exercise therapy reported by people with peripheral artery disease. J Vasc Surg. 2022;77(2):506–14.
28. Dua A, Gologorsky R, Savage D, Rens N, Gandhi N, Brooke B, et al. National assessment of availability, awareness, and utilization of supervised exercise therapy for peripheral artery disease patients with intermittent claudication. J Vasc Surg. 2020;71(5):1702–7.
29. Harwood AE, Smith GE, Cayton T, Broadbent E, Chetter IC. A systematic review of the uptake and adherence rates to supervised exercise programs in patients with intermittent claudication. Ann Vasc Surg. 2016;34:280–9.
30. McDermott MM, Kibbe MR, Guralnik JM, Ferrucci L, Criqui MH, Domanchuk K, et al. Durability of benefits from supervised treadmill exercise in people with peripheral artery disease. J Am Heart Assoc. 2019;8(1):e009380.
31. McDermott MM, Liu K, Guralnik JM, Criqui MH, Spring B, Tian L, et al. Home-based walking exercise intervention in peripheral artery disease: a randomized clinical trial. JAMA. 2013;310(1):57–65.
32. Bearne LM, Volkmer B, Peacock J, Sekhon M, Fisher G, Galea Holmes MN, et al. Effect of a home-based, walking exercise behavior change intervention vs usual care on walking in adults with peripheral artery disease: the MOSAIC randomized clinical trial. JAMA. 2022;327(14):1344–55.
33. Golledge J, Singh TP, Alahakoon C, Pinchbeck J, Yip L, Moxon JV, et al. Meta-analysis of clinical trials examining the benefit of structured home exercise in patients with peripheral artery disease. Br J Surg. 2019;106(4):319–31.
34. McDermott MM, Spring B, Tian L, Treat-Jacobson D, Ferrucci L, Lloyd-Jones D, et al. Effect of low-intensity vs high-intensity home-based walking exercise on walk distance in patients with peripheral artery disease: the LITE randomized clinical trial. JAMA. 2021;325(13):1266–76.
35. Treat-Jacobson D, McDermott MM, Beckman JA, Burt MA, Creager MA, Ehrman JK, et al. Implementation of supervised exercise therapy for patients with symptomatic peripheral artery disease: a science advisory from the American Heart Association. Circulation. 2019;140(13):e700–e10.

36. Thangada ND, McDermott MM. Exercise therapy for peripheral artery disease. Curr Cardiol Rep. 2024;26(5):405–12.
37. McDermott MM. Exercise training for intermittent claudication. J Vasc Surg. 2017;66:1612–20.
38. McDermott MM, Guralnik JM, Tian L, Zhao L, Polonsky TS, Kibbe MR, et al. Comparing 6-minute walk versus treadmill walking distance as outcomes in randomized trials of peripheral artery disease. J Vasc Surg. 2020;71(3):988–1001.
39. McDermott MM, Guralnik JM, Criqui MH, Liu K, Kibbe MR, Ferrucci L. Six-minute walk is a better outcome measure than treadmill walking tests in therapeutic trials of patients with peripheral artery disease. Circulation. 2014;130:61–8.
40. Thangada ND, Zhang D, Tian L, Zhao L, Rejeski WJ, Ho KJ, et al. Home-based walking exercise and supervised treadmill exercise in patients with peripheral artery disease: an individual participant data meta-analysis. JAMA Netw Open. 2023;6(9):e2334590.
41. van den Houten M, Hageman D, Gommans LNM, et al. The effect of supervised exercise, home-based exercise, and endovascular revascularization on physical activity in patients with intermittent claudication: A Network Meta-Analysis. Eur J Vasc Endovasc Surg. 201;58(3):383–392.
42. McDermott MM, Kibbe MR. Improving lower extremity functioning in peripheral artery disease: exercise, endovascular revascularization, or both? JAMA. 2017;317:689–90.
43. Gardner AW, Montgomery PS, Parker DE. Optimal exercise program length for patients with claudication. J Vasc Surg. 2012;55:1346–54.
44. Hammond MM, Tian L, Zhao L, Zhang D, McDermott MM. Attendance at supervised exercise sessions and walking outcomes in peripheral artery disease: results from 2 randomized clinical trials. J Am Heart Assoc. 2022;11(24):e026136.
45. Hirsch AT, Haskal ZJ, Hertzer NR, Bakal CW, Creager MA, Halperin JL, Hiratzka L, Olin JW, Puschett JB, et al. ACC/AHA 2005 Practice Guidelines for the management of patients with arterial disease (lower extremity, renal, mesenteric, and abdominal aortic aneurysm). A collaborative report from the American Association for Vascular Surgery, Society for Cardiovascular Angiography and Intervention, Society for Vascular Medicine and Biology, Society of Interventional Radiology. Circulation. 2006;113:463–654.
46. McDermott MM, Spring B, Berger JS, Treat-Jacobson D, Conte MS, Creager MA, et al. Effect of a home-based exercise intervention of wearable technology and telephone coaching on walking performance in peripheral artery disease: the HONOR randomized clinical trial. JAMA. 2018;319(16):1665–76.
47. Collins TC, Lunos S, Carlson T, Henerson K, Lightbourne M, Nelson B, Hodges JS. Effects of a home-based walking intervention on mobility and quality of life in people with diabetes and peripheral artery disease: a randomized controlled trial. Diabetes Care. 2011;23:2174–8.
48. Collins TC, Lu L, Ahluwalia JS, Nollen NL, Sirard J, Marcotte R, Post S, Zacula R. Efficacy of community-based exercise therapy among African American patients with peripheral artery disease: a randomized clinical trial. JAMA Netw Open. 2019;2(2):e187959.
49. McDermott MM. Walking exercise for peripheral artery disease. JAMA Cardiol. 2023;8(4):310–1.
50. Vermulapalli S, Dolor R, Hasselblad V, Schmitt K, Banks A, et al. Supervised vs. unsupervised exercise for intermittent claudication: a systematic review and meta-analysis. Am Heart J. 2015;69:924–37.
51. Pymer S, Ibeggazene S, Palmer J, et al. An updated systematic review and meta-analysis of home-based exercise programs for individuals with intermittent claudication. J Vasc Surg. 2021;74:2076–85.
52. Stewart KJ, Hiatt WR, Regensteiner JG, Hirsch AT. Exercise training for claudication. N Engl J Med. 2002;347:1941–51.
53. McDermott MM, Dayanidhi S, Kosmac K, et al. Walking exercise therapy effects on lower extremity skeletal muscle in peripheral artery disease. Circ Res. 2021;128:1851–67.
54. van Schaardenburgh M, Wohlwend M, Rognmo O, Mattsson EJR. Calf raise exercise increases walking performance in patients with intermittent claudication. J Vasc Surg. 2017;65:1473–82.

55. Duscha BD, Robbins JL, Jones WS, Kraus WE, Lye RJ, Sanders JM, Allen JD, Regensteiner JG, Hiatt WR, Annex BH. Angiogenesis in skeletal muscle precedes improvement in peak oxygen uptake in peripheral artery disease patients. Arterioscler Thromb Vasc Biol. 2011;31:2742–8.
56. Jones WS, Duscha BD, Robbins JL, et al. Alteration in angiogenic and anti-angiogenic forms of vascular endothelial growth factor-A in skeletal muscle of patients with intermittent claudication following exercise training. Vasc Med. 2012;17:94–100.
57. McGuigan MR, Bronks R, Newton RU, Sharman MJ, Graham JC, Cody DV, et al. Resistance training in patients with peripheral arterial disease: effects on myosin isoforms, fiber type distribution, and capillary supply to skeletal muscle. J Gerontol A Biol Sci Med Sci. 2001;56(7):B302–10.
58. Allen JD, Stabler T, Kenjale A, et al. Plasma nitrite flux predicts exercise performance in peripheral arterial disease after 3 months of exercise training. Free Radic Biol Med. 2010;49:1138–44.
59. Allen JD, Miller EM, Schwark E, Robbins JL, Duscha BD, Annex BH. Plasma nitrite response and arterial reactivity differentiate vascular health and performance. Nitric Oxide. 2009;20(4):231–7. PMID: 19371597. PMCID: PMC2676216.
60. Zwierska I, Walker RD, Choksy SA, Male JS, Pockley AG, Saxton JM. Upper- vs lower-limb aerobic exercise rehabilitation in patients with symptomatic peripheral arterial disease: a randomized controlled trial. J Vasc Surg. 2005;42(6):1122–30.
61. Tew G, Nawaz S, Zwierska I, Saxton JM. Limb-specific and cross-transfer effects of arm-crank exercise training in patients with symptomatic peripheral arterial disease. Clin Sci (Lond). 2009;117(12):405–13.
62. Bronas UG, Treat-Jacobson D, Leon AS. Comparison of the effect of upper body-ergometry aerobic training vs treadmill training on central cardiorespiratory improvement and walking distance in patients with claudication. J Vasc Surg. 2011;53(6):1557–64.
63. Parmenter BJ, Mavros Y, Ritti Dias R, King S, Fiatarone SM. Resistance training as a treatment for older persons with peripheral artery disease: a systematic review and meta-analysis. Br J Sports Med. 2020;54(8):452–61.

Aortoiliac Revascularization for Claudication: Evidence, Outcomes, and Patient Selection

13

Donna Bahroloomi and Donald T. Baril

Introduction

Aortoiliac occlusive disease (AIOD) represents the diverse range of atherosclerotic supra-inguinal vascular disease that can lead to unique debilitating claudication symptoms affecting the lower extremities, thigh and buttocks [1]. In the setting of severe stenosis or occlusion of the aortoiliac system, chronic, progressive atherosclerotic and thrombotic disease often results in severe life-changing claudication first described by Leriche and Morel as a triad of proximal claudication, sexual dysfunction, and absent femoral pulses [2]. Open surgery had previously been the gold standard treatment of severe aortoiliac disease with excellent patency rates, but carries the risk of major complications [3]. With the advent of endovascular technology and less invasive techniques, the percutaneous treatment of AIOD presents the opportunity for treatment of a wider range of patient symptoms and comorbidities with overall fewer clinical consequences, leading to evolving treatment algorithms in patients with claudication [1, 3].

Classification and Pathophysiology

In terms of anatomic lesion morphology, AIOD is primarily described by the distal extent of the disease, with Type 1 limited to the infrarenal abdominal aorta and proximal common iliac arteries, Type 2 involving the external iliac arteries, and Type 3 extending to the femoropopliteal segment [4]. The Trans-Atlantic Inter-Society Consensus (TASC) II guidelines define aortoiliac occlusions as TASC B or higher lesions [5] (Fig. 13.1). While acute occlusions of the native aortoiliac system can occur, these represent a distinct and uncommon disease process associated with

D. Bahroloomi · D. T. Baril (✉)
Division of Vascular Surgery, Cedars-Sinai Medical Center, Los Angeles, CA, USA
e-mail: Donna.Bahroloomi@cshs.org; Donald.Baril@cshs.org

W. P. Robinson III, J. P. Simons (eds.), *The Patient-Centered Approach to Claudication*, https://doi.org/10.1007/978-3-032-02460-2_13

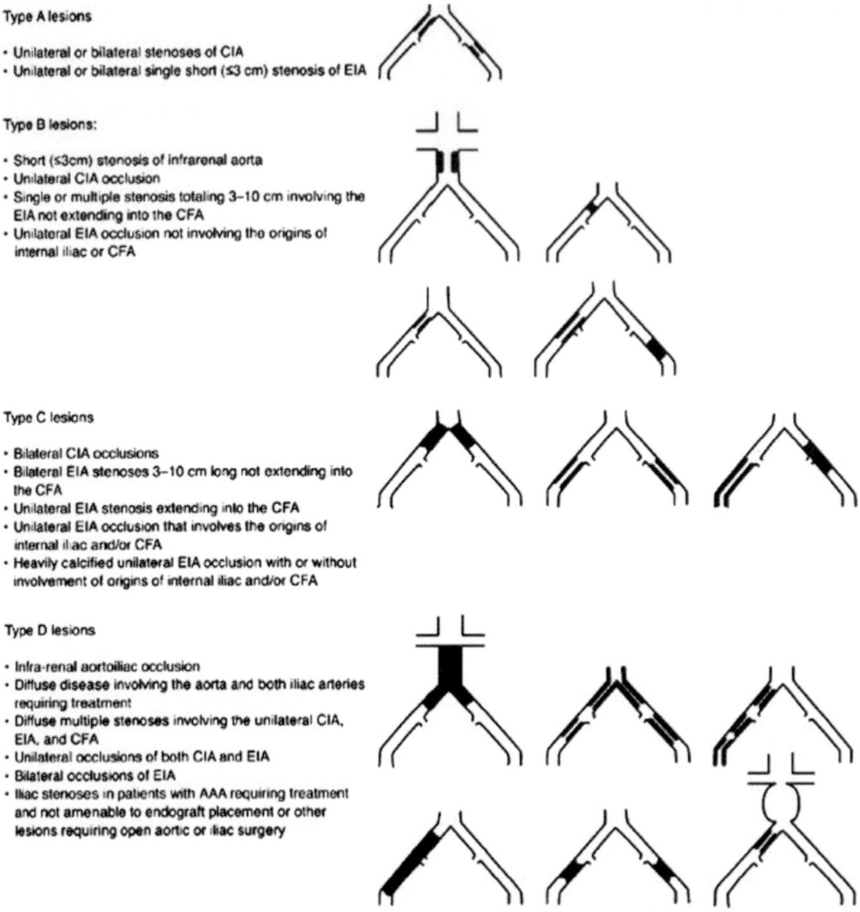

Fig. 13.1 TASC II classification of aortoiliac disease. (The-TASC-II-classification-of-aortoiliac-lesions.png 600 × 680 pixels. https://www.researchgate.net/profile/Bram-Fioole/publication/233723069/figure/fig1/AS:202597035188235@1425314305258/The-TASC-II-classification-of-aortoiliac-lesions.png)

high morbidity and mortality and unique management. Chronic occlusions, by contrast, gradually impair direct inflow to the pelvis and lower extremities, often triggering the development of extensive collateral networks [1, 6, 7]. These networks, involving systemic-systemic pathways (e.g., lumbar, intercostal, epigastric, and circumflex iliac vessels) and visceral-systemic pathways (e.g., branches of the celiac, superior, and inferior mesenteric arteries), can mitigate symptom severity despite advanced disease [1, 6, 7]. When these collaterals are adequate, claudication symptoms are often tolerable and can be successfully managed nonoperatively for years. These collateral networks should also be recognized and preserved during surgical reconstruction.

Prevalence and Clinical Presentation

Patients with AIOD are generally found to have atherosclerotic disease along multiple levels including femoropopliteal and infrageniculate disease [4]. Patients who do present with isolated AIOD are generally younger, are nearly as likely to be female as male, and have higher incidence of smoking and hypercholesterolemia [3, 8]. The prevalence of AIOD has been estimated to range from 15% to 25% in patients older than 70 years [9, 10].

Symptoms of AIOD rarely progress to ischemic rest pain or tissue loss unless there is concomitant atherosclerotic disease in the infrainguinal vessels due to robust collateral networks [4]. Patients with symptomatic isolated AIOD typically present with symptoms of proximal claudication of the thigh, hip, and buttock [1, 6]. Approximately 45–65% of patients present with claudication of the buttocks, thighs, and calves [11–13]. The classic triad of claudication of the buttock and thighs, absent femoral pulses, and impotence described by Leriche is noted in as many as 73% of men with aortoiliac disease [14]. Up to 30% of affected men describe erectile dysfunction likely secondary to inadequate perfusion of internal pudendal arteries [12, 15]. Similarly, AIOD and subsequent decreased iliohypogastric and pudendal perfusion lead to vaginal wall fibrosis and female vaginal vascular insufficiency syndrome [8, 16].

Diagnosis

Patients presenting with symptoms related to aortoiliac disease should undergo a thorough history and physical examination, as variability in presentation and vague pelvic symptoms can often make the diagnosis of claudication secondary to AIOD difficult to distinguish from symptoms of hip arthritis or nerve root irritation due to lumbar disk disease or spinal stenosis [1]. A careful history including a detailed discussion of cardiovascular and pulmonary comorbidities should be performed. As many as 90% of these patients have a smoking history, and almost 60% are still smoking at the time of presentation [14]. Patients with AIOD often have high prevalence of hypertension (65–87%), coronary artery disease (30–60%), chronic obstructive pulmonary disease (13–20%), and chronic renal insufficiency (4–13%) [1–4]. Evaluation of functional status and activities of daily living (ADL) are essential in operative planning [17].

On physical examination, patients will typically have a diminished or absent femoral pulse on the affected side [6, 14]. In many cases, however, the lower extremity may appear well-perfused and, in some cases, there may even be palpable pedal pulses which only diminish or become absent after exercise [4, 6]. A palpable thrill or audible bruit at the lower abdominal or groin level may only become detectable after exertion. Unilateral signs and symptoms point to an iliac lesion, and bilateral issues suggest involvement of the distal aorta and/or its bifurcation. Examination of upper extremity pulse intensity and timing to evaluate for any potential upper extremity disease may impact endovascular access or extra-anatomic surgical reconstruction. A delayed pulse or discrepancy in blood pressure compared to the contralateral extremity may indicate subclavian or a more proximal stenosis [4]. If a discrepancy is found, further imaging is necessary if extra-anatomic bypass is to be considered.

Imaging

All patients presenting with aortoiliac disease should undergo comprehensive noninvasive arterial studies as part of their diagnostic workup and for postoperative comparison [18]. These studies typically include lower extremity segmental pressures and pulse volume recordings, with or without toe pressure measurements, depending on the clinical context and patient-specific indications [19]. Such evaluations provide critical baseline data for both diagnosis and longitudinal monitoring. Exercise ankle-brachial index (ABI) testing is a useful diagnostic tool to detect aortoiliac disease, especially in patients with normal resting ABIs but exercise-induced symptoms like claudication [20]. Exercise ABI involves measuring the ABI before and after treadmill exercise to detect changes in blood flow and identify exercise-induced ischemia. A significant post-exercise drop in ABI indicates vascular obstruction, helping to localize the disease to the aortoiliac or other arterial segments [20]. Exercise treadmill ABI is particularly useful in determining the severity of disease in patients with single-level iliac disease who present with buttock/thigh claudication and preserved pulses [21].

In patients without severe renal insufficiency, computed tomography angiography (CTA) is routinely employed for preprocedural planning [21]. CTA imaging should extend from the abdomen through the lower extremity runoff to allow for a thorough assessment of the aortoiliac disease. This modality is particularly valuable for characterizing the extent and nature of the pathology, including the location of occlusions relative to the renal arteries and the degree of vascular calcification (Fig. 13.1). CTA also provides detailed visualization of significant collateral pathways and coexisting infrainguinal disease that may influence procedural planning [22].

Special attention should be given to the common femoral artery (CFA) and profunda femoris artery, as these vessels serve as critical outflow arteries and primary access points for endovascular interventions addressing aortoiliac occlusions [6]. When the CFA demonstrates stenosis exceeding 50% or significant calcification, a hybrid approach is recommended. This involves performing a CFA endarterectomy followed by patch angioplasty to restore patency and facilitate subsequent endovascular treatment [4]. By integrating advanced imaging and precise anatomical assessment into preoperative planning, clinicians can enhance the efficacy and safety of therapeutic strategies for aortoiliac occlusive disease [3].

Management of Claudication in Aortoiliac Disease

Historically, disabling claudication has been considered a relative indication for treatment of aortoiliac disease. The majority of patients with claudication experience a stable or improving pattern of symptoms with conservative management throughout their lifetime, while 20–30% of AIOD require operation within 5 years of diagnosis due to symptom progression [6]. The degree of lifestyle-limiting disability a patient experiences secondary to AIOD remains subjective and important to assess on an individual level. Conventionally, studies evaluating interventions in AIOD highlighted physician-orientated outcome measures such as patency rates, ankle-brachial pressure index (ABPI), freedom from clinically-driven target lesion revascularization (CD-TLR), and freedom from amputation [23]. However, given the wide range of symptoms experienced by patients, recent literature has emphasized metrics measuring quality of life in patients suffering from claudication secondary to aortoiliac disease in order to highlight the patient's perspective [23]. The annual risk of limb loss is low at approximately 1%, and given that claudication is associated with a higher rate of cardiovascular mortality (5% annually), most patients benefit significantly from risk factor modification and conservative management [1] more so than revascularization (Fig. 13.2). Endovascular options for

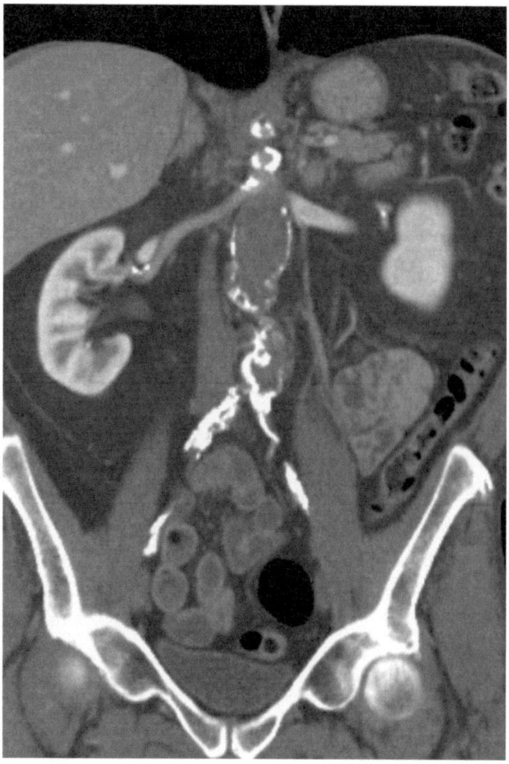

Fig. 13.2 CTA Imaging of Aortoiliac disease

the treatment of AIOD are readily available and associated with high technical success rates. In this setting, The Society for Vascular Surgery Appropriate Use Criteria (AUC) for the management of intermittent claudication was recently published to serve as a comprehensive framework to guide clinicians in the individualized management of aortoiliac disease presenting with intermittent claudication [24]. By integrating patient-specific factors with evidence-based recommendations, these criteria aim to optimize treatment outcomes and enhance patient quality of life.

Initial Management

Initial management for all patients with aortoiliac disease and intermittent claudication begins with non-invasive therapies. Supervised exercise therapy (SET) is the cornerstone of first-line management. This structured approach involves regular, progressive walking sessions, typically performed three times per week for at least 12 weeks, with the goal of walking to near-maximal claudication pain [25]. For patients without access to SET, home-based or technology-assisted exercise programs are acceptable alternatives [25]. Exercise therapy has consistently been shown to improve walking distances and reduce symptoms, making it a foundational intervention for all patients regardless of disease severity [21, 25].

Optimal medical therapy (OMT) is another essential component of initial management and includes the use of lipid-lowering and antiplatelet agents [20, 26]. Statins are prescribed to achieve LDL-C levels aligned with current cardiovascular guidelines, reducing the risk of disease progression and associated cardiovascular events. Antiplatelet therapy, such as aspirin or clopidogrel, is recommended to minimize the likelihood of thrombosis and further ischemic complications [20, 26]. Cilostazol, a phosphodiesterase inhibitor, may be offered to improve walking distances in patients without contraindications, although it is contraindicated for individuals with heart failure [27].

Revascularization Following Optimal Medical Management

For patients who have completed risk factor modification and a trial of exercise therapy but continue to experience significant disability due to claudication, revascularization is often indicated [24]. In straightforward aortoiliac disease, endovascular therapy remains the preferred option due to its minimally invasive nature and high success rates [12, 20, 24]. Open surgical revascularization may be considered in younger, low-risk patients who require durable long-term outcomes [24, 28]. In complex disease, open surgery is generally recommended as the treatment of choice, with endovascular therapy reserved for patients who are not surgical candidates [13, 24].

Factors Influencing Treatment Selection

Several factors influence the choice of revascularization strategy in aortoiliac disease. Nicotine use, for example, is associated with reduced procedural success and increased complication rates, making smoking cessation a critical component of pre-treatment optimization [24, 29]. Patient comorbidities, such as frailty and reduced life expectancy, often tip the balance in favor of less invasive approaches [12, 20, 24]. The complexity of the disease, as classified by TASC II, also plays a pivotal role, with straightforward lesions favoring endovascular interventions and complex lesions often necessitating surgical revascularization [4, 5]. Finally, the severity of lifestyle limitations and walking distances are key determinants, with severe functional impairment favoring more aggressive revascularization strategies [9, 24].

Surveillance and Long-Term Management

Following revascularization, regular surveillance with duplex ultrasonography or other imaging modalities is essential to assess vascular patency and detect restenosis early [20, 24]. Continued adherence to OMT, including statins and antiplatelet agents, is crucial to maintaining vascular health and minimizing the risk of recurrent disease [20]. Lifestyle modifications, particularly smoking cessation, are also vital to optimizing long-term outcomes [20].

The management of claudication in aortoiliac disease requires a nuanced approach that balances the risks and benefits of non-invasive, endovascular, and surgical therapies. For patients requiring revascularization, careful consideration of disease complexity, patient factors, and procedural risks ensures optimal outcomes and quality of life. This comprehensive, patient-centered approach underscores the importance of integrating evidence-based guidelines with clinical expertise to manage this challenging condition effectively.

Open Surgical Treatment for Aortoiliac Disease

Open surgical intervention remains an essential modality in the management of (AIOD), particularly for patients with extensive or complex lesions unsuitable for endovascular approaches. Despite advancements in minimally invasive techniques, open surgical procedures, such as aortoiliac endarterectomy, aortic bypass, and extra-anatomic bypass, continue to provide durable outcomes, especially in physiologically fit individuals with Trans-Atlantic Inter-Society Consensus (TASC) II C and D lesions [5, 6].

Aortoiliac Endarterectomy

Historically, aortoiliac endarterectomy was the standard surgical treatment for AIOD prior to the advent of prosthetic grafts. While less commonly performed today, it remains a viable option for younger patients with focal aortoiliac lesions, where the avoidance of prosthetic materials is desirable [28]. Endarterectomy is most feasible and durable when it is applied to focal stenotic lesions in large-caliber, high-flow vessels. Endarterectomy is particularly effective for exophytic plaques termed "coral reef aorta," which are often characterized by heavy calcification in the visceral segment of the aorta [30]. This condition often presents with chronic mesenteric ischemia, renovascular hypertension, and claudication [30]. Open aortovisceral endarterectomy via a trap-door incision is the standard approach in these complex cases, achieving high rates of symptom relief and long-term patency [31]. Primary patency rates for endarterectomy exceed 94% at 5 years and 78% at 10 years, underscoring its durability in appropriately selected patients [32].

Aortic Bypass

Aortobifemoral bypass (AFB) has conventionally been the preferred surgical intervention for extensive AIOD, particularly in patients with TASC II C and D lesions [24]. AFB demonstrates superior long-term outcomes, with 1- and 5-year patency rates approaching 90%, even for advanced disease [33]. Comparative studies have shown that AFB is associated with lower re-intervention rates and higher overall survival compared to endovascular repair, highlighting its role as the gold standard for physiologically fit patients [34].

Prosthetic conduits, such as Dacron and polytetrafluoroethylene (PTFE), are commonly used in aortic bypass, with no significant differences in long-term patency or complication rates between these materials [35]. The choice of proximal anastomosis configuration (end-to-end versus end-to-side) depends on anatomical considerations. End-to-end anastomosis is preferred in cases involving concomitant abdominal aortic aneurysm repair. Furthermore, it is thought that an end-to-end anastomosis allows for more comprehensive thromboendarterectomy of the proximal stump, better in-line flow pattern, and overall more favorable hemodynamics due to less turbulence. Some studies have demonstrated lower rates of proximal suture line pseudoaneurysm, as well as lower risk of aortoenteric fistula and better long-term patency rates [36, 37] with this configuration. On the other hand, an end-to-side anastomosis is advantageous in patients with occluded or severely diseased external iliac arteries to maintain antegrade pelvic perfusion and prevent pelvic ischemia. In these patients, end-to-side anastomosis helps to preserve antegrade flow to the internal iliac or inferior mesenteric arteries [37]. Alternatively, the inferior mesenteric artery can be reimplanted into a graft whose proximal anastomosis has been performed in end-to-end fashion [6].

The selection of distal anastomotic targets depends on the extent and distribution of disease, but should be no more proximal than the common femoral artery due to risk of disease progression in the external iliac arteries. Aortofemoral bypass is typically favored for ensuring adequate perfusion to the lower extremities and mitigating the risk of graft failure due to disease progression [1]. Additionally, the liberal use of concomitant femoral endarterectomy should be considered to optimize outflow and subsequent patency (Fig. 13.3).

Surgical access for aortic bypass can be achieved through either transperitoneal or retroperitoneal approaches. The transperitoneal approach provides excellent exposure to the infrarenal aorta and bilateral iliofemoral vessels and is achieved via a midline laparotomy [6]. In contrast, the retroperitoneal approach is advantageous for patients with prior abdominal surgeries or abdominal wall reconstruction as it avoids entering the peritoneal cavity and facilitates extension to a thoracoabdominal incision when needed to achieve more proximal aortic control [39].

Extra-anatomic Bypass

When direct aortoiliac reconstruction is contraindicated due to severe comorbidities, infection, or prior surgeries, extra-anatomic bypass serves as a suitable alternative for revascularization [6]. It is worth noting that very careful consideration should be given to the relative benefits of extra-anatomic bypass for claudication in poor surgical candidates.

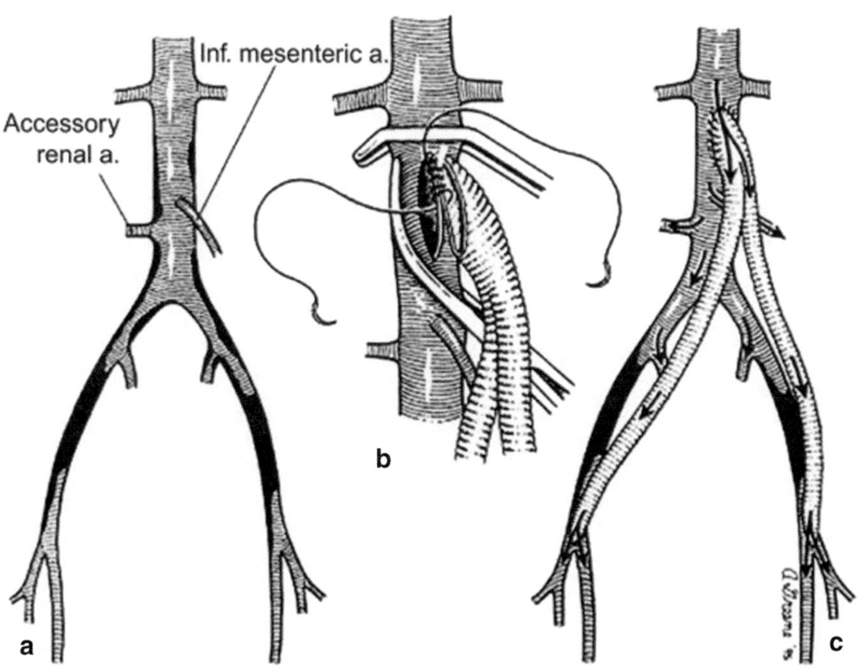

Fig. 13.3 Aortobifemoral bypass [38]

Femoral–femoral crossover bypass is indicated for unilateral iliac occlusive disease or bilateral disease where one side is amenable to endovascular intervention [40]. A prosthetic graft, usually ringed PTFE to prevent kinking, is tunneled subcutaneously between the groins [40]. While technically straightforward, this procedure may offer reduced long-term patency compared to in-line reconstructions.

Axillofemoral bypass (AXFBG) is reserved for patients with significant cardiopulmonary comorbidities or "hostile abdomen" precluding direct aortic reconstruction [41] (Fig. 13.4). Although its use has declined with advancements in endovascular techniques, axillofemoral bypass remains a viable option in select high-risk patients [43]. However, it is associated with inferior patency and higher mortality compared to aortofemoral bypass, with studies reporting mortality rates of 7.3% versus 3.6% and increased rates of re-intervention [44]. Higher rates of morbidity and mortality are likely attributed to patient selection and severity of comorbidities rather than the procedure itself. AXFBG patency rates have varied considerably in the literature, however recent studies have reported 1-year patency of 80–90%, with 5-year patency 60–75% [45]. Preoperative assessment for extra-anatomic bypass includes duplex ultrasonography and computed tomography angiography (CTA) to ensure adequate inflow from the axillary artery [1]. Surgical

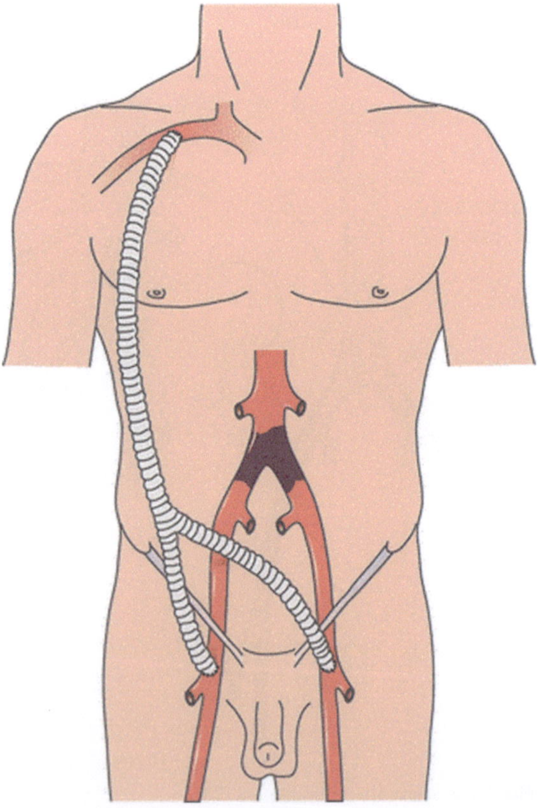

Fig. 13.4 Axillobifemoral bypass [42]

considerations include meticulous tunneling to avoid graft kinking and ensuring sufficient graft length to accommodate movement without tension [46]. Complications of AXFBG include graft thrombosis or infection, seroma, plexus lesions, and arterial steal syndrome [47–49]. Patients may need to undergo a thrombectomy or total graft replacement in order to maintain patency [49]. Complications are most likely to occur within the first 36 months following surgery, with the average being 21.5 months [49].

Open surgical treatment for AIOD remains critical for patients with extensive or complex lesions unsuitable for endovascular repair. Procedures such as aortoiliac endarterectomy, aortic bypass, and extra-anatomic bypass offer durable revascularization with favorable long-term outcomes. Advances in surgical techniques and careful patient selection are pivotal in optimizing the safety and efficacy of these interventions.

Hybrid Treatment for Aortoiliac Disease

The hybrid approach to revascularization for aortoiliac disease is particularly advantageous for patients with TASC II C and D lesions, extensive calcification, or multilevel disease [50] (Fig. 13.5). The existence of concurrent common femoral artery

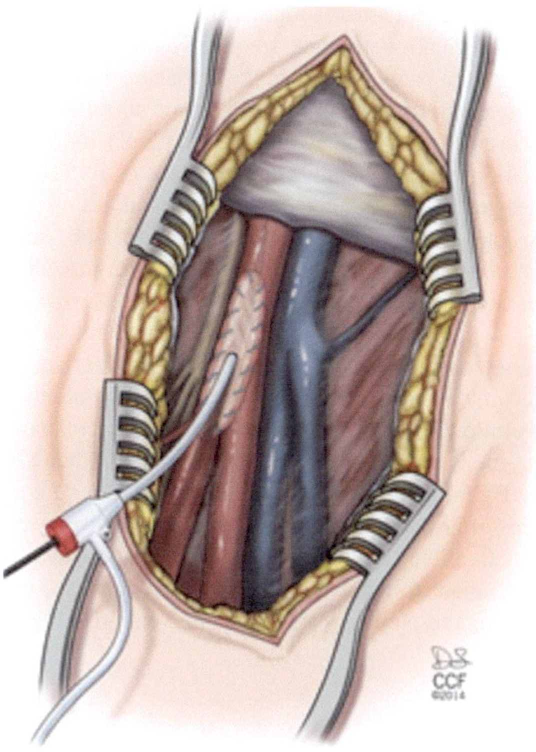

Fig. 13.5 Hybrid approach via common femoral endarterectomy with endovascular revascularization [33]

and aortoiliac disease is a marker of increased systemic atherosclerotic disease burden as patients with concurrent disease also have a higher incidence of symptomatic cardiac disease, hypertension, and hyperlipidemia [50]. It is also a marker of more anatomically diffuse atherosclerotic disease [4]. For patients undergoing treatment for claudication secondary to aortoiliac disease, the hybrid approach is most commonly utilized by performing common femoral endarterectomy in conjunction with iliac angioplasty and stenting [50]. Recent studies have demonstrated that concurrent common femoral endarterectomy in conjunction with iliac artery angioplasty and stenting is a safe, effective, and durable approach to multilevel atherosclerotic disease [50]. Primary patency rates range between 94 and 58% at 1–5 years [50]. These patency rates are enhanced with clinically driven reintervention to obtain an assisted patency rate of 98–79% at 1–5 years for re-stenotic lesions [50]. Recent studies comparing outcomes of hybrid interventions in relation to endovascular revascularization showed a trend toward higher patency rates, although results have not been statistically significant [51, 52]. Therefore, whether the hybrid technique offers more favorable outcomes compared to the endovascular technique remains unclear [50–52].

Endovascular Treatment for Aortoiliac Disease

The aortoiliac arteries represent critical anatomical targets in IC, as the alleviation of proximal obstruction frequently provides symptomatic relief and satisfactory long-term patency, even in the presence of distal disease [4]. Endovascular therapy has transformed the management of aortoiliac disease, providing a less invasive alternative that enables surgeons to adopt a more aggressive approach to revascularization while reducing periprocedural morbidity [11]. With advancements in stent design, drug-eluting technologies, and lesion preparation tools, even complex lesions once considered suitable only for open surgery can now be addressed with endovascular techniques [50]. This shift has allowed interventionalists to treat a broader range of patients—including those with extensive or multi-level disease—while minimizing the risks associated with traditional surgery. The current American Heart Association/American College of Journal Pre-proof Cardiology guidelines recommend endovascular intervention for patients with lifestyle-limiting IC caused by inflow AIOD when conservative medical management fails, provided the disease profile is amenable to percutaneous intervention [20].

By mitigating recovery time and procedural complications, endovascular therapies offer patients with claudication effective symptom relief, and faster return to function. This section reviews the current endovascular techniques, including stenting, atherectomy, and drug-coated balloons, and examines the latest evidence supporting these options as viable interventions for aortoiliac disease.

Access

When treating aortoiliac disease with endovascular techniques, careful attention to procedural and technical aspects is essential for successful outcomes. Access is a critical first step, with common access points including the common femoral artery and, in some cases, brachial or radial access when ipsilateral access is challenging or impossible. In endovascular treatment of aortoiliac disease, femoral artery access is the preferred and most common approach due to its direct path to the iliac arteries, ease of sheath insertion, and ability to accommodate larger devices required for aortoiliac interventions [11]. Studies indicate that common femoral access has a procedural success rate of over 90% in aortoiliac interventions [53]. Bilateral femoral access may be required in complex cases, especially in patients with severe bilateral iliac disease, allowing simultaneous access and crossover techniques [54]. Brachial access provides a longer reach and higher procedural success than radial access in aortoiliac cases, though it carries a slightly higher risk of hematoma or vascular injury, especially in the case of large sheaths [6]. Crossover techniques are often employed when access is limited to one side; in this approach, a catheter is advanced from one femoral artery across the aortic bifurcation to reach the contralateral iliac artery. This requires precise catheter and guidewire manipulation to maintain stability, especially in tortuous or calcified anatomy [54].

Device Selection

Guidewire selection is another important aspect of treatment of aortoiliac disease, and it is highly dependent on lesion characteristics such as length, calcification, and tortuosity. For initial crossing of stenotic or occlusive lesions, soft or intermediate guidewires (e.g., Glidewire Advantage or Glidewire Gold) provide maneuverability and reduced risk of vessel injury [53, 55]. In total occlusions or heavily calcified segments, stiff, high-support guidewires such as the Amplatz Super Stiff or Rosen wire are preferred to maintain stability, facilitate device tracking, and achieve adequate lesion crossing [55]. Utilization of a high-support guidewire in complex lesions increases technical success rates from around 75% to 90% compared to standard guidewires alone, as these wires provide the rigidity needed to advance through resistant areas [55, 56].

For crossing total occlusions, operators may employ subintimal re-entry techniques or specialized re-entry devices like the Outback® Elite Re-Entry Catheter or Pioneer Plus Catheter, which have shown success rates as high as 85% in re-establishing true lumen access after subintimal tracking [57]. These re-entry devices are particularly useful in chronic total occlusions (CTOs) where the guidewire dissects into the subintimal space, allowing precise re-entry into the true lumen and reducing the risk of complications like perforation or extended dissection [58]. This careful selection and technique adjustment based on lesion complexity enhances both the technical success and safety of aortoiliac endovascular procedures.

Balloon angioplasty is typically performed as a pre-stenting step to dilate the lesion and prepare the vessel for stenting, which improves stent deployment and apposition [59]. For heavily calcified lesions, atherectomy devices may be used to debulk plaque and enhance stent expansion, but these devices carry a risk of distal embolization, which can be mitigated by using distal protection devices when feasible [59, 60]. Procedural pitfalls include the risk of dissection, perforation, or embolization, particularly in calcified or tortuous vessels [60]. Operators must also be cautious of access-site complications such as hematomas or pseudoaneurysms, especially in patients with challenging anatomy or those on anticoagulation therapy [53]. When placing kissing stents in the aortic bifurcation, careful deployment is necessary to avoid crushing and ensure optimal flow dynamics at the bifurcation [61]. Managing these technical considerations requires experience and an individualized approach, as a tailored strategy can improve procedural success, mitigate complications, and enhance long-term patency in patients with aortoiliac disease.

Techniques

Primary and Provisional Stenting

Primary stenting has emerged as the first-line endovascular approach to iliac lesions, in part due to their ease of deployment and effectiveness in straightforward lesions [53] (Fig. 13.6). Restenosis of these stents is common, especially in complex or long-segment disease, often necessitating reinterventions [62]. The BRAVISSIMO trial, a large-scale study on BMS use in iliac artery disease, reported a primary patency rate of 83% at 3 years in TASC A and B lesions, decreasing to 65% in TASC C and D lesions [62]. This data suggests BMS are effective for shorter lesions but less so for complex disease [62].

Two trials compared primary Bare-Metal-Stent (BMS) implantation to balloon angioplasty (BA). In the STAG trial for treatment of iliac occlusions (length 54.1 ± 15.8 mm), patency rates did not differ through a 2-year follow-up. The study was halted early due to increased major complications for provisional vs. primary stenting (20% vs. 5%, $P = 0.01$), driven by distal embolization [63]. The Dutch Iliac Stent Trial provided data on patency, reintervention, mortality, and amputation rates up to 72 months post-intervention with no differences in outcomes at all follow-up times [64]. Therefore, little evidence indicates that primary BMS placement outperforms provisional stenting in non-occlusive lesions.

Covered Stents

The use of covered stents in aortoiliac disease has gained attention due to their potential advantages over traditional bare-metal stents (BMS). Covered stents create a physical barrier that may reduce neo-intimal hyperplasia and improve long-term patency by shielding the treated vessel from luminal ingrowth [53]. The COBEST trial, a landmark study in this area, directly compared the performance of covered stents and BMS in patients with complex TASC C and D aortoiliac lesions [65]. The trial reported a 3-year primary patency rate of 90% for covered stents,

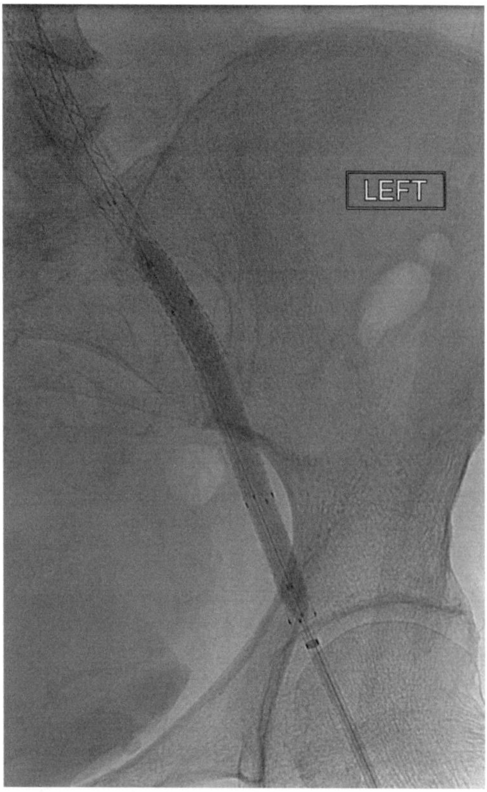

Fig. 13.6 Balloon angioplasty and stenting of left external iliac artery

significantly higher than the 70% observed for BMS [65]. A subsequent meta-analysis by Jongkind et al. reinforced these findings, showing a 5-year primary patency rate of 82% for covered stents compared to 63% for BMS in complex aortoiliac disease [53].

Despite these promising results, certain limitations in the COBEST trial must be acknowledged. Methodological concerns, including reliance on long-term post-hoc analysis, patient attrition during follow-up, and the absence of core laboratory adjudication, complicate the interpretation of these outcomes [65]. Furthermore, mid-term findings from the ICE trial have highlighted potential efficacy advantages of self-expanding BMS, which may mitigate circumferential stress due to lower radial force application [66]. However, the open-label design and lack of core laboratory adjudication in the ICE trial raise questions about the generalizability of these findings to real-world patient populations [66].

These studies underscore the need for further research to elucidate the optimal applications of covered stents in aortoiliac disease. While covered stents demonstrate superior patency in complex lesions, careful patient selection and consideration of study limitations are essential for translating these findings into clinical practice.

Drug-Eluting Stents

The application of drug-eluting stents (DES) in the treatment of aortoiliac disease remains underexplored, with limited data available to define their role. DES function by eluting antiproliferative drugs, such as paclitaxel or sirolimus, to inhibit neointimal proliferation and reduce the risk of in-stent restenosis [67]. While most existing evidence pertains to their use in other vascular territories, extrapolation to aortoiliac disease is supported by studies on drug-coated balloons (DCBs) [67]. For instance, the IN.PACT SFA trial demonstrated a primary patency rate of 89% at 1 year in the superficial femoral artery, underscoring the potential efficacy of antiproliferative drug delivery [68]. Although data specific to the aortoiliac region are scarce, a recent study by Brodmann et al. examined the use of DCBs in iliac arteries and reported a 2-year primary patency rate of 78%, suggesting their potential as an adjunctive therapy in aortoiliac interventions [67]. These findings highlight the need for further research to establish the efficacy and optimal indications for drug-eluting technologies in this vascular bed.

Kissing Stents

The kissing stent technique has become a well-established endovascular approach for treating aortoiliac disease, particularly in patients with bifurcation involvement at the aortic or common iliac level [61] (Fig. 13.7). This method involves the simultaneous deployment of two stents, one in each common iliac artery, extending symmetrically into the aortic bifurcation. It is especially useful for managing bilateral iliac artery stenosis or occlusion, as it preserves patency and flow symmetry at the bifurcation [61, 67]. The procedure is commonly indicated for patients with claudication due to aortoiliac disease, offering a minimally invasive alternative to open surgery [53, 61].

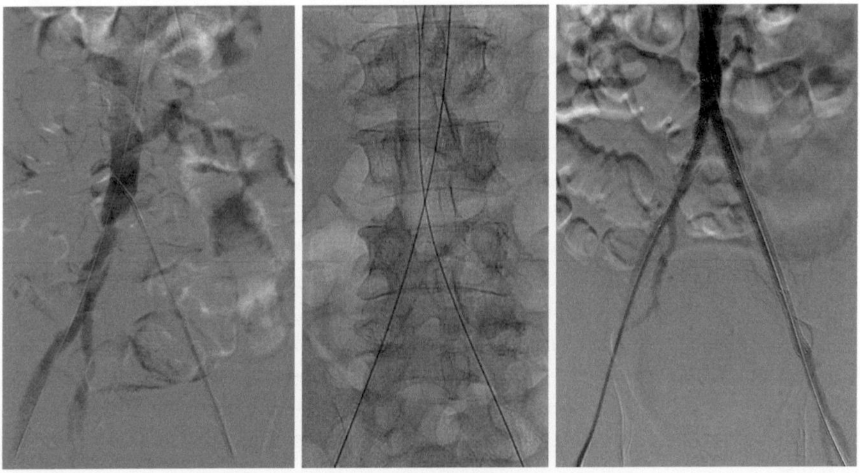

Fig. 13.7 Use of kissing stents for treatment of aortoiliac disease [69]

The technique typically begins with bilateral femoral access, facilitating simultaneous stent deployment in both iliac arteries. Covered stents, such as GORE® VIABAHN® and Cook Medical® iCast®, are frequently preferred due to their superior resistance to restenosis compared to bare-metal stents, particularly in cases with complex, calcified lesions [61, 70]. The precise, simultaneous placement of both stents is critical to prevent complications such as "crushing" or "malapposition" at the aortic bifurcation, which could compromise flow and long-term patency. Optimal stent positioning ensures symmetrical expansion at the bifurcation, promoting durability and reducing the risk of restenosis [70].

Kissing stents have demonstrated favorable outcomes in terms of patency, symptom improvement, and quality of life for patients with claudication due to aortoiliac disease [71]. Primary patency rates have been reported around 88% at 3 years [71]. The study highlighted the technique's effectiveness, particularly in patients with TASC II B and C lesions. More recent studies have demonstrated primary patency at 12, 24, and 60 months to be 89.3%, 78.6%, and 69.0% [71]. These studies underscore the durability of kissing stents as a reliable option for extensive bifurcation involvement. Additionally, compared to open surgery, kissing stents are associated with lower morbidity, shorter recovery times, and fewer postoperative complications [28, 70].

Despite their advantages, kissing stents have potential limitations, including risks of restenosis, re-intervention, and procedural complexity. Restenosis rates range from 10% to 25% over 3 years, depending on lesion complexity and stent type [71]. While covered stents reduce restenosis risk, challenges remain for long-segment or heavily calcified lesions. Procedural precision is essential to avoid stent misalignment or crushing, which can impair patency and necessitate re-intervention. Complex anatomy or severe calcification increases technical challenges and the risk of access-related complications [70]. These findings emphasize the need for meticulous technique and ongoing follow-up in high-risk patients to optimize outcomes and minimize complications.

Atherectomy

The use of atherectomy as a treatment modality for aortoiliac disease in patients with claudication is somewhat controversial. Atherectomy offers targeted plaque modification, particularly advantageous in managing heavily calcified or fibrotic lesions. By enabling plaque debulking and vessel preparation prior to stenting, atherectomy facilitates enhanced luminal gain and optimized stent expansion in cases where severe calcification might otherwise hinder the effectiveness of traditional endovascular techniques [60]. Additionally, by removing plaque burden, atherectomy reduces the need for aggressive post-dilatation with high-pressure balloons, thereby minimizing vessel trauma and decreasing the risk of dissection [59]. Of note, these reported advantages have not been well studied or conclusively proven.

Atherectomy employs several device types, each tailored to specific lesion characteristics and plaque compositions. Directional atherectomy devices, such as

Medtronic®, SilverHawk®, and TurboHawk®, use a side-cutting blade to shave plaque from the vessel wall [72]. This approach is particularly suitable for fibrotic or calcified lesions and is commonly applied in large vessels like the iliac arteries [60]. Rotational atherectomy systems, such as the Phillips® Phoenix® Atherectomy System, use a rotational blade to grind calcified plaque, making them ideal for eccentric calcifications [60]. Orbital atherectomy, exemplified by the Abbott® Diamondback 360® system, uses a diamond-tipped, orbiting crown to sand calcium deposits, particularly in heavily calcified vessels where standard angioplasty might be insufficient [73]. Laser atherectomy employs high-frequency laser energy to vaporize plaque, as seen in devices like Philips® Turbo Elite [60]. Although less commonly used in the aortoiliac region, laser atherectomy remains a viable option in select cases.

Recent studies highlight the efficacy of atherectomy as an adjunctive therapy to stenting in the treatment of complex aortoiliac lesions [60]. The DEFINITIVE LE study demonstrated that directional atherectomy before stenting achieved an average luminal gain of 2.3 mm [74]. Additionally, this approach reduced the reliance on high-pressure ballooning, minimizing vessel trauma and the risk of dissection in calcified iliac arteries [74]. These findings underscore the utility of atherectomy in maintaining vessel patency while reducing procedural complications.

Covered Endovascular Reconstruction of the Aortic Bifurcation (CERAB)

Covered Endovascular Reconstruction of the Aortic Bifurcation (CERAB) has emerged as a minimally invasive alternative to open surgical procedures for treating aortoiliac occlusive disease (AIOD) in patients presenting with claudication. The CERAB technique utilizes covered stents to reconstruct the aortic bifurcation, aiming to restore adequate blood flow while minimizing procedural risks. The technique involves first placing a balloon-expandable aortic stent, followed by flaring the proximal 2/3 portion of the aortic stent, then placing 2 covered iliac stents overlapping in the distal 1/3 of the aortic stent.

A recent review and meta-analysis evaluated outcomes of CERAB compared to standard endovascular treatments (SEV) and open surgery (OS) in patients with extensive AIOD [75]. The study reported that CERAB had a 30-day morbidity rate of 10% and a mortality rate of 0%, which were favorable compared to OS, which had morbidity and mortality rates of 15% and 3%, respectively [75]. Additionally, CERAB demonstrated a 3-year primary patency rate of 82%, comparable to the 78% observed with SEV [75].

Further supporting these findings, a recent study by Taeymans et al. assessed the 3-year outcomes of the CERAB technique in patients with extensive AIOD [76]. The study included 130 patients, predominantly with Trans-Atlantic Inter-Society Consensus II (TASC-II) D lesions, and reported a technical success rate of 97% [76]. At 3 years, the primary patency rate was 82%, with secondary patency reaching 97%. Notably, 96% of patients experienced clinical improvement of at least one Rutherford category, indicating significant symptomatic relief [76].

These studies suggest that CERAB is a viable and effective endovascular option for patients with complex aortoiliac lesions, offering favorable patency rates and clinical outcomes comparable to traditional surgical approaches.

Future Perspectives

The future of aortoiliac disease treatment in patients with claudication is poised to advance through the integration of novel technologies, enhanced imaging techniques, and individualized therapeutic strategies. Drug-eluting devices, including stents and balloons, may play an increasing role, addressing restenosis challenges through targeted drug delivery that inhibits neointimal hyperplasia. Emerging bioresorbable scaffolds, which provide temporary vessel support and degrade over time, offer theoretical advantages by reducing long-term complications such as stent fracture or chronic inflammation. Precision imaging technologies, including intravascular ultrasound (IVUS) and optical coherence tomography (OCT), are expected to enhance lesion assessment and procedural planning, ensuring optimal stent deployment and alignment. Furthermore, artificial intelligence and machine learning algorithms may facilitate real-time decision-making during interventions by integrating patient-specific data to predict outcomes and recommend tailored therapies. Advances in hybrid techniques, combining endovascular and open surgical approaches, may also refine treatment for complex, multilevel disease. Finally, as endovascular options continue to evolve, there is an increasing emphasis on long-term follow-up protocols and registries to monitor outcomes and refine evidence-based practices. These innovations hold promise for improving patency rates, reducing complications, and enhancing the quality of life for patients with claudication due to aortoiliac disease.

References

1. Paisley MJ, Adkar S, Sheehan BM, Stern JR. Aortoiliac occlusive disease. Semin Vasc Surg. 2022;35:162–71.
2. Leriche R, Morel A. The syndrome of thrombotic obliteration of the aortic bifurcation. Ann Surg. 1948;127:193–206.
3. Aorto-iliac reconstruction—PubMed. https://pubmed.ncbi.nlm.nih.gov/157541/
4. Anatomical significance in aortoiliac occlusive disease—Wooten—2014—clinical anatomy—Wiley Online Library. https://onlinelibrary.wiley.com/doi/10.1002/ca.22444
5. Inter-Society Consensus for the Management of Peripheral Arterial Disease (TASC II)—PubMed. https://pubmed.ncbi.nlm.nih.gov/17223489/
6. Rutherford RB, Cronenwett JL, Johnston KW. Rutherford's vascular surgery and endovascular therapy. 8th ed. Elsevier; 2014.
7. Common and rare collateral pathways in aortoiliac occlusive disease: a pictorial essay—PubMed. https://pubmed.ncbi.nlm.nih.gov/21862782/

8. Vasculogenic female sexual dysfunction: the hemodynamic basis for vaginal engorgement insufficiency and clitoral erectile insufficiency—PubMed. https://pubmed.ncbi.nlm.nih.gov/9138056/
9. Olin JW, Sealove BA. Peripheral artery disease: current insight into the disease and its diagnosis and management. Mayo Clin Proc. 2010;85:678–92.
10. Ethnicity and peripheral arterial disease: the San Diego Population Study—PubMed. https://pubmed.ncbi.nlm.nih.gov/16246968/
11. Endovascular management of chronic infrarenal aortic occlusion—Mireille A. Moise, Javier A. Alvarez-Tostado, Daniel G. Clair, Roy K. Greenberg, Sean P. Lyden, Sunita D. Srivastava, Matthew Eagleton, Timur S. Sarac, Vikram S. Kashyap, 2009. https://journals.sagepub.com/doi/abs/10.1583/08-2526.1
12. Clair DG, Beach JM. Strategies for managing aortoiliac occlusions: access, treatment and outcomes. Expert Rev Cardiovasc Ther. 2015;13:551–63.
13. Kashyap VS, et al. The management of severe aortoiliac occlusive disease: endovascular therapy rivals open reconstruction. J Vasc Surg. 2008;48:1451–7, 1457.e1–3.
14. Management and outcome of chronic atherosclerotic infrarenal aortic occlusion—PubMed. https://pubmed.ncbi.nlm.nih.gov/8808961/
15. Tkocz M, Brzęk A, Marcinek M, Skrzypulec-Plinta V, Ziaja D. Pre and postoperative sexual dysfunction in patients with Leriche syndrome—a prospective pilot study. Int J Environ Res Public Health. 2022;19:3091.
16. Female sexual dysfunction: incidence, pathophysiology, evaluation, and treatment options—Urology. https://www.goldjournal.net/article/S0090-4295(99)00230-7/fulltext#BIB18
17. Abelha FJ, Botelho M, Fernandes V, Barros H. Outcome and quality of life after aortobifemoral bypass surgery. BMC Cardiovasc Disord. 2010;10:15.
18. Factors influencing pathological ankle-brachial index values along the chronic kidney disease spectrum: the NEFRONA study | Nephrology Dialysis Transplantation | Oxford Academic. https://academic.oup.com/ndt/article/32/3/513/3059407
19. Allison: ethnicity and risk factors for change in…—Google Scholar. https://scholar.google.com/scholar_lookup?title=Ethnicity%20and%20risk%20factors%20for%20change%20in%20the%20ankle-brachial%20index%3A%20the%20Multi-Ethnic%20Study%20of%20Atherosclerosis&publication_year=2009&author=MA%20Allison&author=M%20Cushman&author=C%20Solomon
20. ACC/AHA 2005 Practice Guidelines for the Management of Patients With Peripheral Arterial Disease (Lower Extremity, Renal, Mesenteric, and Abdominal Aortic): Executive Summary: a collaborative report from the American Association for Vascular Surgery/Society for Vascular Surgery* Society for Cardiovascular Angiography and Interventions, Society for Vascular Medicine and Biology, Society of Interventional Radiology, and the ACC/AHA Task Force on Practice Guidelines (Writing Committee to Develop Guidelines for the Management of Patients With Peripheral Arterial Disease): Endorsed by the American Association of Cardiovascular and Pulmonary Rehabilitation; National Heart, Lung, and Blood Institute; Society for Vascular Nursing; TransAtlantic Inter-Society Consensus; and Vascular Disease Foundation. Circulation. 2006;113:1474–547.
21. Ricco J-B, Bartelink M-LEL. Document covering atherosclerotic disease of extracranial carotid and vertebral, mesenteric, renal, upper and lower extremity arteries endorsed by: the European Stroke Organization (ESO).
22. CT angiography and 3D imaging in aortoiliac occlusive disease: collateral pathways in Leriche syndrome | Abdominal Radiology. https://link.springer.com/article/10.1007/s00261-017-1137-0
23. Review: quality of life in lower limb peripheral vascular surgery—JMW Donker, J de Vries, GH Ho, F Bastos Gonçalves, SE Hoeks, HJM Verhagen, L van der Laan, 2016. https://journals.sagepub.com/doi/10.1177/1708538115578961
24. Woo K. Society for Vascular Surgery appropriate use criteria for management of intermittent claudication. J Vasc Surg. 2022;76:3–22.e1.

25. Supervised exercise therapy for symptomatic peripheral artery disease among medicare beneficiaries between 2017 and 2018: participation rates and outcomes. https://www.ahajournals.org/doi/epub/10.1161/CIRCOUTCOMES.121.007953. https://doi.org/10.1161/CIRCOUTCOMES.121.007953.
26. Collaboration, A. T. Collaborative meta-analysis of randomised trials of antiplatelet therapy for prevention of death, myocardial infarction, and stroke in high risk patients. BMJ. 2002;324:71–86.
27. Systematic review of the efficacy of cilostazol, naftidrofuryl oxalate and pentoxifylline for the treatment of intermittent claudication | British Journal of Surgery | Oxford Academic. https://academic.oup.com/bjs/article-abstract/99/12/1630/6141159?redirectedFrom=fulltext&login=false
28. Antonello M, et al. Open repair versus endovascular treatment of complex aortoiliac lesions in low risk patients. J Vasc Surg. 2019;70:1155–1165.e1.
29. Gordon T, Kannel WB. Predisposition to atherosclerosis in the head, heart, and legs: the Framingham study. JAMA. 1972;221:661–6.
30. Burton JS, Droz NM, Khetarpaul V, Sanchez LA, Ohman JW. Trapdoor endarterectomy for coral reef plaque of the paravisceral aorta in the modern era. J Vasc Surg Cases Innov Tech. 2024;10:101383.
31. Baldaia L, et al. Coral reef aorta: literature review and analysis of the published cases in the last 20 years. Ann Vasc Surg. 2024;98:374–87.
32. Aortoiliac endarterectomy: an 11-year review | British Journal of Surgery | Oxford Academic. https://academic.oup.com/bjs/article-abstract/77/2/190/6171645
33. Smith AH, et al. Comparison of aortobifemoral bypass to aortoiliac stenting with bifurcation reconstruction for TASC II D aortoiliac occlusive disease. Ann Vasc Surg. 2022;82:120–30.
34. Ghoneim B, et al. Outcomes of unibody bifurcated endograft and aortobifemoral bypass for aortoiliac occlusive disease. Vasc Spec Int. 2020;36:216–23.
35. Collagen-versus gelatine-coated Dacron versus stretch PTFE bifurcation grafts for aortoiliac occlusive disease: long-term results of a prospective, randomized multicenter trial—ScienceDirect. https://www.sciencedirect.com/science/article/abs/pii/S0039606003001272
36. Pierce GE, et al. Evaluation of end-to-side v end-to-end proximal anastomosis in aortobifemoral bypass. Arch Surg Chic Ill. 1982;1960(117):1580–8.
37. Functional assessment at the buttock level of the effect of aortobifemoral bypass surgery—PubMed. https://pubmed.ncbi.nlm.nih.gov/18438126/
38. Velazquez-Ramirez G, Rosenberg ML. Chapter 6c—suprainguinal peripheral artery disease: open management. In: Hicks CW, Harris LM, editors. Vascular disease in women. Academic; 2021. p. 185–202.
39. Thoracofemoral bypass outcomes in the Vascular Quality Initiative—ScienceDirect. https://www.sciencedirect.com/science/article/pii/S0741521420325507
40. Femorofemoral Bypass—an overview | ScienceDirect Topics. https://www.sciencedirect.com/topics/medicine-and-dentistry/femorofemoral-bypass
41. Scopus preview—scopus—document details—is axillo bilateral femoral graft an effective substitute for aortic bilateral lliac/femoral graft? An analysis of ten years experience. https://www.scopus.com/record/display.uri?eid=2-s2.0-0017385480&origin=inward&txGid=71a09634c82f85d2bf73b60140b7a544
42. Aboian E, Rao AS. Extra-anatomic bypass. In: Lanzer P, editor. Panvascular medicine. Berlin/Heidelberg: Springer; 2014. https://doi.org/10.1007/978-3-642-37393-0_137-2.
43. Mishall PL, et al. Axillobifemoral bypass: a brief surgical and historical review. Einstein J Biol Med EJBM. 2016;31:6–10.
44. Samson RH, et al. Improved patency after axillofemoral bypass for aortoiliac occlusive disease. J Vasc Surg. 2018;68:1430–7.
45. Martin D, Katz SG. Axillofemoral bypass for aortoiliac occlusive disease. Am J Surg. 2000;180:100–3.
46. Blaisdell FW. Development of femoro-femoral and axillo-femoral bypass procedures. J Vasc Surg. 2011;53:540–4.

47. Passman: comparison of axillofemoral and aortofemoral…—Google Scholar. https://scholar.google.com/scholar_lookup?journal=J%20Vasc%20Surg&title=Comparison%20of%20axillofemoral%20and%20aortofemoral%20bypass%20for%20aortoiliac%20occlusive%20disease&author=MA%20Passman&author=LM%20Taylor&author=GL%20Moneta&author=JM%20Edwards&author=RA%20Yeager&volume=23&issue=2&publication_year=1996&pages=263-269&pmid=8637103&doi=10.1016/s0741-5214(96)70270-7&
48. Ray: axillofemoral bypass: a critical reappraisal…—Google Scholar. https://scholar.google.com/scholar_lookup?journal=Am%20J%20Surg&title=Axillofemoral%20bypass:%20a%20critical%20reappraisal%20of%20its%20role%20in%20the%20management%20of%20aortoiliac%20occlusive%20disease&author=LI%20Ray&author=JB%20O%E2%80%99Connor&author=CC%20Davis&author=DG%20Hall&author=PB%20Mansfield&volume=138&issue=1&publication_year=1979&pages=117-128&pmid=157077&doi=10.1016/0002-9610(79)90251-4&
49. Donaldson: axillofemoral bypass: a tool with a limited role—Google Scholar. https://scholar.google.com/scholar_lookup?journal=J%20Vasc%20Surg&title=Axillofemoral%20bypass:%20a%20tool%20with%20a%20limited%20role&author=MC%20Donaldson&author=JC%20Louras&author=CA%20Bucknam&volume=3&issue=5&publication_year=1986&pages=757–763&pmid=2939265&
50. Kirksey L, et al. Endovascular and hybrid interventions for aortoiliac occlusive disease in patients with intermittent claudication. Ann Vasc Surg. 2025;110:480–9.
51. Gao Z, et al. Comparison of clinical outcomes of endovascular therapy and hybrid surgery in the treatment of trans-Atlantic inter-society consensus II D aortoiliac occlusive disease. Int J Gen Med. 2023;16:2149–56.
52. Chen T-W, et al. Endovascular and hybrid revascularization for complicated aorto-iliac occlusive disease: short-term results in single institute experience. Acta Cardiol Sin. 2018;34:313–20.
53. Jongkind V, Akkersdijk GJM, Yeung KK, Wisselink W. A systematic review of endovascular treatment of extensive aortoiliac occlusive disease. J Vasc Surg. 2010;52:1376–83.
54. Baumann F, et al. Endovascular treatment of common femoral artery obstructions. J Vasc Surg. 2011;53:1000–6.
55. Ünlü Ç, Deloose K, Mees VBME. Guidewire selection and techniques in peripheral arterial interventions. Eur J Vasc Endovasc Surg. 2024;67:1027–30.
56. Tóth GG, Yamane M, Heyndrickx GR. How to select a guidewire: technical features and key characteristics. Heart. 2015;101:645–52.
57. Tsitsiou Y, Ekpe J, Harris L, Kashef E, Hamady M. Use and effectiveness of Pioneer re-entry device for subintimal true lumen re-entry: single-centre data and a review of the literature. CVIR Endovasc. 2021;4:81.
58. Hayakawa N, Kodera S, Arakawa M, Kanda J. Successful re-entry using the outback® elite catheter via retrograde popliteal access with IVUS guidance for femoropopliteal occlusion: a case report. CVIR Endovasc. 2020;3:63.
59. Koeckerling D, et al. Endovascular revascularization strategies for aortoiliac and femoropopliteal artery disease: a meta-analysis. Eur Heart J. 2023;44:935–50.
60. Pinto P, Chaar CIO. Atherectomy—the options, the evidence, and when should it be used. Ann Vasc Surg. 2024;107:127–35.
61. Jebbink EG, Holewijn S, Slump CH, Lardenoije J-W, Reijnen MMPJ. Systematic review of results of kissing stents in the treatment of aortoiliac occlusive disease. Ann Vasc Surg. 2017;42:328–36.
62. de Donato G, et al. 24-month data from the BRAVISSIMO: a large-scale prospective registry on iliac stenting for TASC A & B and TASC C & D Lesions. Ann Vasc Surg. 2015;29:738–50.
63. Randomized clinical trial of stents versus angioplasty for the treatment of iliac artery occlusions (STAG trial) | British Journal of Surgery | Oxford Academic.
64. Klein WM, et al. Dutch iliac stent trial: long-term results in patients randomized for primary or selective stent placement. Radiology. 2006;238:734–44.

65. Mwipatayi BP, et al. Durability of the balloon-expandable covered versus bare-metal stents in the covered versus balloon expandable stent trial (COBEST) for the treatment of aortoiliac occlusive disease. J Vasc Surg. 2016;64:83–94.e1.
66. Krankenberg H, et al. Self-expanding versus balloon-expandable stents for iliac artery occlusive disease: the randomized ICE trial. JACC Cardiovasc Interv. 2017;10:1694–704.
67. Sustainable antirestenosis effect with a low-dose drug-coated balloon. https://www.jacc.org/doi/epdf/10.1016/j.jcin.2018.08.034. https://doi.org/10.1016/j.jcin.2018.08.034.
68. Schneider PA. Sustained durability of IN.PACT™ Admiral™ DCB treatment effect with no late catch-up through 2 years.
69. Taeymans K, Jebbink EG, Holewijn S, Martens JM, Versluis M, Goverde PCJM, Reijnen MMPJ. Three-year outcome of the covered endovascular reconstruction of the aortic bifurcation technique for aortoiliac occlusive disease. J Vasc Surg. 2018;67(5):1438–47.
70. Groot Jebbink E, Holewijn S, Slump CH, Lardenoije J-W, Reijnen MMPJ. Systematic review of results of kissing stents in the treatment of aortoiliac occlusive disease. Ann Vasc Surg. 2017;42:328–36.
71. Sonetto A, et al. Kissing stent technique for TASC C-D lesions of common iliac arteries: clinical and anatomical predictors of outcome. Ann Vasc Surg. 2021;71:288–97.
72. Ettles DF, MacDonald AW, Burgess PA, Nicholson AA, Dyet JF. Directional atherectomy in iliac stent failure: clinical technique and histopathologic correlation. Cardiovasc Intervent Radiol. 1998;21:475–80.
73. Rao S, Martinsen BJ, Higgins J, Dhandhusaria H, Patel D. Orbital atherectomy for treating calcified iliac artery disease to enable large bore device delivery: a case series report. SAGE Open Med Case Rep. 2020;8:2050313X20943068.
74. Lower extremity revascularization using directional atherectomy: 12-month prospective results of the DEFINITIVE LE study. American College of Cardiology.
75. Salem M, et al. Management of extensive aorto-iliac disease: a systematic review and meta-analysis of 9319 patients. Cardiovasc Intervent Radiol. 2021;44:1518–35.
76. Taeymans K, et al. Three year outcome of the covered endovascular reconstruction of the aortic bifurcation (CERAB) technique for aortoiliac occlusive disease. J Vasc Surg. 2018;67:1438–47.

Revascularization: Common Femoral and Profunda Femoris Arteries—Evidence, Techniques, and Patient Selection

14

Momodou L. Jammeh and Peter Rossi

Introduction

Peripheral artery disease (PAD) affects over 200 million people globally, with common femoral artery (CFA) lesions being a significant contributor [1, 2]. Isolated CFA disease is uncommon and often occurs with concomitant aorto-iliac or femoral-popliteal occlusive disease. PAD prevalence increases with age, affecting 10–20% of individuals over 60. Major risk factors include smoking, diabetes, hypertension, hyperlipidemia, and renal failure [3–5]. The predisposing risks also shape the severity and distribution of disease. Smoking predominantly affects large vessels, while diabetes and renal failure contribute to vascular calcification in smaller vessels.

CFA lesions lead to significantly lower extremity hemodynamic disruption and symptomatic PAD [6]. Patients may present with intermittent claudication (calf pain with exertion, relieved by rest). These symptoms result in significant functional impairment and diminished quality of life. This highlights the importance of a thorough evaluation and timely intervention to preserve functionality and improve outcomes.

M. L. Jammeh (✉)
Department of Surgery, Medical College of Wisconsin, Milwaukee, WI, USA
e-mail: mjammeh@mcw.edu

P. Rossi
Division of Vascular and Endovascular Surgery, Medical College of Wisconsin, Milwaukee, WI, USA
e-mail: prossi@mcw.edu

W. P. Robinson III, J. P. Simons (eds.), *The Patient-Centered Approach to Claudication*, https://doi.org/10.1007/978-3-032-02460-2_14

Medical Management

PAD involving common femoral artery (CFA) lesions is associated with a 20–30% 5-year mortality and significant morbidity often from cardiovascular causes (stroke, myocardial infarction, etc.). Management of claudication depends on the degree of functional impairment and lifestyle limitation. In the absence of severe symptoms or chronic limb-threatening ischemia (CLTI), medical management is preferred [4–9]. Evidence suggests early intervention in patients with claudication may accelerate disease progression to CLTI and limb loss [10–13].

Exercise therapy is the foundation of medical management for improving pain-free walking distance [13–15]. The addition of vasodilators such as cilostazol in eligible patients enhances exercise tolerance [16]. Risk factor modification, including emphasis on glycemic control, anti-hypertensive, and statin therapy, is critical to reducing cardiovascular events and mortality [4, 5, 16]. Smoking cessation remains the most impactful modifiable factor, requiring multidisciplinary support through behavioral and pharmacological strategies [17, 18].

For symptomatic PAD, antiplatelet therapy, HMG Co-A reductase inhibitors, smoking cessation, and comprehensive comorbidity management improve symptom severity and reduce risks of major amputation and death [4, 5, 13–18].

Indications for Common Femoral Artery Revascularization

While most individuals presenting with claudication improve with conservative management and optimization of comorbid conditions, 10–15% develop debilitating extremity pain that requires revascularization for immediate symptom relief and quality-of-life improvement [5, 13, 19]. Approximately 1% per year of these patients will progress to chronic limb-threatening ischemia (CLTI), necessitating intervention for limb salvage [20]. Occlusive disease involving the CFA is most often observed in this setting, making CFA revascularization a procedure more frequently performed for rest pain than claudication [7].

Ultimately, the decision to pursue CFA intervention for claudication should be guided by the patient's degree of functional impairment, the anatomical distribution and complexity of disease, and the associated peri-operative risk. According to the most recent appropriate use criteria for the management of claudication with CFA disease, revascularization may be considered after an initial trial of exercise therapy, alongside optimal medical therapy, if the response is inadequate [5]. Among patients requiring revascularization for CFA disease, endarterectomy is preferred over endovascular intervention due to its superior durability, safety, and efficacy in this anatomical region [21–23].

Preoperative Imaging

The clinical evaluation of patients with claudication begins with a focused history to assess the duration and severity of symptoms, alongside a careful characterization of cardiovascular risk factors [24]. A thorough physical examination, with particular attention to the presence or absence of pulses at the femoral, popliteal, and pedal levels, provides valuable insight into the anatomical distribution of disease. The ankle-brachial index (ABI), a simple and non-invasive measure of extremity perfusion, is commonly used as a confirmatory test in patients suspected of having PAD [25, 26]. However, in cases of suspected vasculogenic claudication involving the CFA, ABIs may be normal or only mildly reduced at rest. If suspicion remains high, exercise stress testing of the lower extremities can assess perfusion changes during symptom provocation (e.g., comparing ABI at rest versus post-exercise and monitoring recovery time) [27–29]. Additionally, segmental pulse volume recordings (PVRs) combined with ABIs offer a more precise determination of the level of disease, using waveform data and changes in normal arterial phasicity.

Once physiologic testing confirms the presence and severity of CFA disease, an anatomic assessment is required to guide surgical planning. This evaluation focuses on the aorto-iliac system, including the feasibility of clamp placement for proximal control, the burden of calcific atheroma, the degree of profunda femoris artery (PFA) involvement, and the status of the superficial femoral artery (SFA), popliteal artery, and tibial run-off vessels. Several imaging modalities are available for anatomical assessment, each with unique strengths and limitations:

Duplex Ultrasound (DUS): DUS is performed bedside and offers direct visualization of intraluminal arterial plaque, residual flow lumen diameter, and velocity measurements to quantify hemodynamic significance. While effective, DUS is operator-dependent and may be limited by body habitus or calcific atherosclerotic disease. Additionally, its ability to assess the aorto-iliac segments and mid-to-distal PFA is limited [30, 31].

Computed Tomography Angiography (CTA): CTA provides excellent delineation of arterial disease from the aorta to the pedal arteries in a single contrast-enhanced run. A pre-contrast phase highlights arterial calcification, while a delayed contrast phase outlines distal run-off vessels. However, CTA requires iodinated contrast, which may not be suitable for patients with contraindications such as advanced renal disease [32].

Magnetic Resonance Angiography (MRA): For patients with contraindications to iodinated contrast, newer MRA techniques that do not require contrast administration offer a viable alternative. These approaches allow a detailed evaluation of the anatomic distribution of disease while minimizing risk in vulnerable populations [33].

Digital Subtraction Angiography (DSA): Catheter-directed DSA remains the gold standard for evaluating distal run-off vessels, particularly in cases of extensive femoral-popliteal disease or significant infra-geniculate arterial calcification.

DSA's superior resolution can overcome challenges posed by disrupted contrast timing or excessive artifact from calcification [34].

Common Femoral Endarterectomy

CFA endarterectomy is typically performed under general endotracheal anesthesia. However, regional anesthesia via epidural or spinal block can be utilized in patients deemed to be at high risk for complications from general anesthesia [35]. While regional anesthesia may reduce respiratory morbidity in patients at risk for pulmonary complications, there is no proven 30-day mortality or long-term advantage [36]. Additionally, many patients are unable to tolerate lying supine for more than 2 h, and regional anesthesia has significant variability in efficacy. CFA endarterectomy can be performed with just moderate sedation and local anesthesia, in selected cases; it requires an attentive anesthesiologist.

The external iliac artery (EIA) transitions into the CFA as it passes beneath the inguinal ligament, with the femoral nerve positioned laterally and the femoral vein medially. Bony landmarks such as the anterior superior iliac spine and the pubic tubercle serve as markers for the level of the inguinal ligament and help determine the proximal extent of the skin incision. The CFA gives rise to the profunda femoris artery (PFA) posterior-laterally and transitions into the superficial femoral artery (SFA) along the anterior-medial thigh. In the absence of a palpable pulse and without intraoperative DUS, the CFA can often be identified by palpating a cylindrical mass along the medial aspect of the mid-point of the ligament where the artery should be.

For surgical exposure, a longitudinal incision about one fingerbreadth medial to the midpoint of the inguinal ligament is generally appropriate, with proximal extension to the inguinal ligament. When disease is confined to the CFA without the need for extensive PFA or SFA revascularization, an oblique or transverse incision approximately two finger breadths above the groin crease may suffice. The distal extent of the incision depends on the degree of exposure required for the SFA or PFA. For PFA disease limited to the orifice, proximal control of the main trunk allows for an eversion endarterectomy. In cases of extensive PFA disease, slight anterior-lateral curvature of the incision and ligation of the lateral circumflex femoral vein allows adequate exposure for the main trunk down to its second- and third-order branches [38, 40]. Care must be taken to avoid branches of the femoral nerve, which runs superficial to the mid-distal profunda, crossing laterally to medially.

After arterial exposure proximal and distal to the plaque, systemic heparin is administered at a dose of approximately 80–100 units per kilogram, targeting an activated clotting time (ACT) >250 s, and vascular control is obtained using atraumatic vascular clamps. A longitudinal arteriotomy is made proximal to the plaque or to the level of the inferior epigastric artery and extended distally onto the SFA if profundaplasty can be accomplished via eversion. In the setting of SFA occlusion or extensive PFA disease requiring direct endarterectomy, distal extension is made onto the PFA [41, 42]. An endarterectomy plane is established in the CFA, and complete plaque mobilization is achieved using a freer elevator. Care is taken to ensure clear visibility of distal endpoints, with tacking sutures applied to address any intimal flaps that might cause flow-limiting dissections once antegrade flow is restored. Following a satisfactory endarterectomy, the arteriotomy is closed with a patch angioplasty technique using bovine pericardium, a Dacron patch, or a vein patch, with no single material demonstrating superiority [43–45].

Upon completion of the arteriotomy repair and restoration of flow, continuous-wave Doppler is used to detect any flow-limiting dissections or technical defects, which can be further assessed with intraoperative DUS. Patients with SFA occlusions who are PFA-dependent may not exhibit significant changes in pedal pulse examination but may show a monophasic Doppler signal. Any signs of extremity discoloration, delayed capillary refill, or worsening vascular status in the foot should prompt intraoperative catheter angiography to evaluate both inflow and distal runoff [46, 47].

Postoperative Outcomes After CFA Endarterectomy

In the literature, 30–45% of patients undergoing CFA endarterectomy present with lifestyle-limiting claudication, with high technical success rates and early symptom relief [48–52]. A National Surgical Quality Improvement Program (NSQIP) database study of 1843 CFA endarterectomies recorded a failure rate of only 1.1% at 30 days, with a 1.5% risk of adverse cardiovascular events and a 3.3% pulmonary complication rate [51]. Advanced age remains an independent risk factor for perioperative mortality, with Uhl et al. reporting a 7.6% mortality rate in octogenarians compared to 1.6% in patients under 80 years old [52].

While routine preoperative evaluation for cardiac ischemia is not recommended in patients without symptoms suggestive of coronary artery disease (CAD), most severe PAD patients have some degree of CAD. Maintaining a high index of suspicion for myocardial ischemia is critical, as any new symptoms in the postoperative period must be promptly evaluated and treated. Similarly, PAD patients frequently exhibit smoking-related comorbidities or undiagnosed chronic obstructive pulmonary disease (COPD). Pulmonary complications, ranging from aspiration pneumonitis to respiratory failure requiring reintubation or prolonged ventilation, can significantly contribute to postoperative morbidity [53, 54]. For patients with claudication, this serves as another reason why smoking cessation should be achieved prior to any revascularization.

Early thrombosis after CFA endarterectomy is rare but typically occurs in cases of suboptimal inflow due to untreated iliac artery disease or compromised distal endpoints at the PFA or SFA [55]. Careful review of preoperative imaging is crucial for planning the management of these endpoints. For instance, profunda disease confined to the orifice or proximal few millimeters of the main trunk can often be treated with an eversion endarterectomy, avoiding extensive exposure and patching. Similarly, extensive SFA endarterectomy should generally be avoided due to lack of added benefit. Remote SFA endarterectomy, a hybrid approach combining CFA endarterectomy and long-segment SFA revascularization, has been reported, but its 1-year patency rate of ~60% underscores the importance of prioritizing inflow optimization and addressing any profunda disease for durable outcomes [56, 57].

For active smokers, the risk-benefit ratio of CFA endarterectomy is favorable only in the setting of severe claudication. The importance of perioperative smoking cessation cannot be overstated. A retrospective cohort study of more than 14,000 patients undergoing open or endovascular revascularization demonstrated a 48% increase in postoperative complications in those who smoked within a year of the procedure, largely wound and cardiopulmonary related [58].

CFA endarterectomy is associated with excellent long-term patency rates. In a cohort of 91 limbs, the perioperative mortality rate was 2.2%, with an 8-year primary patency rate of 84% and 91% freedom from target lesion revascularization [59]. Similarly, Ballotta et al. reported a primary patency rate of 91% at 7 years, with 80% revascularization-free survival in 117 patients undergoing CFA endarterectomy [60]. In a large retrospective study of nearly 1000 patients, including octogenarians, 7-year primary patency was 84%, with limb salvage rates of 94% for patients under 80 and 92% for patients over 80 [61].

Management of Groin Infection

Surgical site infection (SSI) remains a significant concern following common femoral artery (CFA) endarterectomy, with an incidence ranging from 5% to 15% [62–65]. Risk factors include smoking, perioperative hyperglycemia, redo groin exposure, and return to the operating room during the same hospitalization. Large systematic reviews have demonstrated that neither antibiotic prophylaxis beyond 24 h nor the use of antibiotic-bonded Dacron patches provides additional benefit in preventing postoperative infections [64]. While CDC guidelines recommend a full-body shower before surgery, studies have shown no significant difference in infection rates between antiseptic and unmedicated bathing for patients undergoing groin exploration [67, 68].

Oblique or transverse incisions have been associated with lower rates of seroma and infection compared to vertical incisions, likely due to reduced lymphatic disruption [69–72]. However, laterally placed vertical incisions, which preserve lymphatic structures, have not shown these increased infection risks [73]. Vertical incisions are often selected for patients with greater comorbidity burden or more extensive arterial reconstruction, where the increased incision size contributes to higher wound morbidity. Regardless of the incision type, negative pressure wound therapy has consistently been shown in multiple randomized clinical trials to significantly reduce groin complications, including infection, particularly in high-risk patients [73–77].

Surgical intervention for groin infection after endarterectomy carries substantial morbidity and mortality. Superficial SSIs are typically treatable with antibiotics alone, while deep SSIs, often associated with seromas or hematomas, frequently require surgical debridement and local wound care. Organ/space (O/S) SSIs, which involve vascular patch or graft infections, are particularly devastating. They can result in thrombosis, limb loss, or catastrophic bleeding caused by infected false aneurysms [78, 79].

A scoring system has been devised to predict patients who would benefit from prophylactic muscle flap coverage [80–83]. Early involvement of plastic surgery is recommended for high-risk patients, as early flap coverage (commonly a pedicled anterolateral thigh myocutaneous flap) can salvage infected patches in low-virulence infections. However, infections involving gram-negative bacteria usually necessitate patch excision, wide debridement, and autogenous reconstruction.

For high-risk patients, sartorius myoplasty may be performed by the vascular surgeon at the time of femoral endarterectomy. This technique involves mobilization of the lateral edge of the sartorius muscle, from the distal extent of the incision up to the tendinous origin at the anterior superior iliac spine (ASIS). After transecting the tendinous insertion at the ASIS, the muscle is rotated medially while preserving its medial arterial blood supply. The muscle is secured cranially to the inguinal ligament and medially to the femoral sheath and surrounding deep soft tissue, ensuring complete coverage of the femoral reconstruction. A closed suction drain is placed in the muscle harvest site, and the incision is closed in layers over the muscle flap. The drain is removed once drainage is less than 30 cc in 24 h for two consecutive days.

Endovascular Therapy

While surgical endarterectomy remains the gold standard for treating common CFA disease, advances in endovascular therapy (EVT) have led to an increasing adoption of fully endovascular approaches [84]. This trend is driven by a growing population of patients with symptomatic peripheral artery disease (PAD) who are elderly and/or have significant comorbidities, rendering them high-risk candidates for surgical revascularization. There is an obvious potential contradiction in this pretense, with deeming a patient too high risk medically for even a regional anesthetic, but vigorous enough to have significant disability from claudication. However, the Society for Vascular Surgery (SVS) appropriate use criteria on intermittent claudication classify endovascular intervention for CFA disease as more risk than benefit in most scenarios [5]. The exception applies to non-nicotine users with severe disease who are on optimal medical therapy, where its efficacy remains indeterminate. By contrast, the 2024 American College of Cardiology/American Heart Association (ACC/AHA) consensus guidelines acknowledge a role for EVT in patients with favorable anatomical factors who are at too high risk for surgery [85]. In general, these procedures should be reserved for the highest-risk patients with either CLTI or debilitating lower extremity claudication symptoms. Patients with multiple prior groin operations, prior wound complications, and/or muscle flaps may be considered for EVT.

Endovascular access to the CFA is typically achieved through the contralateral femoral artery or via the upper extremity. Both approaches allow for profunda femoris artery (PFA) intervention, although a contralateral femoral approach provides the most flexibility for choosing among angioplasty, atherectomy, or stenting. As radial and pedal intervention tools become more versatile, the limitations of upper extremity access may diminish over time. A retrospective study from the Vascular Quality Initiative involving 1014 patients reported a 30-day mortality of 1.6% and a 1-year re-intervention-free survival rate of 88% [84]. In this cohort, chronic obstructive pulmonary disease (COPD), case urgency, and prior bypass surgery were significant predictors of re-intervention. Similarly, a multicenter propensity-matched study comparing EVT and surgical thromboendarterectomy found fewer perioperative complications and shorter hospital stays in the EVT group. However, 1-year primary patency was significantly lower in EVT patients (82% vs. 97% in the surgical group) [86].

Among EVT modalities, angioplasty alone—whether with plain or drug-coated balloons—carries a nine-fold higher risk of restenosis, while stenting reduces this to a four-fold increase compared to surgical revascularization. The presence of nodular calcification is strongly associated with early restenosis, while the use of intravascular ultrasound (IVUS) has shown no significant impact on restenosis risk [87, 88].

Intravascular lithotripsy (IVL) is increasing in popularity as an adjunct for vessel preparation prior to angioplasty or stenting in cases of eccentric calcific stenosis. A case series with 18-month follow-up reported technical success rates with <30% restenosis and a target lesion revascularization-free survival rate of 81% [89, 90]. Similarly, the Disrupt PAD trial showed improved 2-year patency rates with IVL (70%) compared to vessel preparation with plain balloon angioplasty (51%) before drug-coated balloon angioplasty [91–93].

Atherectomy, another modality for vessel preparation and plaque debulking prior to angioplasty or stenting, has seen increasing adoption despite mixed evidence supporting its added clinical benefit [94–98]. Devices employing rotational, directional, orbital, or laser ablation have become commercially available, with directional atherectomy often preferred for CFA disease due to the burden of eccentric calcific stenosis [99–101]. While limited data suggest 1-year patency rates >90% when combined with drug-coated balloon angioplasty and/or selective stenting, the risks of pseudoaneurysm formation, perforation, and distal embolization are significant. Distal embolic protection is recommended in all atherectomy cases due to the high technical difficulty of distal outflow vessel rescue when embolization occurs [102–105].

Stenting of the CFA is generally avoided due to the artery's mobility near the inguinal ligament, which increases the risk of stent fracture and thrombosis. Stenting also risks "jailing" the profunda, potentially compromising its patency as a key outflow vessel. While stenting can reduce vessel recoil during the initial intervention, 1-year patency rates remain at 80–85%, lower than those of endarterectomy [106]. A study by Martin et al. reported 80% patency at 2 years for nitinol stenting of the CFA, which improved to 96% with secondary interventions [107].

Antithrombotic therapy is essential following intervention. According to the 2024 ACC/AHA consensus guidelines, dual antiplatelet therapy with aspirin and a P2Y12 inhibitor is recommended after EVT [85]. For patients requiring anticoagulation for other indications, single antiplatelet therapy is advised. Recent clinical trials have shown that adding low-dose rivaroxaban to aspirin significantly reduces major adverse cardiovascular and limb events compared to aspirin alone, with similar benefits observed in patients at high baseline risk for cardiovascular complications [108, 109].

Hybrid Techniques

CFA occlusive disease is rarely an isolated phenomenon, as coexisting iliac, aortic, and distal occlusive disease is common. Femoral endarterectomy alone is unlikely to succeed in patients with severe inflow disease. In such cases, a hybrid approach that combines inflow angioplasty and stenting with femoral endarterectomy and profundaplasty may be necessary.

In a retrospective study of consecutive cases, Boulitrop et al. reported a 48% rate of iliac stenting in conjunction with CFA endarterectomy, with a 30-day mortality rate of 3% and an 8% overall complication rate, consistent with other studies [110, 111]. Long-term primary patency was 82% at 2 years, improving to 95% with secondary interventions. While there is a relative increase in ipsilateral hypogastric artery occlusion following combined interventions, cases of symptomatic pelvic ischemia have not been reported.

When adjunctive iliac artery stenting is required, or when balloon inflow occlusion is preferable to clamping an extensively diseased external iliac artery, the pre-arteriotomy guidewire access (PAGA, Fig. 14.1a) technique can be highly beneficial [112–114]. Although not always necessary, PAGA offers advantages by avoiding retrograde dissection, which can occur when attempting to access the iliac artery retrogradely after CFA endarterectomy if a plaque shelf is left in the distal external iliac artery.

In the PAGA technique, patients with patent but diseased CFA and external iliac arteries undergo surgical exposure of the CFA. The artery is accessed retrograde with a micropuncture set, followed by the placement of a sheath. A guidewire and catheter are advanced into the aorta, and the intraluminal location is confirmed. A stiff guidewire (e.g., Storq, Amplatz) is then advanced into the proximal aorta, allowing a balloon to be positioned in the external iliac artery for inflow occlusion (Fig. 14.1b).

Variations of this technique exist depending on the adjunctive procedures planned. If iliac inflow stenting is anticipated, the balloon catheter and wire are left exiting through the side of the patch closure. Once the patch closure is near completion and the proximal and distal sutures are brought around the balloon catheter, they are secured with a Rummel tourniquet to prevent bleeding at the exit site. The deflated balloon is then removed over the wire, and a sheath is placed to perform inflow stenting, including into the patch if needed. After the endovascular procedure, the sheath and wire are removed, and the sutures are tied down. Reinforcing U-stitches of 5-0 polypropylene may be required to secure hemostasis.

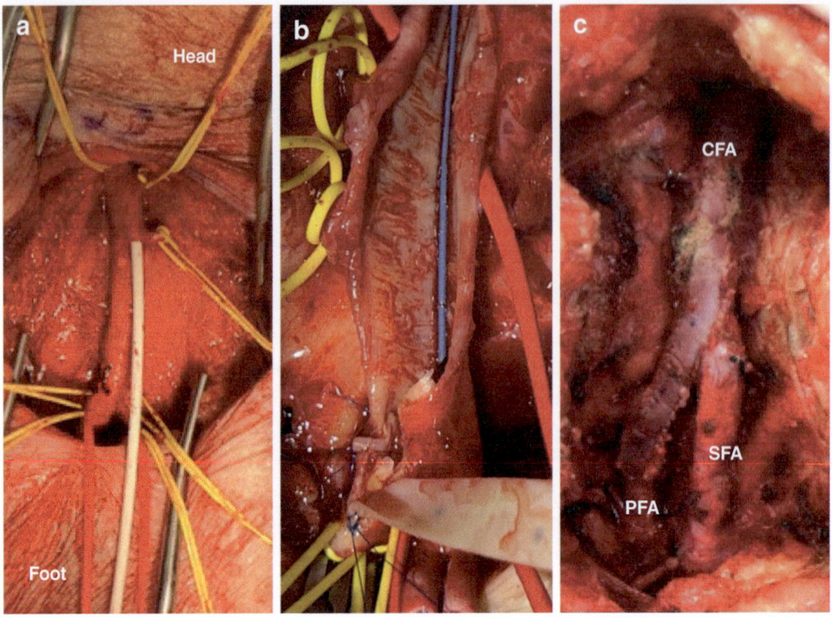

Fig. 14.1 Surgical revascularization of the common femoral artery with (**a**) pre-arteriotomy guide wire access (PAGA) for concurrent iliac artery endovascular revascularization or balloon occlusion for proximal control, (**b**) as demonstrated here with the endarterectomized common femoral artery with patch anchored distally and stiff guidewire in place, and (**c**) finally, the completed patch after common femoral artery (CFA) to main trunk profunda femoris artery (PFA) endarterectomy with bovine pericardial patch angioplasty in the setting of superficial femoral artery (SFA) occlusion

For patients with occluded iliac arteries, the PAGA technique is similar but involves retrograde recanalization using a glidewire and crossing catheter. Percutaneous contralateral access is another option, allowing balloon inflow occlusion from the external iliac artery. After patch closure is complete, the balloon is removed, and additional procedures are performed. This method is especially useful for patients requiring concomitant superficial femoral artery (SFA) intervention, as it avoids the ergonomic challenges of antegrade patch access for SFA procedures.

CFA revascularization with profundaplasty is generally sufficient to relieve symptoms of claudication (Fig. 14.1c). This is true even in the presence of severe femoropopliteal disease if there is robust collateralization through the PFA to the infra-geniculate vessels. While the proximal several centimeters of the PFA can be reconstructed using extensive endarterectomy, severe mid-to-distal PFA disease with disrupted collateralization to the tibial vessels is challenging to address. In such cases, inline flow restoration through the femoropopliteal segment may be necessary. Hybrid techniques, such as SFA recanalization from a pedal approach with externalization of the wire through the endarterectomy site followed by antegrade intervention, have shown proven technical success in these rare situations [115, 116].

Summary

Patients with claudication due to common femoral and/or profunda occlusive disease should receive counseling for risk factor modification, smoking cessation, and exercise therapy as first-line treatment. For those who continue to experience lifestyle-limiting functional walking impairment, a discussion of revascularization may be warranted. While open, endovascular, and hybrid techniques have all been described, common femoral endarterectomy with profundaplasty remains the gold standard. The Achilles heel of this operation remains the risk of wound dehiscence and SSI. Efforts such as transverse incisions, impeccable sterile technique, and adherence to all SSI-reducing best practices should be considered.

References

1. Fowkes FGR, Rudan D, Rudan I, Aboyans V, Denenberg JO, McDermott MM, Criqui MH, Sampson UK, Norman PE, Mills JL. Comparison of global estimates of prevalence and risk factors for peripheral artery disease in 2000 and 2010: a systematic review and analysis. Lancet. 2013;382(9901):1329–40.
2. Criqui MH, Aboyans V. Epidemiology of peripheral artery disease. Circ Res. 2015;116(9):1509–26.
3. Shammas NW. Epidemiology, classification, and modifiable risk factors of peripheral arterial disease. Vasc Health Risk Manag. 2007;3(2):229–34. https://doi.org/10.2147/vhrm.2007.3.2.229.
4. Gerhard-Herman MD, Gornik HL, Barrett C, Barshes NR, Corriere MA, Drachman DE, Fleisher LA, Fowkes FGR, Hamburg NM, Kinlay S. 2016 AHA/ACC guideline on the management of patients with lower extremity peripheral artery disease: executive summary. Circulation. 2017;135(12):e686–725.
5. Woo K, Siracuse JJ, Klingbeil K, Kraiss LW, Osborne NH, Singh N, Tan TW, Arya S, Banerjee S, Bonaca MP, Brothers T, Conte MS, Dawson DL, Erben Y, Lerner BM, Lin JC, Mills JL Sr, Mittleider D, Nair DG, O'Banion LA, Patterson RB, Scheidt MJ, Simons JP, Society for Vascular Surgery Appropriateness Committee. Society for Vascular Surgery appropriate use criteria for management of intermittent claudication. J Vasc Surg. 2022;76(1):3–22.e1.
6. McDermott MM, Liu K, Greenland P, Guralnik JM, Celic L, Criqui MH, Schneider JR. Functional decline in peripheral arterial disease: associations with the ankle-brachial index and leg symptoms. JAMA. 2004;292(4):453–61.
7. Norgren L, Hiatt WR, Dormandy JA, Nehler MR, Harris KA, Fowkes FGR. Inter-society consensus for the management of peripheral arterial disease (TASC II). J Vasc Surg. 2007;45(1):S5–S67.
8. Bonaca MP, Creager MA. Pharmacological treatment and current management of peripheral artery disease. Circ Res. 2015;116(9):1579–98.
9. Conte MS, Bradbury AW, Kolh P, White JV, Dick F, Fitridge R, Mills JL, Ricco J-B, Suresh KR, Murad MH. Global vascular guidelines on the management of chronic limb-threatening ischemia. J Vasc Surg. 2019;69(6):3S–125S.
10. Sorber R, Dun C, Kawaji Q, Abularrage CJ, Black JH 3rd, Makary MA, Hicks CW. Early peripheral vascular interventions for claudication are associated with higher rates of late interventions and progression to chronic limb threatening ischemia. J Vasc Surg. 2023;77(3):836–847.e3.
11. Golledge J, Moxon JV, Rowbotham S, Pinchbeck J, Yip L, Velu R, Quigley F, Jenkins J, Morris DR. Risk of major amputation in patients with intermittent claudication undergoing early revascularization. Br J Surg. 2018;105(6):699–708.

12. Madabhushi V, Davenport D, Jones S, Khoudoud SA, Orr N, Minion D, Endean E, Tyagi S. Revascularization of intermittent claudicants leads to more chronic limb-threatening ischemia and higher amputation rates. J Vasc Surg. 2021;74(3):771–9.
13. Society for Vascular Surgery Lower Extremity Guidelines Writing Group, Conte MS, Pomposelli FB, Clair DG, Geraghty PJ, JF MK, Mills JL, Moneta GL, Murad MH, Powell RJ, Reed AB, Schanzer A, Sidawy AN, Society for Vascular Surgery. Society for Vascular Surgery practice guidelines for atherosclerotic occlusive disease of the lower extremities: management of asymptomatic disease and claudication. J Vasc Surg. 2015;61(3 Suppl):2S–41S.
14. Hiatt WR, Regensteiner JG. Exercise in the management of peripheral arterial disease. Vasc Med. 1993;1(2):65–73.
15. McDermott MM, Ades P, Guralnik JM, Dyer A, Ferrucci L, Liu K, Nelson M, Lloyd-Jones D, Van Horn L, Garside D, Kibbe M, Criqui MH. Treadmill exercise and resistance training in patients with peripheral arterial disease with and without intermittent claudication: a randomized controlled trial. JAMA. 2009;301(2):165–74.
16. Beebe HG, Dawson DL, Cutler BS, Herd JA, Strandness DE Jr, Berman SS, Rapp JH, Bakal CW. A new pharmacological treatment for intermittent claudication: results of a randomized, multicenter trial. Arch Intern Med. 1999;159(18):2041–50.
17. Creager MA, Matsushita M, Arya S, Hamburg NM. Risk factor modification in patients with lower extremity peripheral artery disease: a scientific statement from the American Heart Association. Circulation. 2018;137(8):e493–522.
18. Bonaca MP, Hamburg NM, Creager MA. Contemporary medical management of peripheral artery disease. Circ Res. 2021;128(12):1868–84.
19. Steg PG, Bhatt DL, Wilson PW, D'Agostino R, Ohman EM, Röther J, Liau CS, Hirsch AT, Mas JL, Ikeda Y, Pencina MJ, Goto S. One-year cardiovascular event rates in outpatients with atherothrombosis. JAMA. 2007;297(11):1197–206.
20. Dormandy J, Heeck L, Vig S. The natural history of claudication: risk to life and limb. Semin Vasc Surg. 1999;12(2):123–37.
21. Boufi M, Ejargue M, Gaye M, Boyer L, Alimi Y, Loundou AD. Systematic review and meta-analysis of endovascular versus open repair for common femoral artery atherosclerosis treatment. J Vasc Surg. 2021;73(4):1445–55.
22. Ng JJ, Choong AMTL. More randomized controlled trials are needed to support the use of endovascular treatment in common femoral artery atherosclerotic lesions. J Vasc Surg. 2021;74(1):345–6.
23. Soga Y, Nakano M, Yokoi H, Shiraki T. Long-term outcome of endovascular therapy for common femoral artery lesions. Circ J. 2015;79(11):2422–9.
24. Wennberg PW. Approach to the patient with peripheral arterial disease. Circulation. 2013;128(20):2241–50.
25. Aboyans V, Criqui MH, Abraham P, Allison MA, Creager MA, Diehm C, Fowkes FGR, Hiatt WR, Norgren L. Measurement and interpretation of the ankle-brachial index: a scientific statement from the American Heart Association. Circulation. 2012;126(24):2890–909.
26. Hiatt WR, Marshall JA, Baxter J, Sandoval R, Hildebrandt W, Kahn LR, Hamman RF. Diagnostic methods for peripheral arterial disease in the San Luis Valley Diabetes Study. J Clin Epidemiol. 1990;43(6):597–606.
27. Davidson BP, Hodovan J, Mason OR, Moccetti F, Gupta A, Muller M, Belcik JT, Annex BH, Lindner JR. Limb perfusion during exercise assessed by contrast ultrasound varies according to symptom severity in patients with peripheral artery disease. J Am Soc Echocardiogr. 2019;32(9):1086–1094.e3.
28. Dawson DL, Cutler BS, Hiatt WR, Hobson RW, Martin JD, Berman SS. A comparison of segmental arterial Doppler pressures and pulse volume recordings in peripheral arterial disease detection. J Vasc Surg. 1997;26(6):923–9.
29. Crawford F, Welch K, Andras A, Chappell FM. Ankle brachial index for the diagnosis of lower limb peripheral arterial disease. Cochrane Database Syst Rev. 2016;9(9):CD010680.
30. Gao M, Hua Y, Zhao X, Jia L, Yang J, Liu B. Optimal ultrasound criteria for grading stenosis of the superficial femoral artery. Ultrasound Med Biol. 2018;44(2):350–8.

31. Macharzina RR, Schmid SF, Beschorner U, Noory E, Rastan A, Vach W, Schwarzwälder U, Sixt S, Bürgelin K, Neumann FJ, Zeller T. Duplex ultrasound assessment of native stenoses in the superficial femoral and popliteal arteries: a comparative study examining the influence of multisegment lesions. J Endovasc Ther. 2015;22(2):254–60.
32. White CM, Armstrong PJ. Computed tomography angiography in the management of peripheral arterial disease. Semin Intervent Radiol. 2009;26(2):86–101.
33. Edelman RR, Koktzoglou I, Lovrencic M. Non-contrast MR angiography for the assessment of peripheral arterial disease. Radiology. 2018;287(2):570–80.
34. Gupta R, Sedgwick JF. Digital subtraction angiography: techniques, applications, and practical tips. J Postgrad Med. 2002;48(4):333–40.
35. Ghanami RJ, Hurie J, Andrews JS, Harrington RN, Corriere MA, Goodney PP, Hansen KJ, Edwards MS. Anesthesia-based evaluation of outcomes of lower-extremity vascular bypass procedures. Ann Vasc Surg. 2013;27(2):199–207.
36. Johnson OW, Branche JA, Coleman DM. Regional anesthesia in vascular surgery: a critical analysis of benefits, outcomes, and controversies. Semin Vasc Surg. 2018;31(3–4):116–22.
37. Creager MA, Belkin M, Auster M. Vascular anatomy and exposure. In: Surgery of the aorta and its branches. W.B. Saunders; 2004.
38. Wain RA, White GH. Techniques for common femoral artery reconstruction. J Cardiovasc Surg. 2012;53(3):283–94.
39. Schneider PA, Caps MT. Common femoral endarterectomy: indications and operative technique. Tech Vasc Endovasc Surg. 2013;16(1):24–30.
40. Black JH, Sicard GA. Arterial exposure and endarterectomy. In: Current techniques in vascular surgery. New York: McGraw-Hill; 2003.
41. Towne JB, Rollins DL. Profundaplasty: its role in limb salvage. Surg Clin North Am. 1986;66(2):403–14.
42. Taylor LM Jr, Baur GM, Eidemiller LR, Porter JM. Extended profundaplasty. Indications and techniques with results of 46 procedures. Am J Surg. 1981;141(5):539–42.
43. Biasi G, Mingoli A, Simonetti G. Patch angioplasty in femoral artery surgery: materials and results. Eur J Vasc Endovasc Surg. 2005;30(5):547–54.
44. Nasr B, Carret M, Pluchon K, Bezon E. Common femoral artery endarterectomy by eversion versus prosthetic patch angioplasty: a propensity-matched study. J Cardiovasc Surg. 2023;64(3):279–86.
45. Oldenburg WA, Almerey T, Selim M, Farres H, Hakaim AG. Durability of carotid endarterectomy with bovine pericardial patch. Ann Vasc Surg. 2018;50:218–24.
46. Normahani P, Khan B, Sounderajah V, Poushpas S, Anwar M, Jaffer U. Applications of intraoperative Duplex ultrasound in vascular surgery: a systematic review. Ultrasound J. 2021;13(1):8.
47. Miller A, Campbell DR, Gibbons GW, Pomposelli FB Jr, Freeman DV, Jepsen SJ, Lees RS, Isaacsohn JL, Purcell D, Bolduc M, et al. Routine intraoperative angioscopy in lower extremity revascularization. Arch Surg. 1989;124(5):604–8.
48. Nguyen BN, Amdur RL, Abugideiri M, Rahbar R, Neville RF, Sidawy AN. Postoperative complications after common femoral endarterectomy. J Vasc Surg. 2015;61(6):1489–94.e1.
49. Ballotta E, Gruppo M, Mazzalai F, Da Giau G. Common femoral artery endarterectomy: a prospective evaluation of 108 consecutive cases. Ann Vasc Surg. 2010;24(4):465–73.
50. Darling RC 3rd, Lumsden AB. Common femoral artery reconstruction: techniques and outcomes. Ann Surg. 1997;225(4):434–9.
51. Neville RF, Sidawy AN, Katz B, Kumer S. Outcomes of common femoral endarterectomy: insights from the NSQIP database. J Vasc Surg. 2010;52(4):80S–6S.
52. Uhl C, Hohmann C. Perioperative outcomes in elderly patients undergoing femoral artery surgery. Eur J Vasc Endovasc Surg. 2016;51(6):755–62.
53. Siracuse JJ, Gill HL, Schneider DB, Graham AR, Connolly PH, Jones DW, Meltzer AJ. Assessing the perioperative safety of common femoral endarterectomy in the endovascular era. Vasc Endovasc Surg. 2014;48(1):27–33.

54. Sarfati M, Mouquet C. Pulmonary complications after vascular surgery. Eur J Vasc Endovasc Surg. 2017;53(3):347–52.
55. Kang JL, Patel VI, Conrad MF, Lamuraglia GM, Chung TK, Cambria RP. Common femoral artery occlusive disease: contemporary results following surgical endarterectomy. J Vasc Surg. 2008;48(4):872–7.
56. Antoniou GA, Koutsias S, Antoniou SA, Giannoukas AD. Remote endarterectomy for long segment superficial femoral artery occlusive disease. A systematic review. Eur J Vasc Endovasc Surg. 2008;36(3):310–8.
57. Malkawi AH, Hinchliffe RJ, Loftus IM. Remote superficial femoral artery endarterectomy: long-term outcomes. Eur J Vasc Endovasc Surg. 2008;36(5):545–50.
58. Reitz KM, Althouse AD, Meyer J, Arya S, Goodney PP, Shireman PK, Hall DE, Tzeng E. Association of smoking with postprocedural complications following open and endovascular interventions for intermittent claudication. JAMA Cardiol. 2022;7(1):45–54.
59. Hashimoto T, Yamamoto S, Kimura M, Sano M, Sato O, Deguchi J. Long-term outcomes following common femoral endarterectomy. J Clin Med. 2022;11(22):6873.
60. Ballotta E, Gruppo M, Mazzalai F, Da Giau G. Common femoral artery endarterectomy for occlusive disease: an 8-year single-center prospective study. Surgery. 2010;147(2):268–74.
61. Uhl C, Götzke H, Zeman F, Woronowicz S, Betz T, Töpel I, Steinbauer M. Long-term outcome of common femoral artery endarterectomy in octogenarians and non-octogenarians. Scand J Surg. 2021;110(3):400–6.
62. Derksen WJ, Verhoeven BA, van de Mortel RH, Moll FL, de Vries JP. Risk factors for surgical-site infection following common femoral artery endarterectomy. Vasc Endovasc Surg. 2009;43(1):69–75.
63. Greenblatt DY, Rajamanickam V, Mell MW. Predictors of surgical site infection after open lower extremity revascularization. J Vasc Surg. 2011;54(2):433–9.
64. Amato B, Compagna R, De Vivo S, Rocca A, Carbone F, Gentile M, Cirocchi R, Squizzato F, Spertino A, Battocchio P. Groin surgical site infection in vascular surgery: systemic review on peri-operative antibiotic prophylaxis. Antibiotics (Basel). 2022;11(2):134.
65. McGinigle KL, Spangler EL, Ayyash K, Arya S, Settembrini AM, Thomas MM, Dell KE, Swiderski IJ, Davies MG, Setacci C, Urman RD, Howell SJ, Garg J, Ljungvist O, de Boer HD. A framework for perioperative care for lower extremity vascular bypasses: a consensus statement by the Enhanced Recovery after Surgery (ERAS®) Society and Society for Vascular Surgery. J Vasc Surg. 2023;77(5):1295–315.
66. Robbins JM, Courtney J, Hingorani A. Systematic review of groin incision surgical site infection preventative measures in vascular surgery. J Vasc Surg. 2023;77(6):1835–1850.e2.
67. Mangram AJ, Horan TC, Pearson ML, Silver LC, Jarvis WR. Guideline for prevention of surgical site infection, 1999. Infect Control Hosp Epidemiol. 1999;20(4):247–80.
68. Webster J, Osborne S. Preoperative bathing or showering with skin antiseptics to prevent surgical site infection. Cochrane Database Syst Rev. 2015;2015(2):CD004985.
69. Roberts JR, Walters GK, Zenilman ME, Jones CE. Groin lymphorrhea complicating revascularization involving the femoral vessels. Am J Surg. 1993;165(3):341–4.
70. Ng JJ, Tan JKH, Lee JWK, Choong AMTL. Longitudinal versus transverse incision for common femoral artery exposure: a systematic review and meta-analysis. ANZ J Surg. 2021;91(5):822–31.
71. Canteras M, Baptista-Silva JC, do Carmo Novaes F, Cacione DG. Transverse versus vertical groin incision for femoral artery approach. Cochrane Database Syst Rev. 2020;4(4):CD013153.
72. Swinnen J, Chao A, Tiwari A, Crozier J, Vicaretti M, Fletcher J. Vertical or transverse incisions for access to the femoral artery: a randomized control study. Ann Vasc Surg. 2010;24(3):336–41.
73. Ploeg AJ, Lardenoye JW, Peeters MP, Hamming JF, Breslau PJ. Wound complications at the groin after peripheral arterial surgery sparing the lymphatic tissue: a double-blind randomized clinical trial. Am J Surg. 2009;197(6):747–51.
74. Kostiuk V, Fereydooni S, Setia O, Loh SA, Strosberg D, Tonnessen BH, Ochoa Chaar CI, Aboian E. Comparative analysis of negative pressure wound therapy (PICO)

and standard dressing application after arterial vascular reconstructions. Vascular. 2024;2024:17085381241296606.
75. Kwon J, Staley C, McCullough M, Goss S, Arosemena M, Abai B, Salvatore D, Reiter D, DiMuzio P. A randomized clinical trial evaluating negative pressure therapy to decrease vascular groin incision complications. J Vasc Surg. 2018;68(6):1744–52.
76. Murphy P, Lee K, Dubois L, DeRose G, Forbes T, Power A. Negative pressure wound therapy for high-risk wounds in lower extremity revascularization: study protocol for a randomized controlled trial. Trials. 2015;16:504.
77. Boll G, Callas P, Bertges DJ. Meta-analysis of prophylactic closed-incision negative pressure wound therapy for vascular surgery groin wounds. J Vasc Surg. 2022;75(6):2086–2093.e9.
78. Walker H, Chana MS, Mandalia K, Kulkarni SR, Paravastu SCV. Observational study on the risk of surgical site infection in patients undergoing common femoral endarterectomy in conjunction with an endovascular procedure compared with common femoral endarterectomy alone. EJVES Vasc Forum. 2024;61:116–20.
79. Sapienza P, Napoli F, Tartaglia E, Venturini L, Sterpetti AV, Brachini G, Gazzanelli S, Mingoli A. Infection of prosthetic patches after femoral endarterectomy: an unreported complication. Ann Vasc Surg. 2019;56:11–6.
80. Fischer JP, Nelson JA, Rohrbach JI, Wu LC, Woo EY, Kovach SJ, Low DW, Serletti JM, Kanchwala S. Prophylactic muscle flaps in vascular surgery: the penn groin assessment scale. Plast Reconstr Surg. 2012;129(6):940e–9e.
81. Wallace AB, Piper ML, Holland M, Lee S, Orringer M, Eichler C, Kim EA, Hansen SL. Prophylactic muscle flaps in primary vascular procedures of the groin. Ann Vasc Surg. 2022;78:77–83.
82. Fischer JP, Nelson JA, Mirzabeigi MN, Wang GJ, Foley PJ 3rd, Wu LC, Woo EY, Kanchwala S. Prophylactic muscle flaps in vascular surgery. J Vasc Surg. 2012;55(4):1081–6.
83. Fischer JP, Nelson JA, Shang EK, Wink JD, Wingate NA, Woo EY, Jackson BM, Kovach SJ, Kanchwala S. Predicting the need for muscle flap salvage after open groin vascular procedures: a clinical assessment tool. J Plast Surg Hand Surg. 2014;48(6):389–95.
84. Siracuse JJ, Van Orden K, Kalish JA, Eslami MH, Schermerhorn ML, Patel VI, Rybin D, Farber A, Vascular Quality Initiative. Endovascular treatment of the common femoral artery in the Vascular Quality Initiative. J Vasc Surg. 2017;65(4):1039–46.
85. Writing Committee Members, Gornik HL, Aronow HD, Goodney PP, Arya S, Brewster LP, Byrd L, Chandra V, Drachman DE, Eaves JM, Ehrman JK, Evans JN, Getchius TSD, Gutiérrez JA, Hawkins BM, Hess CN, Ho KJ, Jones WS, Kim ESH, Kinlay S, Kirksey L, Kohlman-Trigoboff D, Long CA, Pollak AW, Sabri SS, Sadwin LB, Secemsky EA, Serhal M, Shishehbor MH, Treat-Jacobson D, Wilkins LR. 2024 ACC/AHA/AACVPR/APMA/ABC/SCAI/SVM/SVN/SVS/SIR/VESS Guideline for the Management of Lower Extremity Peripheral Artery Disease: a report of the American College of Cardiology/American Heart Association Joint Committee on Clinical Practice Guidelines. J Am Coll Cardiol. 2024;83(24):2497–604.
86. Nakama T, Takahara M, Iwata Y, Fujimura N, Yamaoka T, Suzuki K, Obunai K, CAULIFLOWER Study Investigators. 1-year outcomes of thromboendarterectomy vs endovascular therapy for common femoral artery lesions: CAULIFLOWER study results. JACC Cardiovasc Interv. 2022;15(14):1453–63.
87. Kuo TT, Chen PL, Huang CY, Lee CY, Shih CC, Chen IM. Outcome of drug-eluting balloon angioplasty versus endarterectomy in common femoral artery occlusive disease. J Vasc Surg. 2019;69(1):141–7.
88. Imran HM, Hyder ON, Soukas PA. Efficacy and safety of adjunctive drug-coated balloon therapy in endovascular treatment of common femoral artery disease. Cardiovasc Revasc Med. 2019;20(3):210–4.
89. Brodmann M, Schwindt A, Argyriou A, Gammon R. Safety and feasibility of intravascular lithotripsy for treatment of common femoral artery stenoses. J Endovasc Ther. 2019;26(3):283–7.

90. Baig M, Kwok M, Aldairi A, Imran HM, Khan MS, Moustafa A, Hyder ON, Saad M, Aronow HD, Soukas PA. Endovascular intravascular lithotripsy in the treatment of calcific common femoral artery disease: a case series with an 18-month follow-up. Cardiovasc Revasc Med. 2022;43:80–4.
91. Tepe G, Brodmann M, Bachinsky W, Holden A, Zeller T, Mangalmurti S, Nolte-Ernsting C, Virmani R, Parikh SA, Gray WA. Intravascular lithotripsy for peripheral artery calcification: mid-term outcomes from the randomized disrupt PAD III trial. J Soc Cardiovasc Angiogr Interv. 2022;1(4):100341.
92. Brodmann M, Holden A, Zeller T, et al. Intravascular lithotripsy for treatment of calcified peripheral artery lesions: 12-month results of the DISRUPT PAD III trial. JACC Cardiovasc Interv. 2020;13(2):2681–93.
93. Scheinert D, Zeller T. DISRUPT PAD III: results from the prospective randomized trial of intravascular lithotripsy versus angioplasty. J Vasc Surg. 2021;73(5):1785–95.
94. Akkus NI, Abdulbaki A, Jimenez E, Tandon N. Atherectomy devices: technology update. Med Devices (Auckl). 2014;8:1–10.
95. Parikh K, Chandra P, Choksi N, Khanna P, Chambers J. Safety and feasibility of orbital atherectomy for the treatment of calcified coronary lesions: the ORBIT I trial. Catheter Cardiovasc Interv. 2013;81(7):1134–9.
96. Shammas NW, Lam R, Mustapha J, Ellichman J, Aggarwala G, Rivera E, Niazi K, Balar N. Comparison of orbital atherectomy plus balloon angioplasty vs. balloon angioplasty alone in patients with critical limb ischemia: results of the CALCIUM 360 randomized pilot trial. J Endovasc Ther. 2012;19(4):480–8.
97. Dave RM, Patlola R, Kollmeyer K, Bunch F, Weinstock BS, Dippel E, Jaff MR, Popma J, Weissman N, CELLO Investigators. Excimer laser recanalization of femoropopliteal lesions and 1-year patency: results of the CELLO registry. J Endovasc Ther. 2009;16(6):665–75.
98. Tran T, Brown M, Lasala J. An evidence-based approach to the use of rotational and directional coronary atherectomy in the era of drug-eluting stents: when does it make sense? Catheter Cardiovasc Interv. 2008;72(5):650–62.
99. Picazo F, Kwok RCH, Hockley JA, Garbowski MW, Samuelson SD, Jansen SJ. Directional atherectomy of the common femoral artery: complications and outcomes. Ann Vasc Surg. 2020;66:621–30.
100. Stavroulakis K, Schwindt A, Torsello G, Beropoulis E, Stachmann A, Hericks C, Bollenberg L, Bisdas T. Directional atherectomy with antirestenotic therapy vs drug-coated balloon angioplasty alone for common femoral artery atherosclerotic disease. J Endovasc Ther. 2018;25(1):92–9.
101. Sauguet A, Philippart R, Honton B. Directional atherectomy with antirestenotic therapy for the treatment of no-stenting zones. J Cardiovasc Surg. 2019;60(2):198–204.
102. Mendes BC, Oderich GS, Fleming MD, Misra S, Duncan AA, Kalra M, Cha S, Gloviczki P. Clinical significance of embolic events in patients undergoing endovascular femoropopliteal interventions with or without embolic protection devices. J Vasc Surg. 2014;59(2):359–367.e1.
103. Suri R, Wholey MH, Postoak D, Hagino RT, Toursarkissian B. Distal embolic protection during femoropopliteal atherectomy. Catheter Cardiovasc Interv. 2006;67(3):417–22.
104. Fereydooni A, Bai H, Baril D, Chandra V, Ochoa Chaar CI. Embolic protection devices are not associated with improved outcomes of atherectomy for lower extremity revascularization. Ann Vasc Surg. 2022;86:168–76.
105. Ochoa Chaar CI, Kim TI, Shebl FM, Dardik A. The use of embolic protection devices during lower extremity peripheral vascular interventions. Ann Vasc Surg. 2020;69:9–16.
106. Bath J, Avgerinos E. A pooled analysis of common femoral and profunda femoris endovascular interventions. Vascular. 2016;24(4):404–13.
107. Martin R, Vanesa GDC, Raleigh JV, Jose C, Vadim K, Maynar M, Zander T. Common femoral artery stenting: computed tomography angiography based long-term patency. Vasc Endovasc Surg. 2021;55(6):571–6.
108. Bonaca MP, Bauersachs RM, Anand SS, Debus ES, Nehler MR, Patel MR, Fanelli F, Capell WH, Diao L, Jaeger N, Hess CN, Pap AF, Kittelson JM, Gudz I, Mátyás L, Krievins DK,

Diaz R, Brodmann M, Muehlhofer E, Haskell LP, Berkowitz SD, Hiatt WR. Rivaroxaban in peripheral artery disease after revascularization. N Engl J Med. 2020;382(21):1994–2004.
109. Steffel J, Eikelboom JW, Anand SS, Shestakovska O, Yusuf S, Fox KAA. The COMPASS trial: net clinical benefit of low-dose rivaroxaban plus aspirin as compared with aspirin in patients with chronic vascular disease. Circulation. 2020;142(1):40–8.
110. Boulitrop C, Jayet J, Duprey A, Pellenc Q, Roussel A, Cerceau P, Ben Abdallah I, Castier Y. From the aortic bifurcation to the groin: long-term outcomes of covered kissing stent placement in combination with iliofemoral reconstruction for extensive iliofemoral occlusive disease. Ann Vasc Surg. 2020;64:11–6.
111. Inahara T, Yamamoto T. Hybrid strategies in the management of complex aortoiliac and femoral occlusive disease. Vasc Endovasc Surg. 2019;53(7):528–34.
112. Schneider PA, Laird JR. Pre-arteriotomy guidewire access: an essential tool in complex hybrid procedures. J Endovasc Ther. 2016;23(5):655–62.
113. Hinchliffe RJ, Loftus IM. Techniques for iliac stenting in conjunction with common femoral endarterectomy. Vasc Surg. 2014;12(4):271–6.
114. Kashyap VS, Clair DG. Combining open and endovascular techniques for complex aortoiliac and femoral disease. J Vasc Surg. 2013;58(6):1537–44.
115. Soga Y, Hirano K. Retrograde guidewire techniques in lower limb interventions: tips and tricks for success. J Endovasc Ther. 2015;22(3):413–9.
116. Dake MD, Scheinert D, Schmidt A. Hybrid interventions in the management of advanced femoropopliteal occlusive disease. J Endovasc Ther. 2019;26(3):371–82.

Revascularization: Infrainguinal—Evidence, Techniques, and Patient Selection

15

Reginald Nkansah and Gale Tang

Introduction

The overall natural history of intermittent claudication is slowly progressive and benign with respect to limb loss; less than 5% of patients develop chronic limb threatening ischemia (CLTI) and risk of major amputation with medical optimization. With regard to intervention, the Society for Vascular Surgery [1] recommends surgical treatment or endovascular therapy for intermittent claudication in patients with lifestyle-limiting disability with a reasonable likelihood of improvement who have already been medically optimized and have failed supervised exercise therapy (1B recommendation). There are no specific recommendations on the modality (1C recommendation).

Many studies have documented sustained benefit in patients with treatment of aorto-iliac occlusive disease and isolated proximal femoral disease. However, the outcomes of treatment of the femoropopliteal segment and the infrainguinal arterial tree are mixed, and treatment for intermittent claudication in these anatomic areas is more controversial. This chapter will specifically discuss open and endovascular therapy for infrainguinal disease as they relate to claudication. Patient selection for these procedures and outcomes of various stand-alone combined therapies are reviewed.

R. Nkansah
Division of Vascular Surgery, University of Washington, Seattle, WA, USA

G. Tang (✉)
Division of Vascular Surgery, Section Chief Vascular Surgery VAPSHCS, Department of Surgery, University of Washington, Seattle, WA, USA
e-mail: gtang@uw.edu

W. P. Robinson III, J. P. Simons (eds.), *The Patient-Centered Approach to Claudication*, https://doi.org/10.1007/978-3-032-02460-2_15

Patient Selection

There are numerous revascularization strategies to treat patients with intermittent claudication. This chapter reviews both open and endovascular options including open femoral endarterectomy, femoral to popliteal and tibial artery bypasses with various conduits as well as endovascular therapy including angioplasty, stenting, lithotripsy, atherectomy, and the DETOUR procedure. However, patient and procedural selection is imperative to achieve treatment success from the patient's perspective.

In patients with serious comorbidities, it has generally been considered prudent to pursue endovascular-first therapy. However, any intervention should be questioned if the severity of comorbidities is thought to be this high, particularly in the context of true benefit to the patient, as these patients are likely to be more limited by their other comorbidities than by their intermittent claudication. In those who are smoking or have a history of hypercoagulability, an open approach may be better, although revascularization in patients with claudication who have not achieved abstinence from smoking is controversial given increased rates of periprocedural complications [2] and long-term amputation rates as well as decreased overall survival [3].

Anatomic challenges based on significant arterial calcification and runoff should also impact approach as certain patterns of arterial disease such as popliteal occlusion or limited tibial runoff will significantly affect longer-term patency of endovascular revascularizations. Finally, the patient's smoking status should not be taken lightly as many of the recent trial data and Vascular Quality Initiative data indicate that a significant proportion of patients undergoing therapy for intermittent claudication were active smokers [4]. This may cause early graft thrombosis after intervention or particularly stent thrombosis of endovascular implants leading to acute limb ischemia. The ideal patient for revascularization in either case is likely a highly functional, medically optimized, non-smoking patient with lifestyle-limiting claudication.

Revascularization Evidence and Outcomes

Although the Global Limb Anatomic Staging System (GLASS) [5] was developed for patients with CLTI, assessing patients using the staging system with its prediction for immediate technical failure and limb-based patency may be helpful to determine whether a patient is more likely to have a durable result via open or endovascular approach. Lesion length, degree of calcification, and location (isolated to the SFA or including popliteal disease) as well as quality of tibial runoff all affect long-term patency for endovascular interventions. GLASS staging should therefore be taken into consideration in addition to the patient's preference, available vein conduit, and comorbidities when determining open vs endovascular approach.

Isolated Open Therapies

There are a number of isolated open strategies for infra-inguinal revascularization of the lower extremity including femoral thromboendarterectomy and patch angioplasty, femoral-popliteal, or femoral-tibial bypass of which many conduits can be used including native vein, prosthetic with Dacron or expanded polytetrafluoroethylene (ePTFE), cryopreserved allograft, as well as newer conduits including tissue-engineered grafts (Humacyte). Many would argue that more distal bypasses are inappropriate for treatment of intermittent claudication, as these are more effective for treatment of CLTI and less effective at providing in-line flow to the gastrocnemius muscles most affected by intermittent claudication.

Femoral Endarterectomy and Profundaplasty

Common femoral endarterectomy with profundaplasty is a well-described procedure and is widely used to treat both claudication and CLTI. It has durable results, and treatment of this segment of the infrainguinal arterial tree is often thought best treated with an open procedure given the undesirability of long-term stent implantation in an area with frequent eccentric calcified plaque and frequent flexion. Many studies describe good long-term patency [6, 7]. At times this can be combined with iliac stenting, which has also been shown to be durable in the long term [8, 9]. Long-term patency rates including freedom from target lesion revascularization in the setting of common femoral endarterectomy have been demonstrated to be as great as 90%. This demonstrates a durable open option for patients with intermittent claudication who are otherwise medically optimized and have failed exercise therapy particularly in the setting of preserved tibial runoff [7, 10].

There are more recent studies that compare endovascular treatment of the common femoral region especially with helical nitinol stents with improved flexibility but generally, patency remains better with open surgery [10, 11].

Femoropopliteal and Tibial Bypass

VQI data from 2003 to 2018 recorded 5347 infrainguinal bypasses completed and codified in the database for intermittent claudication; 22% were to tibial arteries and 78% to popliteal arteries. In this cohort, the major demographic differences among those undergoing tibial bypasses included higher male gender, increased prior and current smoking history, ambulatory status, higher prevalence of COPD, and increased previous history of ipsilateral bypass. For both groups less than 75% of patients were recorded as being treated with preoperative aspirin and statin. Of those undergoing tibial artery bypasses, they had worse perioperative outcomes with higher rates of 1-year reintervention, 1-year bypass occlusion/death, and 1-year major amputation [12, 13].

Conduits

Single Segment Great Saphenous Vein

Single segment great saphenous vein (SS-GSV) has long been thought to be the conduit of choice for open surgical bypass. Per the literature it boasts 3-year patency of greater than 87% which is superior to alternative vein conduits, which have highly variable patency rates depending on their construction. This suggests that great saphenous vein is a durable option for bypass in the setting of both claudication and CLTI [14].

Spliced Vein

Studies suggest that in the absence of SS-GSV, spliced arm vein or small saphenous vein may be suitable conduits for lower extremity revascularization [15]. [16] Multiple single-center studies exist reporting highly variable patency rates between 10% and 80% [15, 17, 18], all of which are inferior to single-segment great saphenous vein patency. The secondary patency is often lower. In addition, harvest of these veins limits the patient's IV access for other procedures as well as future creation of dialysis access if needed [13, 15, 17].

Prosthetic

Heparin-bonded expanded polytetrafluoroethylene (ePTFE) is the most often used prosthetic bypass for claudication with equivalent 1- and 2-year patency rates (>90%) to great saphenous vein for above-knee popliteal targets [19]. Dacron has been reported to have equivalent or higher levels of patency to ePTFE for above-knee targets [20]. EPTFE is also the most often used prosthetic conduit for infra-popliteal level distal targets; however, vein grafts have improved primary patency as compared to prosthetic below the knee. The use of vein patches or cuffs has been demonstrated to improve compliance mismatch between the prosthetic and target vessel with an approximately 10% improvement in long-term patency rates over prosthetic without vein patch or cuff. A recent meta-analysis demonstrated equivalent 4-year patency of heparin-bonded ePTFE to the below-knee popliteal artery when compared to SS-GSV [21]. Long-term patency for tibial level prosthetic bypasses is exceedingly poor [12, 22]. Given these limited patency rates, the use of prosthetic to a below-knee popliteal target for claudication should be very carefully considered. The benefits of tibial bypass with prosthetic for claudication are not outweighed by the risks.

Cryopreserved Cadaveric Allograft

Cryopreserved cadaveric allograft has been used in the absence of suitable autogenous conduit for lower extremity bypass. Cryopreserved cadaveric allograft is not recommended for claudication, and there is no significant long-term data on the utilization of this conduit for this pathology. Based on the literature that exists for CLTI patients, 3-year patency is less than 25%, and results of either open or endovascular reintervention on these conduits are undesirable [23]. They are often used in last ditch maneuvers for limb salvage, especially in the setting of prosthetic graft infection, and in this situation have reasonable results; however, we overall would not recommend utilization of cryopreserved allograft in patients with intermittent claudication, especially as it is significantly more expensive than ePTFE [24, 25].

Human Acellular Vessel

Human acellular vessel is a bioengineered decellularized human blood vessel (Fig. 15.1) that is available off-the-shelf and can be used as a replacement conduit for arterial bypass grafting. It is currently undergoing a phase 2 clinical trial evaluation through the FDA. It is utilized as a conduit for vascular repair or replacement in patients with symptomatic PAD. For the primary portion of the trial, 20 patients were enrolled at 3 sites between October 2013 and June 2014 and underwent single-segment human acellular vessel implantation [26]. For 17 patients the proximal anastomosis was performed to the common femoral artery, while 3 patients had

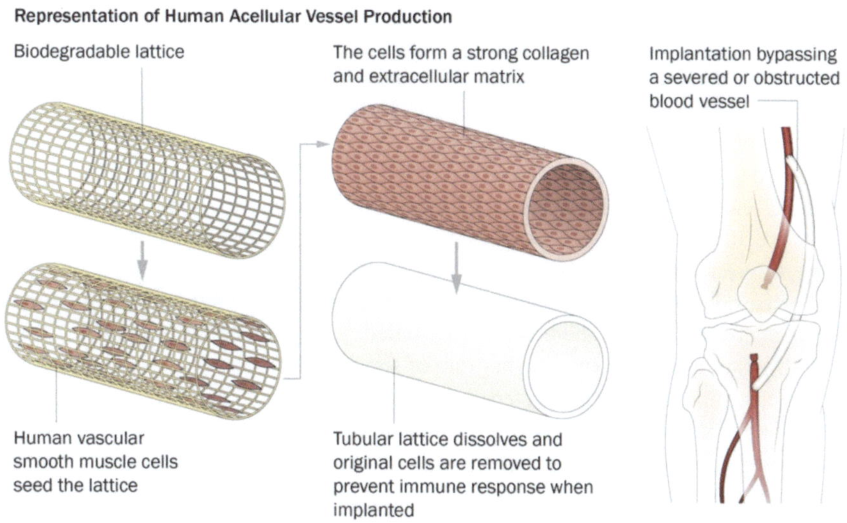

Fig. 15.1 DVIDS—News—Surgeons perform first bioengineered blood vessel transplant in military patient

their proximal anastomosis at the proximal superficial femoral artery. The distal anastomosis was at the superficial femoral artery for 11 patients and the above-knee popliteal for 9 patients. Of the 20 patients, seven had short-distance claudication less than 50 m, five had claudication at less than 20 m, and two patients had rest pain. Seven patients withdrew prior to 24 months, of which four experienced graft occlusion. Three patients died unrelated to the surgery per study report. The 24-month data indicated that there was 58% primary patency for this conduit including 58% primary assisted patency and 74% secondary patency. The patients were followed in a secondary study for midterm and long-term results. This included monitoring for up to 10 years after implantation. Of the 13 remaining patients, one died of a cerebrovascular accident greater than 12 months out from implantation of the conduit. Of the remaining 12 patients, three have died, four lost patency, and five remained patent without intervention. Overall, their secondary patency rate at 72 months was 60%, higher than that of some reports of prosthetic above-knee bypasses though more recent studies seem to indicate comparatively higher patency for above-knee bypasses particularly with heparin-bonded ePTFE [21]. They reported no acute mechanical failure such as rupture of the conduit.

This study demonstrates early results for an alternative conduit to utilize in peripheral arterial disease. The study population predominantly included patients with severe lifestyle-limiting claudication. The surviving patients reported good quality of life with no ischemic rest pain or tissue loss at 72 months. They had varying levels of claudication; however, all were improved from prior to their intervention [27]. Further data that demonstrated better outcomes would be needed to recommend the use of this conduit for claudication.

Isolated Endovascular Therapies

There is limited randomized trial data for endovascular interventions in the setting of intermittent claudication. However, we do know that among the modalities of intervention, angioplasty plus stenting increases overall patency in the short term compared with angioplasty alone. The incremental benefit of paclitaxel drug-eluting balloons and stents has been suggested [28]. More recent iterations of drug-eluting stents are advertised as delivering drug up to 6 months post-implantation. The primary difference seen among drug-eluting stents versus non-drug-eluting stents is the decreased need for early reintervention within 6 months. With regard to covered versus uncovered stents, there is a higher patency rate among covered stents; however, this is complicated by a higher rate of stent thrombosis [29].

Various studies have suggested that long-term endovascular revascularization patency rates are better when chronic total occlusions are crossed via the true lumen as opposed to subintimal. Improvement in endovascular techniques such as retrograde pedal access with or without the use of subintimal arterial flossing with antegrade-retrograde intervention (also known as SAFARI) as well as the use of re-entry devices have increased technical success for endovascular revascularization over time. These techniques also assist in limiting antegrade dissection and re-entry into segments significantly distal to where the true lumen reconstitutes, which decreases the risk of threatening distal bypass targets.

Atherectomy

The use of atherectomy is quite controversial due to the inherent risk of complication of distal embolization leading to loss of runoff vessels and reported high rates of restenosis. However, this remains a tool to treat peripheral arterial disease particularly in the outpatient setting. A recent Johns Hopkins study identified that in the 2019 Medicare database, 59.6% of peripheral vascular interventions done for atherectomy were in patients with claudication. They also identified that there was a reintervention rate 33% higher for atherectomy as compared to non-atherectomy interventions for intermittent claudication. There was also evidence of shorter time to claudication recurrence. There was not, however, any evidence indicating a higher risk of amputation as compared to other endovascular therapies. Based on available data, this represents short-term efficacy with frequent endovascular reintervention, which may lead to hastening of major amputation among these patients [30, 31].

Intravascular Lithotripsy

Intravascular lithotripsy is typically used for the treatment of highly calcific disease and can be used both in the femoral-popliteal segment and the tibial segment. It utilizes low-pressure balloons and sound waves to disrupt laminated medial calcifications and is often utilized in conjunction with angioplasty and/or stenting. The Disrupt PAD III trial (2021) compared treatment of femoral-popliteal artery calcifications with intravascular lithotripsy versus percutaneous transluminal angioplasty prior to drug-coated balloon angioplasty for symptomatic peripheral arterial disease. The results were primarily geared toward anatomic outcomes including decreased residual stenosis and freedom from major adverse events. As compared to plain angioplasty (which is not the present-day standard of care), they reported technical success; however, there was no significant report of long-term outcomes of patients with claudication, and thus data is limited in the evaluation of use of intravascular lithotripsy for this pathology [32].

DETOUR Procedure

The Endologix PQ bypass DETOUR system (Fig. 15.2) was developed as an alternative to open surgical bypass for above-knee long-segment femoral-popliteal occlusions. This utilizes a percutaneous approach and places a covered stent from the superficial femoral artery proximally to the popliteal artery distally. It is deployed through a transvenous route. The DETOUR1 trial included patients with symptomatic PAD including severe short-distance claudication or rest pain and excluding

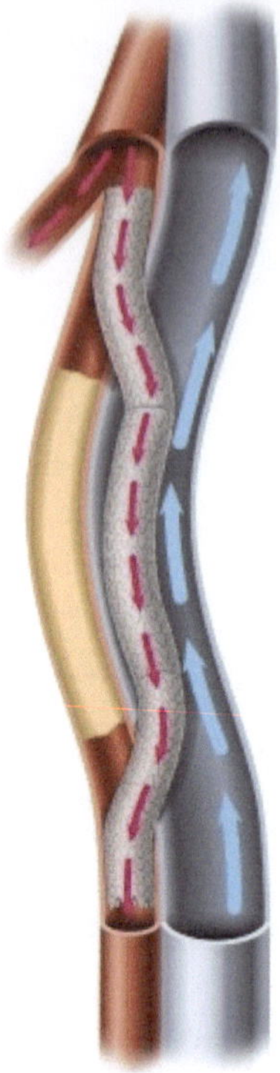

Fig. 15.2 PQ bypass receives FDA breakthrough device designation for the Detour system—Interventional News

those with lesser degrees of intermittent claudication. This was designed as a single-arm multicenter international premarket trial enrolling 78 patients (82 limbs) at 8 sites over a 24-month period. Their primary safety endpoint was 1-month major adverse events and primary effectiveness outcome was 6-month patency. Their results included no deaths within the first month achieving their primary safety outcome. Kaplan-Meir analysis demonstrated 1-year primary, primary assisted patency, and secondary patency rates of 81%, 82%, and 90% respectively. Patients had an ABI increase of >0.2 and 1-year freedom from stent thrombosis of 84%. Patient had improved Rutherford class in 77 of 80 limbs (96%) and 65 out of the 80 limbs were asymptomatic (81%) after treatment. DVT developed in 2 limbs with no documented occurence of pulmonary embolism [33]. The DETOUR2 Trial included a similar patient population with long-segment SFA occlusion or near occlusion and found 72.1% primary patency at 12 months in a study population of 200 treated patients. 97% of patients improved their Rutherford status within 1 year [34]. The role for this therapy in patients with claudication remains unclear at this time, with no satisfactory controls for comparison reported in the literature.

Drug-coated Balloon Angioplasty

The concept of "leaving nothing behind" (angioplasty without stent placement) as a way to remove the nidus for restenosis has gained interest recently. However, it has been well documented that plain old balloon angioplasty (POBA) has inferior outcomes to POBA with stenting. For these reasons, isolated claudication with nonocclusive lesions of the femoral-popliteal segment, plain balloon angioplasty (POBA), followed by drug-coated balloon (DCB) angioplasty, has been proposed as an alternative to stenting. This is demonstrated to have excellent short-term patency especially for shorter lesion lengths; however, there is a continuously growing body of evidence in the literature that there is restenosis of treated lesions that may eventually require stenting. Drug-coated balloon angioplasty has been demonstrated to be superior to plain balloon angioplasty and many pivotal trials, with an approximate 20–30% improvement in primary patency and a decrease in target lesion revascularization up to 3 years [35]. However, there has not been a comparison to angioplasty with stenting, which limits interpretation of the results. The role for DCB angioplasty in patients with claudication due to femoropopliteal disease remains somewhat uncertain, though likely not inferior to POBA or stenting.

Femoropopliteal Stenting

Numerous descriptions of angioplasty and stenting for disease of the superficial femoral artery have been reported; this is a well-accepted modality for treating these lesions in patients with claudication. Self-expanding stents are used, generally after a pre-dilation balloon angioplasty, followed by a second, brief balloon angioplasty to ensure the stent is brought to profile. There is no clearly documented role for covered stents for SFA occlusive disease. Stenting of the femoral-popliteal segment can be extended down to the popliteal artery. Primary popliteal artery stenting is rarely used for isolated claudication; however, in instances of short-distance claudication and occlusive popliteal lesions, stenting may be warranted. Typically, this is done with uncovered stents as opposed to covered stents used for popliteal aneurysm repair [29]. Some studies indicate long-term durability of popliteal stents; however, at the level of Hunter's canal and behind the knee, there are significant muscular compression and torsion forces that can lead to recurrent in-stent stenosis or occlusion [36]. Given failure may lead to acute limb ischemia in the absence of sufficient collateral vessels, popliteal stenting may be better reserved for the setting of chronic limb-threatening ischemia [37].

Hybrid Therapies

Any of these therapies can be combined to treat multilevel disease, however this is less likely to be necessary in patients with intermittent claudication, since claudication is generally caused by (and treated for) single-level disease. Following the principles of treating inflow disease prior to treating outflow disease, significant common femoral artery stenosis should be addressed either concomitantly or prior to treating superficial femoral artery disease. Given the influence of patent tibial runoff on improving durability of endovascular SFA and popliteal interventions, some practitioners will perform concomitant endovascular tibial interventions in an effort to improve tibial runoff. There is no current data to support this practice, and the relatively poor durability of tibial interventions suggests that this will not provide long-term patency benefits and may increase risks.

Conclusions

Intermittent claudication affects a large proportion of symptomatic vascular patients worldwide; given the increasing prevalence of comorbidities and advanced age, we can expect the incidence of this pathology to increase. There are a number of open and endovascular therapies that can be utilized to treat claudication (Table 15.1). Open surgical revascularization based on studies related to both claudication and CLTI demonstrates longer durability, particularly with single-segment great saphenous vein. However, similar to endovascular interventions, alternative conduits have relatively limited patency. Utilization of these conduits in patients with claudication is not generally recommended, the one exception being above-knee popliteal targets in the absence of SS-GSV. The durability of endovascular therapies in the infrainguinal segment is limited; angioplasty and stenting of the SFA demonstrates acceptable results out to 2 years, but durability is less for other endovascular infrainguinal therapies. Given that the overall risk for medically optimized patients with claudication for experiencing limb loss is less than 5% over a 5-year period, and cardiovascular mortality rates that exceed that, it may be prudent to limit significant endovascular intervention for a non-limb-threatening indication.

Intermittent and short-distance claudication can be debilitating for many patients. This can affect their livelihood, mental health, relationships, and overall quality of life. The outcome of intervention can be variable ranging from a new lease on life to accelerated risk of major amputation and early death. Ultimately, the decision for

Table 15.1 Summary of recommendations for infrainguinal interventions for intermittent claudication by arterial segment

Disease segment	Recommendations
Common femoral and profunda femoris	Open revascularization with femoral endarterectomy and profundaplasty demonstrates good long-term durability Endovascular options haven't shown good long-term durability
Femoropopliteal	Short-segment disease can be treated with endovascular therapy Long-segment chronic occlusions can be treated with single-segment GSV or prosthetic bypass to above-knee targets, but single-segment GSV is best for any below-knee target
Tibial and inframalleolar	Treatment is not recommended

intervention is between the patient and their doctor though the above-stated risks should be well understood [38].

References

1. Woo K, et al. Society for vascular surgery appropriate use criteria for the management of intermittent claudication. J Vasc Surg. 2022;76(1):3–22.e1. PMID: 35470016.
2. Reitz KM, Althouse AD, Meyer J, et al. Association of smoking with postprocedural complications following open and endovascular interventions for intermittent claudication. JAMA Cardiol. 2022;7(1):45–54. https://doi.org/10.1001/jamacardio.2021.3979.
3. Patel RJ, Zarrintan S, Jagadeesh V, Vootukuru NR, Gaffey A, Malas MB. Long-term outcomes after lower extremity bypass in the actively smoking claudicant. J Vasc Surg. Elsevier Inc. 2023;78:1003–1011. https://doi.org/10.1016/j.jvs.2023.05.047.
4. Levin SR, Hawkins SS, Farber A, et al. Association of state tobacco control policies with active smoking at the time of intervention for intermittent claudication. J Vasc Surg. Mosby Inc. 2021;73:1759–68.e1. https://doi.org/10.1016/j.jvs.2020.08.156.
5. Conte MS, Bradbury AW, Kolh P, et al. Global vascular guidelines on the management of chronic limb-threatening ischemia. Eur J Vasc Endovasc Surg. 2019;58(1):S1–S109.e33. https://doi.org/10.1016/j.ejvs.2019.05.006.
6. Park S, Ku T, Hwang D, Yun WS, Kim HK, Huh S. Outcomes of isolated endarterectomy and patch angioplasty of the common femoral artery according to current inclusion criteria for endovascular treatment. Vasc Spec Int. 2022;38 https://doi.org/10.5758/vsi.220040.
7. Hashimoto T, Yamamoto S, Kimura M, Sano M, Sato O, Deguchi J. Long-term outcomes following common femoral endarterectomy. J Clin Med. 2022;11(22) https://doi.org/10.3390/jcm11226873.
8. Uhl C, Götzke H, Zeman F, et al. Long-term outcome of common femoral artery endarterectomy in octogenarians and non-octogenarians. Scand J Surg. 2021;110(3):400–6. https://doi.org/10.1177/1457496920907733.
9. Kim JH, So BJ, Byun SJ, Kim KY. The advantage of common femoral endarterectomy alone or combined with endovascular treatment. Vasc Spec Int. 2018;34(3):65–71. https://doi.org/10.5758/vsi.2018.34.3.65.
10. Nakama T, Takahara M, Iwata Y, et al. 1-year outcomes of thromboendarterectomy vs endovascular therapy for common femoral artery lesions: CAULIFLOWER study results. JACC Cardiovasc Interv. 2022;15(14):1453–63. https://doi.org/10.1016/j.jcin.2022.03.010.
11. Boufi M, Ejargue M, Gaye M, Boyer L, Alimi Y, Loundou AD. Systematic review and meta-analysis of endovascular versus open repair for common femoral artery atherosclerosis treatment. J Vasc Surg. 2021;73(4):1445–55. https://doi.org/10.1016/j.jvs.2020.10.026.
12. Levin SR, Farber A, Osborne NH, et al. Tibial bypass in patients with intermittent claudication is associated with poor outcomes. J Vasc Surg. 2021;73(2):564–571.e1. https://doi.org/10.1016/j.jvs.2020.06.118.
13. Pereira CE, Albers M, Romiti M, Brochado-Neto FC, Pereira CAB. Meta-analysis of femoropopliteal bypass grafts for lower extremity arterial insufficiency. J Vasc Surg. 2006;44(3) https://doi.org/10.1016/j.jvs.2006.04.054.
14. Farber A, Menard MT, Conte MS, et al. Surgery or endovascular therapy for chronic limb-threatening ischemia. N Engl J Med. 2022;387(25):2305–16. https://doi.org/10.1056/nejmoa2207899.
15. Chang BB, Clement R, Iii D, Bock DEM, Shah DM, Leather RP. The use of spliced vein bypasses for infrainguinal arterial reconstruction. J Vasc Surg. 1995;21(3):403–10; discussion 410–2.

16. Kreienberg PB, Darling RC, Chang BB, et al. Early results of a prospective randomized trial of spliced vein versus polytetrafluoroethylene graft with a distal vein cuff for limb-threatening ischemia. J Vasc Surg. 2002;35(2):299–306. https://doi.org/10.1067/mva.2002.121208.
17. Thompson J, Li R, Pomy BJ, et al. Spliced-vein conduit offers better patency and limb salvage than prosthetic graft for femoral-tibial bypasses in critical limb-threatening ischemia. Ann Vasc Surg. 2025;110:82–90. https://doi.org/10.1016/j.avsg.2024.07.118.
18. Pascarella L, Mureebe L, Cox MW, McCann RL. Spliced arm vein grafts for critical lower limb ischemia. J Vasc Surg. 2012;56(6):1826. https://doi.org/10.1016/j.jvs.2012.10.047.
19. Daenens K, Schepers S, Fourneau I, Houthoofd S, Nevelsteen A. Heparin-bonded ePTFE grafts compared with vein grafts in femoropopliteal and femorocrural bypasses: 1- and 2-year results. J Vasc Surg. 2009;49(5):1210–6. https://doi.org/10.1016/j.jvs.2008.12.009.
20. Rychlik IJ, Davey P, Murphy J, O'Donnell ME. A meta-analysis to compare Dacron versus polytetrafluroethylene grafts for above-knee femoropopliteal artery bypass. J Vasc Surg. 2014;60(2):506–15. https://doi.org/10.1016/j.jvs.2014.05.049.
21. Dexter DJ, O'Neill F, Neville RF. Systematic literature review comparing clinical utility of heparin-bonded expanded polytetrafluoroethylene graft with autologous saphenous vein graft for the management of below-the-knee peripheral arterial disease. J Vasc Surg. Published online December 1, 2024. https://doi.org/10.1016/j.jvs.2024.07.023.
22. Ambler GK, Twine CP. Graft type for femoro-popliteal bypass surgery. Cochrane Database Syst Rev. 2018;2018(2) https://doi.org/10.1002/14651858.CD001487.pub3.
23. Harris L, O'Brien-Irr M, Ricotta JJ. Long-term assessment of cryopreserved vein bypass grafting success. J Vasc Surg. 2001;33(3):528–32. https://doi.org/10.1067/mva.2001.111729.
24. Zehr BP, Niblick CJ, Downey H, Ladowski JS. Limb salvage with CryoVein cadaver saphenous vein allografts used for peripheral arterial bypass: role of blood compatibility. Ann Vasc Surg. 2011;25(2):177–81. https://doi.org/10.1016/j.avsg.2010.07.020.
25. O'Banion LA, Wu B, Eichler CM, Reilly LM, Conte MS, Hiramoto JS. Cryopreserved saphenous vein as a last-ditch conduit for limb salvage. Vasc Surg. Mosby Inc. 2017;66:844–49. https://doi.org/10.1016/j.jvs.2017.03.415.
26. Gutoswki P, et al. Arterial reconstruction with human bioengineered acellular blood vessels in patients with peripheral arterial disease. J Vasc Surg. 2020;72(4):1247–58. PMID: 32093913.
27. Gutowski P, Guziewicz M, Ilzecki M, et al. Six-year outcomes of a phase II study of human-tissue engineered blood vessels for peripheral arterial bypass. JVS Vasc Sci. 2023;4:100092. https://doi.org/10.1016/j.jvssci.2022.11.001.
28. Müller-Hülsbeck S, Benko A, Soga Y, et al. Two-year efficacy and safety results from the IMPERIAL randomized study of the eluvia polymer-coated drug-eluting stent and the zilver PTX polymer-free drug-coated stent. Cardiovasc Intervent Radiol. 2021;44(3):368–75. https://doi.org/10.1007/s00270-020-02693-1.
29. Müller AM, Löhn-Kannengießer L, Bradaric C, et al. Outcomes of endovascular treatment for popliteal artery disease. Vasa Eur J Vasc Med. 2023;52(6):386–93. https://doi.org/10.1024/0301-1526/a001096.
30. Wardle BG, Ambler GK, Radwan RW, Hinchliffe RJ, Twine CP. Atherectomy for peripheral arterial disease. Cochrane Database Syst Rev. 2020;2020(9) https://doi.org/10.1002/14651858.CD006680.pub3.
31. Kawaji Q, Dun C, Walsh C, et al. Index atherectomy peripheral vascular interventions performed for claudication are associated with more reinterventions than nonatherectomy interventions. J Vasc Surg. Elsevier Inc. 2022;76:489–98.e4. https://doi.org/10.1016/j.jvs.2022.02.034.
32. Tepe G, Brodmann M, Werner M, et al. Intravascular lithotripsy for peripheral artery calcification: 30-day outcomes from the randomized disrupt PAD III trial. JACC Cardiovasc Interv. 2021;14(12):1352–61. https://doi.org/10.1016/j.jcin.2021.04.010.
33. Krievins DK, Halena G, Scheinert D, et al. One-year results from the DETOUR I trial of the PQ bypass DETOUR system for percutaneous femoropopliteal bypass. J Vasc Surg. 2020;72(5):1648–1658.e2. https://doi.org/10.1016/j.jvs.2020.02.043.

34. Lyden SP, Soukas PA, De A, et al. DETOUR2 trial outcomes demonstrate clinical utility of percutaneous transmural bypass for the treatment of long segment, complex femoropopliteal disease. J Vasc Surg. Elsevier Inc. 2024;79:1420–27.e2. https://doi.org/10.1016/j.jvs.2024.02.004.
35. Caradu C, Lakhlifi E, Colacchio EC, et al. Systematic review and updated meta-analysis of the use of drug-coated balloon angioplasty versus plain old balloon angioplasty for femoropopliteal arterial disease. J Vasc Surg. 2019;70(3):981–995.e10. https://doi.org/10.1016/j.jvs.2019.01.080.
36. Lammer J, Zeller T, Hausegger KA, et al. Heparin-bonded covered stents versus bare-metal stents for complex femoropopliteal artery lesions: the randomized VIASTAR trial (viabahn endoprosthesis with propaten bioactive surface [VIA] versus bare nitinol stent in the treatment of long lesions in superficial femoral artery occlusive disease). J Am Coll Cardiol. 2013;62(15):1320–7. https://doi.org/10.1016/j.jacc.2013.05.079.
37. Katsanos K, Al-Lamki SAM, Parthipun A, et al. Peripheral stent thrombosis leading to acute limb ischemia and major amputation: incidence and risk factors in the aortoiliac and femoropopliteal arteries. Cardiovasc Intervent Radiol. 2017;40(3):351–9. https://doi.org/10.1007/s00270-016-1513-0.
38. O'Banion LA, Saadi S, Hasan B, et al. Lack of patient-centered evaluation of outcomes in intermittent claudication literature. J Vasc Surg. 2023;78(3):828–36. https://doi.org/10.1016/j.jvs.2023.03.497.

16 Revascularization for Claudication in the Setting of Multi-level and/or Bilateral Disease: How Many Levels to Treat and How

Michael S. Conte

Introduction

Intermittent claudication (IC) is the most prevalent symptom of peripheral artery disease (PAD). Anatomic patterns of disease in PAD are varied and strongly associated with risk factors such as smoking and diabetes [1, 2]. Occlusive disease of the aorto-iliac and/or femoro-popliteal segments are recognized causes of IC. Bilateral and multi-level involvement of atherosclerosis in the lower extremities is common. Thus, the question of how much disease to treat in patients with disabling IC, and in what order, is frequently encountered in clinical practice. Despite this, multi-level and bilateral disease is not directly addressed in any of the contemporary clinical practice guidelines or appropriate use criteria (AUC) for claudication treatment [3–6]. In this chapter, we will address this decision-making within the context of a good risk patient with disabling, lifestyle-limiting IC, who has discontinued smoking, is compliant with optimal medical therapy (OMT), and has failed to improve despite at least 3 months of a regular exercise regimen.

The physiologic goal of revascularization in patients with IC is to increase blood flow to the symptomatic muscle beds to improve exercise tolerance and reduce or eliminate pain in the limb. The "open artery hypothesis" provides the anatomic rationale—i.e., elimination or reduction of flow-limiting lesions leads to hemodynamic improvement which is the pre-requisite for clinical effectiveness in IC. However, the presumed direct relationship between anatomy, physiology, and clinical symptoms that underlies the rationale for revascularization is poorly understood—and not always predictable. IC is not a limb-threatening condition but may severely impact quality of life across multiple domains. A fundamental principle of

For: The Patient Centered Approach to Claudication (Robinson W, Simons J, Eds.)

M. S. Conte (✉)
Division of Vascular and Endovascular Surgery, University of California at San Francisco, San Francisco, CA, USA
e-mail: Michael.conte2@ucsf.edu

W. P. Robinson III, J. P. Simons (eds.), *The Patient-Centered Approach to Claudication*, https://doi.org/10.1007/978-3-032-02460-2_16

revascularization for IC is to minimize the risk of accelerating the disease to chronic limb-threatening ischemia (CLTI) and the potential risk of major amputation. Durability of the intervention, which is linked to sustained anatomic patency, is likewise a critical consideration. Minimization of risk, invasiveness, and the need for additional downstream procedures are also highly valued by patients in shared decision-making conversations about the treatment choices.

Clinical Evaluation, Patient Goals, and Setting Expectations

A clear understanding of the patient's PAD symptoms and history is foremost to developing a treatment strategy to best address their goals—where is the pain with ambulation primarily felt (hip, buttock, thigh, calf)?; how severe is the disability?; are symptoms unilateral or bilateral?; if bilateral is one side more severe than the other?; have there been prior interventions?; if so, did these initially produce symptom relief? While proximal muscle group symptoms (e.g., hip, buttock, thigh) strongly implicate aorto-iliac (AI) or common femoral artery (CFA) involvement, calf claudication can result from any combination of femoro-popliteal (FP), AI, and/or CFA disease. Infra-popliteal artery disease is an infrequent cause of IC, particularly in isolation.

It bears mention here that exertional limb pain and poor exercise tolerance are complex symptoms that are often multi-factorial in nature. The PAD population is older and has a high prevalence of relevant comorbidities including cardiopulmonary disease, musculo-skeletal conditions, spine disease, and general frailty. Trying to dissect out the component that is likely vascular in nature—and hence potentially improved by revascularization—can be challenging and nuanced. But it is critical to do so to fully engage the patient in an understanding of the achievable outcomes and possible modes of failure. This is most relevant in cases with complex anatomy such as multi-level disease.

The unilateral versus bilateral nature of symptoms, as well as their localization to muscle groups, is central to the clinical evaluation of patients with IC (Fig. 16.1). Patients with bilateral severe calf claudication will almost always require a staged revascularization approach. If their symptoms are equal or near equal in both limbs, they may experience limited benefit in walking performance unless or until both limbs are successfully addressed. In a similar fashion, the clinical durability of the treatment plan may be reduced in proportion to the product of anatomic patency of the interventions in both limbs. Stated another way, success in one limb and failure in the other may be seen subjectively as an overall failure if exertional symptoms quickly recur or function is not meaningfully improved. The same calculus is relevant to multi-level intervention in the same limb. These are important elements to address frankly with patients, who may frequently underestimate the complexity of the overall undertaking.

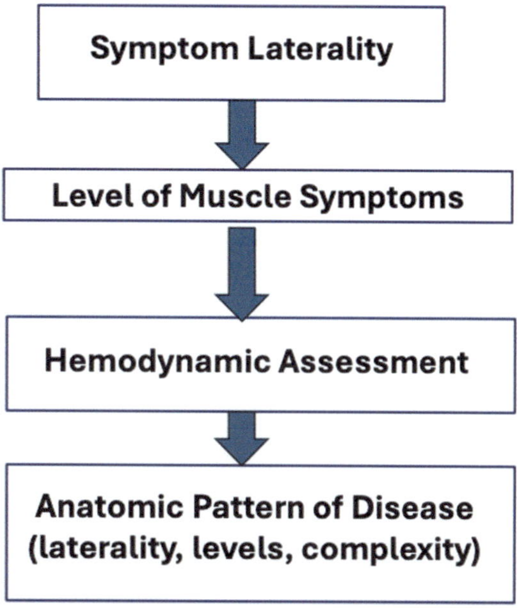

Fig. 16.1 Clinical evaluation of patients with IC includes a thorough assessment of symptom laterality and localization, as well as hemodynamic studies and imaging to understand the atherosclerotic disease pattern. Full understanding of these factors is critical to formulating a treatment plan and evaluating revascularization options

Hemodynamic and Imaging Studies

Non-invasive studies such as segmental limb pressures, Doppler waveforms, and ankle-brachial index play an important role in the diagnosis of PAD and assessment of its severity. Some discordance between hemodynamic measurements and the patient's expression of symptoms is common in IC but should always prompt a close examination of alternative mechanisms of leg pain such as spine disease. Exercise studies can be particularly valuable in such instances. A full review of the diagnostic approaches to IC is outside of the scope of the present chapter, but the hemodynamic assessment gives important information about both the laterality and the multi-level nature of the underlying atherosclerotic disease. For example, if a patient is complaining of unilateral calf claudication but the noninvasive studies suggest symmetric hemodynamic compromise in both limbs, they should be made aware of the possibility that a successful intervention in the symptomatic limb could soon be followed by an unmasking of the problem on the contralateral side. Demonstration of the total burden of disease also helps to emphasize the critical importance of smoking cessation, lifestyle modification, and compliance with optimal medical therapy as foundational elements of the PAD treatment plan.

In IC patients who fit the above criteria to consider revascularization, initial non-invasive imaging studies are essential to characterize the disease pattern and to engage the patient in the decision-making process. Duplex ultrasound is frequently employed as a first-line tool and can provide good resolution of levels of involvement and their severity (e.g., stenosis versus occlusion). Axial imaging studies such as computed tomography angiography (CTA) give a higher level of resolution and can also be more easily shown to patients as the treatment choices and tradeoffs are considered. They allow for more precise assessment of factors that are known to strongly impact interventional outcomes such as presence of occlusions, vessel size, length of lesions, and calcification. CTA is thus the current imaging modality of choice for revascularization planning in suitable patients with IC.

A fundamental consideration for any revascularization procedure, be it for IC or for CLTI, is the determination of adequate inflow and outflow. This mandates a proximal-to-distal approach when there are lesions at multiple levels. Careful judgment is required in these settings, and direct hemodynamic data (e.g., pull back pressures with or without vasodilator administration during angiography) can be highly useful in settings of mild or moderate stenoses by imaging. While it is imperative to insure hemodynamically adequate inflow for any reconstruction, it is far less clear how outflow disease—or its treatment—impacts the effectiveness of interventions for IC. More of this will be discussed below in the individual scenarios.

In some specific circumstances, it may be relevant to consider the advantage of a combined multi-level approach purely based on technical (e.g., access) factors. A common example is when treatment of severe common femoral artery (CFA) disease by endarterectomy and patch angioplasty is performed. In this setting, direct surgical access may simplify a hybrid approach to either upstream AI or downstream FP disease that may be more difficult if staged. However, these considerations should not be generally prioritized over the rational physiologic factors described above and below.

How to Incorporate Available Data into the Treatment Plan

Endovascular interventions are the predominant revascularization approach in contemporary practice, particularly when the indication for treatment is IC. The overall safety and minimal invasiveness of these procedures is highly attractive for a quality-of-life indication. There is ample data demonstrating the relationships between lesion location and severity attributes on technical failures, reinterventions, anatomic patency, and clinical outcomes for specific endovascular approaches [7, 8]. These data should be meaningfully incorporated into the treatment plan discussions. The data linking these outcomes to quality of life and functional improvement in IC, and long-term clinical effectiveness, is far more limited and of lower quality [9]. It should be evident from the above that the education process required for optimal decision-making in IC requires real time and investment from both the patient and the vascular specialist. The payoff for this time spent is a realistic understanding of the likelihood of achieving the desired treatment goals, the potential modes of failure, and the importance of follow-up surveillance and OMT.

In the current era, emphasis is often misplaced on the initial technical/procedural success of the intervention. Many regulatory trials and observational studies demonstrate high levels of initial technical success, and low rates of serious complications, for peripheral interventions in patients with IC. These studies are generally limited by strict inclusion criteria for patient risk and lesion severity. Thus, the true incidence of technical failure in more complex disease patterns is unclear, and likely underestimated. More germane is that technical success is necessary—but not sufficient—for clinical effectiveness, and an overestimation of its relevance may contribute to an aggressive posture with attendant risks of longer-term harm in patients with IC. Revascularization in any form is not curative for PAD, and unfortunately even the most effective vascular interventions are limited in long-term durability as compared to, e.g., hip arthroplasty, a relevant contrast. Expectations of treatment durability may vary across individual patients and settings, but for IC, the temporal perspective should be in years and the risks associated with repetitive interventions honestly assessed up front. The Society for Vascular Surgery has suggested a >50% estimated likelihood of sustained clinical benefit for at least 2 years as a benchmark for interventions in IC [3]. Recent data from the Vascular Quality Initiative and other sources suggest that contemporary outcomes may fall significantly below this desired threshold [10, 11]. Multiple observational studies demonstrate that the risks of acute limb ischemia, progression to CLTI, amputation, and overall cardiovascular events are increased among PAD patients who have undergone repetitive limb interventions [12–15]. Both the patient and the provider should thus be wary of the risk of entering a "treatment trap" of repetitive interventions for IC with downstream adverse consequences.

A number of studies demonstrate that greater disease severity, and particularly multi-level disease, is associated with worsened outcomes in patients with IC. Anatomic patency and freedom for reintervention are significantly greater for aorto-iliac (AI) as compared to femoro-popliteal (FP) interventions. Combined AI and FP interventions, chronic occlusions, longer lesion lengths (e.g., >10 or 20 cm) and treatment of infra-popliteal (IP) disease are all associated with higher risk for adverse limb outcomes [16–19]. Patient factors such as increased age, presence of diabetes, cardiac or renal disease, and a history of prior interventions are likewise associated with higher risk of major adverse limb events (MALE) [8]. Patients with one or more of these factors need to be well counseled, and as the factors are additive the risk/benefit ratio becomes increasingly adverse and favors either a conservative or a carefully staged interventional strategy.

Considerations in Specific Anatomic Settings

A ladder of anatomic complexity (Fig. 16.2) presents a paradigm for decision-making in IC patients with multi-level disease. For this discussion, the definitions of segmental complexity employed by the Society for Vascular Surgery Appropriate Use Criteria are considered to be relevant [4]. Going up this ladder, procedural success, freedom from reintervention, MALE and MACE, and long-term clinical durability are progressively reduced—and thus greater caution is warranted.

Staging of interventions in IC patients offers a number of significant advantages. Safety and efficacy of procedures is improved when only a single level of disease or a single limb is the focus. Most importantly, many patients may not require or desire additional treatment to meet their symptomatic and functional goals. Time can be

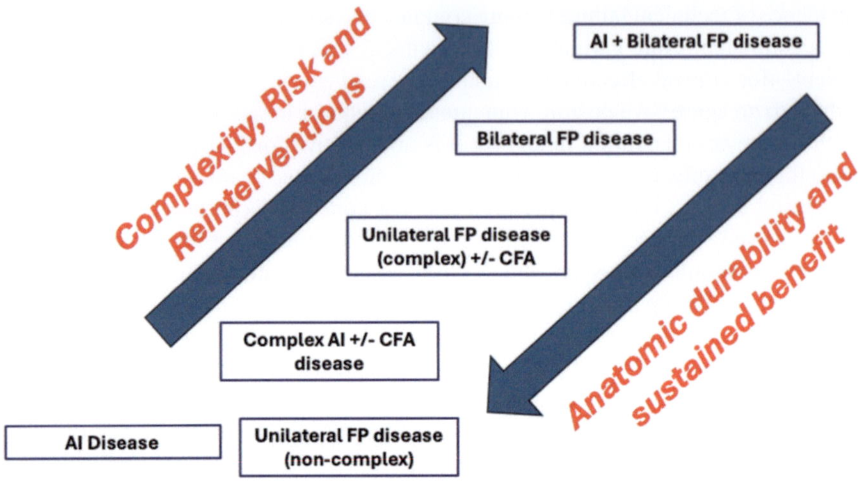

Fig. 16.2 A ladder of complexity is useful for considering the risks and benefits of revascularization in IC patients with multi-level and/or bilateral disease. AI disease (most patterns) and non-complex (i.e., TASC A/B) unilateral FP disease are at the lower end. Increasing the complexity of either the AI or the unilateral FP disease, with or without CFA involvement, moves up the scale. Bilateral severe FP disease, with or without AI disease, presents the greatest level of complexity. Escalation on the ladder is associated with increased procedural risk, greater incidence of re-interventions, and a declining likelihood of sustained clinical benefit. Staging should be increasingly employed as complexity increases

allowed to see how much improvement is realized from the initial intervention. An observation period of 1–3 months is useful to gage the treatment response, the patient's compliance with ongoing medical therapy, smoking cessation, and exercise, and an early signal on restenosis in the treated segment. Many patients may achieve significant improvement with treatment of inflow disease alone, regardless of the severity of downstream infrainguinal disease. Selected good risk patients can be successfully treated with a staged multi-level approach in even the more complex patterns—but considerable judgment and experience is needed, along with full buy-in from the patient for every step along the way.

Bilateral AI Disease

Simultaneous treatment of bilateral AI disease is common, safe, and effective in well-selected patients with disabling IC. Endovascular interventions play a dominant role and have demonstrated good to excellent long-term results in low, intermediate, and even complex disease patterns [20, 21]. Bilateral groin access facilitates these interventions at a single setting. Patients with disease at the aortic bifurcation, even if their symptoms are unilateral, often require bilateral stent placement for technical success. In good risk patients with long segment occlusions, small or severely calcified arteries, or those with prior endovascular failures aorto-bifemoral bypass grafting is a highly durable surgical alternative.

Bilateral AI plus CFA Disease

The presence of severe CFA disease is an important consideration. CFA disease is frequently calcific and extends to the bifurcation. Optimal CFA treatment in good-risk patients remains open femoral endarterectomy and patch angioplasty, though other technologies continue to make advances. Ignoring severe CFA disease while treating upstream AI lesions may severely limit clinical effectiveness. It is important to recognize that the hemodynamic assessment of AI disease via pressure gradients may be falsely negative when there is a severe obstruction at the CFA level. Hybrid open CFA endarterectomy and upstream AI endovascular interventions are well described, commonly employed, and are both safe and effective [22, 23]. One important consideration is whether to perform simultaneous or staged procedures when there is bilateral CFA disease. Risks of surgical groin complications are amplified by a simultaneous bilateral operation. Thus, the author favors reserving single-staged, bilateral CFA endarterectomy to low-risk patients with normal or thin body habitus, good groin hygiene, primary procedures, and severe bilateral symptoms.

AI plus FP Disease (Unilateral)

When there is significant FP disease present along with AI involvement, the risk/benefit analysis becomes more challenging. In general, the anatomic outcomes for treatment of FP disease are inferior to AI interventions. Most importantly this includes the incidence and severity of restenosis, and the need for re-interventions. Thus, the severity of the FP disease becomes a dominant factor in considering the overall treatment strategy. Factors associated with patency of endovascular interventions in the FP segment include the presence, location, and length of total occlusions, the overall length of disease to be treated, vessel size, and calcification [8, 24]. The TASC classification system remains useful for predicting endovascular outcomes in the FP segment, with a notable decline in anatomic patency and freedom from reintervention for TASC C/D lesions compared to low/intermediate complexity (TASC A/B) disease. Long-segment occlusions (e.g., 20 cm or greater) have markedly inferior outcomes; open bypass, particularly with great saphenous vein, may be considered in good risk, highly symptomatic patients.

If the FP disease is of low or intermediate complexity, simultaneous treatment of unilateral inflow disease is reasonable based on a number of technical factors. When there is significant CFA disease, combining femoral endarterectomy with a downstream SFA intervention or femoro-popliteal bypass can be a useful hybrid approach in appropriately selected patients. If both the inflow disease and the FP disease are complex, and the CFA is spared, a staged approach is recommended for the reasons outlined above.

Bilateral FP Disease

Patients with bilateral symptoms secondary to femoropopliteal disease require the most careful consideration, particularly when the anatomic complexity is high, e.g., bilateral long-segment occlusions, severe calcification, or small vessel caliber. Optimal medical therapy, smoking cessation, and a 3- to 6-month trial of exercise (either supervised or, if not available, home-based) should be pressed. If one limb is more symptomatic than the other, this may be a consideration for a staged intervention. However, the patient should be counselled that walking symptoms may transfer to the contralateral limb and thus clinical gains may be limited. Restenosis rates following endovascular intervention for TASC C/D lesions are significant, approaching 30–50% by 2 years [8, 18]. Accordingly, if clinical effectiveness depends on sustained bilateral patency, there is a high likelihood of failing to meet the minimal SVS 2-year threshold with bilateral long-segment FP interventions.

If bilateral FP disease is to be treated in well-selected patients with IC, it should always be staged. An observation period of 1–3 months, as outlined, is recommended in all but the most severely disabled patients with bilateral symptoms. In some highly compliant low-risk patients, staged bilateral femoro-popliteal bypass can provide durable effectiveness, especially when performed with autogenous vein in the presence of good runoff.

Tibial Disease

The relevance of tibial disease to IC symptoms is unclear, whether in isolation or in combination with upstream disease. In addition, results of tibial interventions or bypass are inferior, and risks of MALE and progression to CLTI are increased [6, 8, 25, 26]. High-grade disease of the tibioperoneal trunk deserves careful consideration in the overall treatment strategy. As complexity rises, the rationale for intervention in IC becomes less grounded. There is no data to support prophylactic intervention to reduce the likelihood of progression to CLTI; in contradistinction the risk rises when IP interventions are performed. As a result, current SVS practice guidelines recommend against treatment of tibial disease in patients with IC; the SVS appropriate use criteria also deem tibial interventions to have risks outweighing the benefits [4, 6].

Conclusions

Multi-level and/or bilateral disease is common among patients with disabling IC being considered for revascularization. When symptoms are unilateral or of greater severity in one limb, contralateral disease can be monitored in a staged fashion. A ladder of complexity provides a useful model for shared decision-making with patients and development of a goal-oriented treatment strategy. Treatment of multi-level disease requires careful judgment and as anatomic complexity rises, the risks and benefits of intervention become less favorable. Staging provides an increased margin of safety, procedural efficiency, and time to assess the patient's response. Despite high rates of technical success, long-term clinical effectiveness is limited by restenosis rates that are multiplied for each segment treated. An overaggressive approach may lead to higher rates of reintervention, MALE, and disease progression to CLTI.

References

1. Diehm N, Shang A, Silvestro A, Do D-D, Dick F, Schmidli J, Mahler F, Baumgartner I. Association of cardiovascular risk factors with pattern of lower limb atherosclerosis in 2659 patients undergoing angioplasty. Eur J Vasc Endovasc Surg. 2006;31:59–63.
2. Haltmayer M, Mueller T, Horvath W, Luft C, Poelz W, Haidinger D. Impact of atherosclerotic risk factors on the anatomical distribution of peripheral arterial disease. Int Angiol. 2001;20:200–7.
3. Conte MS, Pomposelli FB, Clair DG, Geraghty PJ, McKinsey JF, Mills JL, Moneta GL, Murad MH, Powell RJ, Reed AB, et al. Society for Vascular Surgery practice guidelines for atherosclerotic occlusive disease of the lower extremities: management of asymptomatic disease and claudication. J Vasc Surg. 2015;61:2S–41S. https://doi.org/10.1016/j.jvs.2014.12.009.
4. Woo K, Siracuse JJ, Klingbeil K, Kraiss LW, Osborne NH, Singh N, Tan TW, Arya S, Banerjee S, Bonaca MP, et al. Society for Vascular Surgery appropriate use criteria for management of intermittent claudication. J Vasc Surg. 2022;76(3–22):e21. https://doi.org/10.1016/j.jvs.2022.04.012.
5. Gornik HL, Aronow HD, Goodney PP, Arya S, Brewster LP, Byrd L, Chandra V, Drachman DE, Eaves JM, Ehrman JK, et al. 2024 ACC/AHA/AACVPR/APMA/ABC/SCAI/SVM/SVN/SVS/SIR/VESS Guideline for the Management of Lower Extremity Peripheral Artery Disease: a report of the American College of Cardiology/American Heart Association Joint Committee on Clinical Practice Guidelines. Circulation. 2024;149:e1313–410. https://doi.org/10.1161/CIR.0000000000001251.
6. Conte MS, Aulivola B, Barshes NR, Bertges DJ, Corriere MA, Murad MH, Powell RJ, Reed AB, Robinson WP 3rd, Simons JP. Society for Vascular Surgery Clinical Practice Guideline on the management of intermittent claudication: focused update. J Vasc Surg. 2025; https://doi.org/10.1016/j.jvs.2025.04.041.
7. DeRubertis BG, Pierce M, Chaer RA, Rhee SJ, Benjeloun R, Ryer EJ, Kent C, Faries PL. Lesion severity and treatment complexity are associated with outcome after percutaneous infra-inguinal intervention. J Vasc Surg. 2007;46:709–16.
8. Saadi S, Nayfeh T, Rajjoub R, Hasan B, Firwana M, Jawaid T, Hazem W, Shah S, Alsawaf Y, Seisa MO, et al. A systematic review supporting the Society for Vascular Surgery guideline update on the management of intermittent claudication. J Vasc Surg. 2025; https://doi.org/10.1016/j.jvs.2024.12.135.

9. Vogel TR, Braet DJ, Kruse RL, Bath J, Wang J, Gosch K, Smolderen KG. Level of disease and association with health status in patients presenting with claudication from the PORTRAIT registry. J Vasc Surg. 2020;72:2017–26. https://doi.org/10.1016/j.jvs.2020.03.042.
10. Bath J, Lawrence PF, Neal D, Zhao Y, Smith JB, Beck AW, Conte M, Schermerhorn M, Woo K. Endovascular interventions for claudication do not meet minimum standards for the Society for Vascular Surgery efficacy guidelines. J Vasc Surg. 2021;73(1693–1700):e1693. https://doi.org/10.1016/j.jvs.2020.10.067.
11. Smolderen KG, Romain G, Cleman J, Callegari S, Peri-Okonny PA, Mena-Hurtado C. Twelve-month health status response after peripheral vascular intervention for femoropopliteal lesions using Zilver PTX databases focusing on the role of preprocedural health status, comorbid risks, and global setting. J Vasc Surg. 2025;81(210–220):e217. https://doi.org/10.1016/j.jvs.2024.08.035.
12. Hess CN, Huang Z, Patel MR, Baumgartner I, Berger JS, Blomster JI, Fowkes FGR, Held P, Jones WS, Katona B, et al. Acute limb ischemia in peripheral artery disease. Circulation. 2019;140:556–65. https://doi.org/10.1161/CIRCULATIONAHA.119.039773.
13. Hess CN, Debus ES, Nehler MR, Anand SS, Patel MR, Szarek M, Capell WH, Hsia J, Beckman JA, Brodmann M, et al. Reduction in acute limb ischemia with rivaroxaban versus placebo in peripheral artery disease after lower extremity revascularization: insights from VOYAGER PAD. Circulation. 2021;144:1831–41. https://doi.org/10.1161/CIRCULATIONAHA.121.055146.
14. Bauersachs RM, Szarek M, Brodmann M, Gudz I, Debus ES, Nehler MR, Anand SS, Patel MR, Hess CN, Capell WH, et al. Total ischemic event reduction with rivaroxaban after peripheral arterial revascularization in the VOYAGER PAD trial. J Am Coll Cardiol. 2021;78:317–26. https://doi.org/10.1016/j.jacc.2021.05.003.
15. Szarek M, Hess C, Patel MR, Jones WS, Berger JS, Baumgartner I, Katona B, Mahaffey KW, Norgren L, Blomster J, et al. Total cardiovascular and limb events and the impact of polyvascular disease in chronic symptomatic peripheral artery disease. J Am Heart Assoc. 2022;11:e025504. https://doi.org/10.1161/JAHA.122.025504.
16. Peri-Okonny PA, Romain G, Callegari S, Cleman J, Vashist A, Smolderen KG, Mena-Hurtado C. Prediction of health status in patients undergoing lower extremity intervention for claudication. Ann Vasc Surg. 2025;110:314–22. https://doi.org/10.1016/j.avsg.2024.08.016.
17. Peri-Okonny PA, Romain G, Rambhujun V, Callegari S, Vashist A, Cleman J, Smolderen KG, Mena-Hurtado C. Factors associated with sustained improvement after peripheral vascular intervention in patients with claudication. Vasc Med. 2024;29:718–9. https://doi.org/10.1177/1358863X241261369.
18. Connors G, Todoran TM, Engelson BA, Sobieszczyk PS, Eisenhauer AC, Kinlay S. Percutaneous revascularization of long femoral artery lesions for claudication: patency over 2.5 years and impact of systematic surveillance. Catheter Cardiovasc Interv. 2011;77:1055–62. https://doi.org/10.1002/ccd.22802.
19. Torsello G, Stavroulakis K, Brodmann M, Micari A, Tepe G, Veroux P, Benko A, Choi D, Vermassen FEG, Jaff MR, et al. Three-year sustained clinical efficacy of drug-coated balloon angioplasty in a real-world femoropopliteal cohort. J Endovasc Ther. 2020;27:693–705. https://doi.org/10.1177/1526602820931477.
20. Jongkind V, Akkersdijk GJ, Yeung KK, Wisselink W. A systematic review of endovascular treatment of extensive aortoiliac occlusive disease. J Vasc Surg. 2010;52:1376–83. https://doi.org/10.1016/j.jvs.2010.04.080.
21. Ye W, Liu CW, Ricco JB, Mani K, Zeng R, Jiang J. Early and late outcomes of percutaneous treatment of TransAtlantic Inter-Society Consensus class C and D aorto-iliac lesions. J Vasc Surg. 2011;53:1728–37. https://doi.org/10.1016/j.jvs.2011.02.005.
22. Nelson PR, Powell RJ, Schermerhorn ML, Fillinger MF, Zwolak RM, Walsh DB, Cronenwett JL. Early results of external iliac artery stenting combined with common femoral artery endarterectomy. J Vasc Surg. 2002;35:1107–13. https://doi.org/10.1067/mva.2002.124374.

23. Chang RW, Goodney PP, Baek JH, Nolan BW, Rzucidlo EM, Powell RJ. Long-term results of combined common femoral endarterectomy and iliac stenting/stent grafting for occlusive disease. J Vasc Surg. 2008;48:362–7. https://doi.org/10.1016/j.jvs.2008.03.042.
24. Krankenberg H, Tubler T, Sixt S, Fischer M, Schmiedel R, Schulte KL, Balzer JO, Kieback A, Fiehn E, Wittenberg G, et al. German multicenter real-world registry of stenting for superficial femoral artery disease: clinical results and predictive factors for revascularization. J Endovasc Ther. 2014;21:463–71. https://doi.org/10.1583/13-4625R.1.
25. Bose S, Dun C, Solomon AJ, Black JH 3rd, Conte MS, Kalbaugh CA, Woo K, Makary MA, Hicks CW. Editor's choice—infrapopliteal peripheral vascular interventions for claudication are performed frequently in the USA and are associated with poor long term outcomes. Eur J Vasc Endovasc Surg. 2025;69:89–101. https://doi.org/10.1016/j.ejvs.2024.06.017.
26. Bose S, McDermott KM, Dun C, Mao J, Solomon AJ, Black JH, Columbo JA, Conte MS, Deery SE, Goodney PP, et al. Infrapopliteal endovascular interventions for claudication are associated with poor long-term outcomes in medicare-matched registry patients. Ann Surg. 2024; https://doi.org/10.1097/SLA.0000000000006368.

Risks of Revascularization: The So-Called Treatment Trap

17

Laura T. Boitano

Introduction

The goals of treatment for intermittent claudication are to improve walking distance, functional status, and quality of life while reducing cardiovascular risk. Treatment strategies include conservative management with exercise therapy and management of cardiovascular comorbidities. Revascularization may be utilized and options range from open surgical to endovascular interventions. While such surgical and endovascular treatments can offer immediate symptomatic relief and improve walking distance, there has been an increased awareness of the limited durability and risks associated with intervention.

The natural history of intermittent claudication is overall benign with only a small subset of patients progressing to chronic limb-threatening ischemia, about 1% per year [1]. However, cardiovascular comorbidity is not insignificant with resultant 5-year all-cause mortality as high as 20% [2]. Guidelines for the management of intermittent claudication stress the importance of a structured walking program and risk factor management including smoking cessation, diabetes management, cholesterol management, and blood pressure control. Consideration of treatment should carefully weigh patient selection and risk management. Risks associated with revascularization are greatest when conservative measures have not been optimized and the strategies focus on short-term symptomatic relief rather than long-term durability [2–4]. Given this, there is an increased awareness of what has been termed the "treatment trap," which includes the overuse or premature use of invasive interventions in patients with intermittent claudication. Such patients succumb to early treatment failures and multiple revascularizations which may lead to chronic limb-threatening ischemia and amputation [3].

L. T. Boitano (✉)
Division of Vascular and Endovascular Surgery, University of Massachusetts, T.H. Chan School of Medicine, Worcester, MA, USA

W. P. Robinson III, J. P. Simons (eds.), *The Patient-Centered Approach to Claudication*, https://doi.org/10.1007/978-3-032-02460-2_17

This chapter aims to identify the components associated with the treatment trap of intervention and explore the outcomes of revascularization in patients presenting with intermittent claudication due to peripheral artery disease.

Decision to Revascularize

The natural history of claudication suggests that majority of patients will either develop slow functional decline or maintain their level of activity [4]. A minority of patients will develop severe disability despite conservative management; this minority may warrant intervention. Such individuals should have lifestyle- or occupation-limiting functional impairment. There should be a significant impairment on the quality of life. They should have failed conservative measures including a structured walking program for at least 12 weeks and be optimized on medical therapy. The goal of intervention is to improve function and should not be done prophylactically or to avoid limb loss.

For patients presenting with bilateral claudication, significant functional improvement can only be achieved by successfully treating disease in both legs. As such, there should be a higher threshold to treat patients with bilateral symptoms. Similarly, the durability of intervention is lower when infrainguinal disease is treated versus aortoiliac disease, so treatment threshold should be higher in this circumstance also. Current Society for Vascular Surgery (SVS) guidelines recommend an individualized approach to select an invasive treatment for intermittent claudication. The modality offered should provide a reasonable likelihood of sustained benefit to the patient (>50% likelihood of clinical efficacy for at least 2 years) [4].

Components of the Treatment Trap

Overuse of Invasive Procedures

Current guidelines recommend 12 weeks of conservative therapy including optimal medical strategies and a structured exercise program prior to intervention for claudication. Despite this, many patients are being directed toward revascularization procedures prematurely after only a brief trial of conservative therapy [4, 5]. Furthermore, the indication to treat should be based on incapacitating claudication after failure of conservative therapy. Tibial interventions for patients with claudication are rarely, if ever, indicated [6, 7].

Despite societal recommendations and data supporting a conservative approach, researchers have noted that patients with claudication are undergoing interventions too soon and tibial interventions persist [5, 6, 8]. Bose et al. conducted a retrospective analysis of Medicare data from 2017 to 2019 and found that of the almost 60,000 patients undergoing peripheral vascular intervention for claudication, nearly 30% received a tibial intervention with a significant proportion of these being isolated tibial interventions [8]. In a Vascular Quality Initiative study of infrainguinal bypasses for claudication, one-fifth of bypasses were to tibial targets and non-saphenous vein conduit was used in 22% of these cases [9]. Studies have suggested that high volume outpatient settings among physicians with high reimbursement practices are driving this practice [5, 8]. Further study is warranted to understand these findings.

Short-Term Versus Long-Term Outcomes

It is important to consider durability of intervention and long-term outcomes when offering a patient with claudication an intervention. Societal guidelines stress the importance of long-term benefit of intervention and suggest a minimum threshold of a >50% likelihood of sustained efficacy for at least 2 years as a benchmark [4]. Many studies evaluating outcomes of invasive treatments for claudication have failed to meet this benchmark. McCready et al. performed a systematic review of patients with intermittent claudication treated conservatively or with revascularization and demonstrated that the early symptomatic improvement with intervention was lost as early as 6 months following intervention [6]. Similarly, Bath et al. evaluated over 16,000 patients with claudication from the Vascular Quality Initiative treated with endovascular procedures and only 32% were symptom-free at 2 years, falling well below the 50% threshold [10]. The IRONIC trial demonstrated initial quality of life improvements in the revascularization cohort were not sustained, and after 5 years, there was no improvement in quality of life or walking ability compared to those managed conservatively [11]. These studies and others demonstrate the lack of durability among many procedures used to treat patients with claudication. Importantly, tibial interventions are particularly nondurable, and according to the SVS appropriate use criteria for the management of intermittent claudication, invasive intervention in the infrapopliteal segment provides unclear benefit and could be harmful [7].

Progression to Worse Outcomes

There are many studies supporting progression to worse outcomes including progression to chronic limb-threatening ischemia and amputation. This will be discussed in detail in this chapter.

Risks Associated with Revascularization for Intermittent Claudication

Progression to Chronic Limb-Threatening Ischemia (CLTI) and Amputation

One of the significant risks of revascularization for intermittent claudication is altering the disease's natural course, transforming it from a generally benign condition into one that progresses to CLTI. In severe cases, this includes progression to amputation. Several contemporary series have highlighted this. Madabhushi et al. performed a retrospective cohort study of 1051 patients diagnosed with intermittent claudication, of whom 328 underwent revascularization and 723 were treated medically [3]. Patients undergoing revascularization had a significantly higher risk of progressing to CLTI; 5-year progression rates to CLTI were 18% in the revascularization group compared to 8% in the medically managed group. At 10 years, the rates were 27% versus 10%, respectively. Following a similar trend, amputation rates at 5 and 10 years were significantly higher for those in the revascularization cohort (5 years: 6% vs. 1%, 10 years: 11% vs. 2%). Consistent with these findings, Golledge et al. evaluated patients undergoing initial early intervention or initial conservative treatment for management of intermittent claudication; amputation rates at 5 years were significantly higher in the revascularization cohort (6.2%) versus the conservative cohort (0.7%) [12]. McCready et al. conducted a systematic review comparing the outcomes of conservative therapy with revascularization and found that, with one exception, all studies evaluating ≥ 5-year outcomes reported amputation rates exceeding 5% in patients undergoing revascularization [6].

Studies evaluating the treatment of the infrapopliteal segment for intermittent claudication raise even greater concerns [6, 13]. Mukherjee et al. reported a major amputation rate of 5% and 8.5% among patients undergoing tibial atherectomy in the OBL and hospital setting, respectively, within 12 months of the initial procedure [13]. According to the SVS Appropriate Use Criteria, there was unanimous agreement by the rating panel that infrapopliteal interventions distal to a more proximal intervention pose a greater risk than benefit for patients with intermittent claudication [7]. The consensus was based on the extremely low probability that infrapopliteal disease contributes to claudication symptoms, coupled with higher failure rates and potentially more harmful consequences of tibial interventions compared to treatment of proximal arterial segments. Many consider amputation after treatment for intermittent claudication a "never event." [9]

There are several factors that contribute to the progression to CLTI and amputation following revascularization. Revascularization often necessitates repeat procedures due to restenosis or graft failure, which increases the risk of ischemic events. This is particularly true for nondurable procedures. Patients requiring repeat interventions are at higher risk for progression to CLTI. Kim et al. conducted a retrospective review at a single institution among patients who underwent revascularization for disabling claudication between 2013 and 2016 [14]. Undergoing two or more interventions was an independent risk factor for progression to CLTI (OR 2.9).

Other risks identified in this study included congestive heart failure, prior open revascularization, and history of stroke. Similarly, in a retrospective analysis of 187,442 Medicare beneficiaries newly diagnosed with intermittent claudication between 2015 and 2017, Sorber et al. demonstrated that early peripheral intervention initiated a cycle of repeated interventions, with worsening outcomes over time [15].

Invasive procedures may also disrupt collateral circulation which can result in further disease progression. Johnston et al. conducted a retrospective single-center study on 87 limbs treated with Viabahn stent grafts from 2005 to 2010; 56% of the cohort presented with claudication [16]. The authors suggest that coverage of visible distal collaterals in downstream reconstituted segments may predispose patients to increased risk of subsequent thrombosis and clinical deterioration.

Acute Limb Ischemia

In addition to chronic limb-threatening ischemia and amputation, patients undergoing revascularization for intermittent claudication are at higher risk for acute limb ischemia than those treated nonoperatively [17]. In a subgroup analysis of the EUCLID trial, the risk of developing acute limb ischemia was four times higher in the revascularized group compared to patients who had not undergone revascularization [17]. Similarly, there are several mechanisms which contribute to progression to acute limb ischemia after revascularization. Acute thrombosis in an area of intervention or stenosis may result in acute limb ischemia. Revascularization resulting in collateral vessel disruption may ultimately result in acute limb ischemia should the revascularization fail. Technical problems during the intervention can also contribute including arterial dissection and distal embolization resulting in outflow disruption. Acute limb ischemia is an important complication because of the associated need for prolonged hospitalization, high incidence of limb loss, disability, and death, none of which would be expected with conservative management of claudication [18].

Major Cardiovascular Events (MACE)

Patients with PAD are considered a high-risk population at baseline with elevated risk of major adverse cardiac events including cardiovascular death, myocardial infarction (MI), and ischemic stroke [19]. The risk is even greater among patients with concomitant coronary artery disease. In a post hoc analysis of the EUCLID trial which compared the efficacy of ticagrelor versus clopidogrel in patients with PAD, patients with previous revascularization had a 30% higher risk of MI compared to those without such history [17]. In a similar sub-analysis of patients in the EUCLID trial which evaluated outcomes of patients with PAD and those with PAD with concomitant disease in other vascular beds (polyvascular disease), the rate of lower extremity revascularization increased with each additional diseased vascular bed [19]. In this study, the patients with concomitant coronary artery disease experienced the highest rates of cardiovascular death and MI, and patients with PAD and cerebrovascular disease experienced the highest rates of ischemic stroke. The coronary artery disease and cerebrovascular disease were linked to a heightened risk of revascularization.

Increased Risk of Reinterventions

An aspect of the treatment trap includes a cycle of repeated interventions which undermines the potential benefit of the initial revascularization. Revascularization for intermittent claudication is associated with reintervention rates as high as 43% at 10-year follow-up [6]. Regardless of type of intervention, percutaneous or open surgical, there is an association with high rates of repeated revascularization. Atherectomy, in particular, appears to carry a higher risk of reintervention compared to other forms of percutaneous intervention. In a study evaluating tibial atherectomy performed in an outpatient-based laboratory setting, over 45% of patients with claudication required repeat intervention within 1 year [13]. A study evaluating outcomes following lower extremity bypass and infrainguinal endovascular intervention for claudication identified two key independent predictors of major adverse limb events: history of ipsilateral prior open bypass on the same arterial segment and revascularization of an infrageniculate artery. The authors conclude that tibial and redo revascularizations for claudication should be undertaken with caution. These findings underscore the need for adherence to guidelines that emphasize durable intervention strategies [4, 20].

Comparison with Conservative Management

Current Guidelines

Supervised exercise therapy with risk factor modification is the first-line treatment for intermittent claudication [4]. Guidelines emphasize the superior efficacy in improving walking distance and quality of life with exercise compared with invasive interventions. Even if the magnitude of effect were similar with exercise or intervention, the risks are clearly higher with intervention. Revascularization should be reserved for incapacitating claudication that is lifestyle limiting or interferes with the ability to perform one's job. There have been a number of trials comparing conservative management with intervention. The Claudication: Exercise Versus Endoluminal Revascularization (CLEVER) trial compared supervised exercise, primary stenting and optimal medical therapy for patients with aortoiliac occlusive disease resulting in claudication, and demonstrated greatest change in peak walking time at 6 months in the supervised exercise therapy cohort followed by the stenting and optimal medical therapy cohorts [21]. Quality of life evaluation revealed significant improvements in both the supervised exercise and stenting groups compared to pharmacologic therapy alone. Supervised exercise therapy avoided the procedural risks associated with stenting, making it a safer initial option for patients with lifestyle-limiting claudication. The Edinburgh walking study further revealed no significant difference in maximal walking distance, treadmill distance to onset of claudication, or improvement in walking ability between patients undergoing endovascular interventions versus patients offered noninvasive medical management [22]. Again, this study supported the benefits of conservative therapy and provided further evidence for noninvasive therapies as the first-line management for intermittent claudication. The limiting factor in conservative treatments remains noncompliance and drug tolerance.

Long-Term Benefits of Conservative Therapy

Conservative therapy remains a viable treatment strategy long-term without the associated procedural risks. The Invasive Revascularization or Not in Intermittent Claudication (IRONIC) trial was a randomized controlled study to compare the long-term effectiveness and cost-effectiveness of revascularization combined with best medical therapy and structured exercise versus best medial therapy and structured exercise therapy, alone [11]. This study demonstrated, at 5 years, there were no significant differences between the revascularization and non-revascularization groups in terms of treadmill walking distances or health related quality of life. In fact, the early improvements in walking ability and quality of life noted with revascularization in the first 2 years were not sustained over the long term. Conservative therapy is not only the first-line therapy but remains an effective long-term treatment strategy.

Exercise Therapy and Risk Factor Modification

Exercise therapy, when combined with risk factor modification like smoking cessation and statin use, improves walking performance and cardiovascular health [20, 23]. Smoking cessation and diabetes control reduces the progression of PAD and lowers the risk of adverse cardiovascular events [6, 23].

Patient-Reported Outcomes and Satisfaction

Patient-reported outcomes often favor conservative management. While revascularization can offer short-term improvements, long-term satisfaction and quality of life measures are often higher among patients undergoing conservative treatments [22, 25, 26]. The CLEVER trial demonstrated improved quality of life and functional measures in the stenting cohort in the short term, but these benefits were not sustained beyond the first year, particularly in comparison to the supervised exercise therapy [22]. Devine et al. reported significant improvements in patient-reported outcomes like walking distance and pain reduction within 12 months of revascularization, but these gains declined over time [24]. Furthermore, Holeman et al. observed no significant differences in long-term physical function between patients undergoing revascularization and those treated with medical therapy [25]. In addition, the satisfaction in social roles and activities was higher in the non-revascularization group, likely due to the lack of repeat interventions and complications. Factors influencing satisfaction may include lower complication rates, lower costs, and alignment with patient goals that value treatment options that emphasize long-term health and independence from frequent medical interventions [10]. These findings underscore the importance of patient-centered care.

Strategies to Avoid the Treatment Trap

Shared Decision-Making

Patient-centered care must emphasize the importance of individualized success. Technical success and clinical success may not be the same. Shared decision-making is vital to align treatment plans with patient values. Patients must be informed of the potential risks of revascularization, including the possibility of multiple reinterventions, CLTI progression, and increased amputation risk [6, 23].

Emphasize Conservative Treatments

Physicians should stress the importance of conservative treatment strategies including structured exercise programs, appropriate pharmacotherapy, and lifestyle modifications.

Appropriate Patient Selection

Patient selection is a critical factor when considering revascularization for patients with claudication. Patients selected for intervention should demonstrate a severe disability with appropriate risk factor modification suggesting a favorable risk-benefit ratio for revascularization. It is important to ensure control of modifiable patient risk factors including diabetes and smoking. Among patients with PAD, current smoking is associated with higher rates of amputation, death, and MI compared to patients who have successfully quit. In addition, such comorbidities contribute to poorer outcomes after revascularization [3]. Additionally, interventions in patients with advanced frailty or significant systemic disease often result in higher morbidity and mortality, highlighting the importance of patient selection [27].

Long-Term Follow-Up and Monitoring

For those undergoing intervention, continued surveillance is essential to ensure continued success of intervention, risk factor optimization, and exercise. This will allow detection of complications early, which will help to improve the long-term outcomes [20].

Summary

First-line management of intermittent claudication is risk factor modification with optimal medical therapy including aspirin and statin and a structured exercise program. Ideally, 12 weeks of conservative therapy should be documented prior to consideration of any revascularization strategy. Patients unable to tolerate an exercise regimen due to comorbid conditions are unlikely to benefit from revascularization. Patients should be properly informed of the risks associated with revascularization including the risk of repeated interventions, major cardiovascular events, and progression to CLTI and amputation. Furthermore, patients should be informed that the risk of non-intervention has a very low likelihood of progression to CLTI or amputation. Revascularization should only be considered in those who have failed conservative therapy, demonstrate disabling symptoms, and have favorable anatomy. Long-term follow-up is essential for treatment success. Early intervention, resulting in early treatment failures and repeated interventions, can result in the so-called "treatment trap."

References

1. Gerhard-Herman MD, Gornik HL, Barrett C, et al. 2016 AHA/ACC guideline on the management of patients with lower extremity peripheral artery disease: executive summary. Circulation. 2017;135:e686–725.
2. Bhatt DL, Eagle KA, Ohman EM, et al., REACH Registry Investigators. Comparative determinants of 4-year cardiovascular event rates in stable outpatients at risk of or with atherothrombosis. JAMA. 2010;304:1350–7. https://doi.org/10.1001/jama.2010.1322.
3. Madabhushi V, Davenport D, Jones S, et al. Revascularization of intermittent claudicants leads to more chronic limb-threatening ischemia and higher amputation rates. J Vasc Surg. 2021;74:771–9. https://doi.org/10.1016/j.jvs.2021.02.045.
4. Conte MS, Pomposelli FB, Clair DG, et al. Society for Vascular Surgery practice guidelines for atherosclerotic occlusive disease of the lower extremities: management of asymptomatic disease and claudication. J Vasc Surg. 2015;61:2S–41S. https://doi.org/10.1016/j.jvs.2014.12.009.
5. Hicks CW, Holscher CM, Wang P, Black JH III, Abularrage CJ, Makary MA. Overuse of early peripheral vascular interventions for claudication. J Vasc Surg. 2020;71:121–30. https://doi.org/10.1016/j.jvs.2019.05.005.
6. McCready RA, Brown OW, Kiell CS, et al. Revascularization for claudication: changing the natural history of a benign disease. J Vasc Surg. 2024;79:159–66. https://doi.org/10.1016/j.jvs.2023.07.066.

7. Woo K, Siracuse JJ, Klingbeil K, et al. Society for Vascular Surgery appropriate use criteria for management of intermittent claudication. J Vasc Surg. 2022;76:3–22. https://doi.org/10.1016/j.jvs.2022.04.012.
8. Bose S, Dun C, Sorber R, et al. Practice patterns surrounding the use of tibial interventions for claudication in the Medicare population. J Vasc Surg. 2023;77:454–462.e1. https://doi.org/10.1016/j.jvs.2022.08.033.
9. Levin SR, Farber A, Cheng TW, et al. Patients undergoing interventions for claudication experience low perioperative morbidity but are at risk for worsening functional status and limb loss. J Vasc Surg. 2020;72:241–9. https://doi.org/10.1016/j.jvs.2019.08.278.
10. Bath J, Lawrence PF, Neal D, Zhao Y, et al. Endovascular interventions for claudication do not meet minimum standards for the Society for Vascular Surgery efficacy guidelines. J Vasc Surg. 2021;73:2132–2139.e1. https://doi.org/10.1016/j.jvs.2020.10.067.
11. Djerf H, Millinger J, Falkenberg M, et al. Absence of long-term benefit of revascularization in patients with intermittent claudication: five-year results from the IRONIC randomized controlled trial. Circ Cardiovasc Interv. 2020;13:e008450. https://doi.org/10.1161/CIRCINTERVENTIONS.119.008450.
12. Golledge J, Moxon JV, Rowbotham S, et al. Risk of major amputation in patients with intermittent claudication undergoing early revascularization. Br J Surg. 2018;105:699–708. https://doi.org/10.1002/bjs.10765.
13. Mukherjee D, Contos B, Emery E, Collins DT, Black JH III. High reintervention and amputation rates after outpatient atherectomy for claudication. Vasc Endovasc Surg. 2018;52:427–33. https://doi.org/10.1177/153857441877245.
14. Kim TI, Kiwan G, Mohamedali A, et al. Multiple reinterventions for claudication are associated with progression to chronic limb-threatening ischemia. Ann Vasc Surg. 2021;72:166–74. https://doi.org/10.1016/j.avsg.2020.10.004.
15. Sorber R, Dun C, Kawaji Q, et al. Early peripheral vascular interventions for claudication are associated with higher rates of late interventions and progression to chronic limb-threatening ischemia. J Vasc Surg. 2023;77:836–47. https://doi.org/10.1016/j.jvs.2022.10.02.
16. Johnston PC, Vartanian SM, Runge SJ, et al. Risk factors for clinical failure after stent graft treatment for femoropopliteal occlusive disease. J Vasc Surg. 2012;56:998–1007. https://doi.org/10.1016/j.jvs.2012.03.010.
17. Jones WS, Baumgartner I, Hiatt WR, et al. Ticagrelor compared with clopidogrel in patients with prior lower extremity revascularization for peripheral artery disease. Circulation. 2017;135:241–50. https://doi.org/10.1161/CIRCULATIONAHA.116.025880.
18. Bonaca MP, Bauersachs RM, Anand SS, et al. Rivaroxaban in peripheral artery disease after revascularization. N Engl J Med. 2020;382:1994–2004. https://doi.org/10.1056/NEJMoa2000052.
19. Gutierrez JA, Mulder H, Jones WS, et al. Polyvascular disease and risk of major adverse cardiovascular events in peripheral artery disease: a secondary analysis of the EUCLID trial. JAMA Netw Open. 2018;1:e185239. https://doi.org/10.1001/jamanetworkopen.2018.5239.
20. Beckman JA, Schneider PA, Conte MS. Advances in revascularization for peripheral artery disease: revascularization in PAD. Circ Res. 2021;128:1885–912. https://doi.org/10.1161/CIRCRESAHA.121.318261.
21. Murphy TP, Cutlip DE, Regensteiner JG, et al., CLEVER Study Investigators. Supervised exercise versus primary stenting for claudication resulting from aortoiliac peripheral artery disease: six-month outcomes from the claudication: exercise versus endoluminal revascularization (CLEVER) study. Circulation. 2012;125:130–9. https://doi.org/10.1161/CIRCULATIONAHA.111.075770.
22. Whyman MR, Fowkes FG, Kerracher EM, Gillespie IN, Lee AJ, Housley E, et al. Is intermittent claudication improved by percutaneous transluminal angioplasty? A randomized controlled trial. J Vasc Surg. 1997;26:551–7. https://doi.org/10.1016/s0741-5214(97)70052-1.
23. Norgren L, Hiatt WR, Dormandy JA, Nehler MR, Harris KA, Fowkes FG, TASC II Working Group. Inter-Society Consensus for the management of peripheral arterial disease (TASC II). J Vasc Surg. 2007;45(Suppl S):S5A–S67A. https://doi.org/10.1016/j.jvs.2006.12.037.

24. Devine EB, Alfonso-Cristancho R, Yanez ND, et al. Comparative Effectiveness Research Translation Network (CERTAIN) Collaborative. Effectiveness of a medical vs revascularization intervention for intermittent leg claudication based on patient-reported outcomes. JAMA Surg. 2016;151:e162024. https://doi.org/10.1001/jamasurg.2016.2024.
25. Holeman TA, Chester C, Hales JB, et al. Long-term patient-reported outcomes among patients undergoing revascularization versus medical therapy for intermittent claudication. J Vasc Surg. 2024;80:466–77. https://doi.org/10.1016/j.jvs.2024.03.455.
26. O'Banion LA, Saadi S, Hasan B, et al. Lack of patient-centered evaluation of outcomes in intermittent claudication literature. J Vasc Surg. 2023;78:828–36. https://doi.org/10.1016/j.jvs.2023.03.497.
27. Saraidaridis JT, Ergul EA, Clouse WD, et al. The natural history and outcomes of endovascular therapy for claudication. Ann Vasc Surg. 2017;44:34–40. https://doi.org/10.1016/j.avsg.2017.04.021.

A Brief Primer on Shared Decision-Making and Applications to Claudication

18

Xiaoyi Teng and Matthew A. Corriere

Introduction

Although clinical practice guidelines recommend shared decision-making (SDM) for treatment of claudication [1], many clinicians who support this notion might struggle to define this concept or how to implement SDM within clinical practice. Since the field of SDM for claudication is still in its relative infancy, this process is rarely approached in a standard or measurable fashion and clinicians may find it difficult to define when, how, and to what extent the discussion took place.

Contemporary clinical practice has expanded patient access to medical information (including misinformation) that the patient may reference before, after, or even during a clinic visit. This is a major shift from previous decades, where patients instead relied primarily on the clinician as a source of medical information. Pressure on clinicians to shorten clinic visits, to see more patients, and increased documentation requirements are significant roadblocks to effective SDM from the provider standpoint. A computer screen may also be competing with the patient for face time from the clinician tasked with documentation, order entry, and scheduling instructions during the visit. Given these time constraints and competing demands, it should not be assumed that SDM will take place by chance.

Integrating SDM into clinical practice therefore may seem like a daunting task. The benefits of SDM, however, can be rewarding to both patients and clinicians. If the patient and clinician have partnered through SDM, both have "skin in the game" for the treatment plan, adherence, and outcomes. Patients who perceive that they have partnered in development of their own strategy may view their treatment as

X. Teng · M. A. Corriere (✉)
Division of Vascular Diseases & Surgery, Department of Surgery, The Ohio State University, Columbus, OH, USA
e-mail: Xiaoyi.Teng@osumc.edu; Matthew.Corriere@osumc.edu

W. P. Robinson III, J. P. Simons (eds.), *The Patient-Centered Approach to Claudication*, https://doi.org/10.1007/978-3-032-02460-2_18

consistent with their personal goals and preferences. This perspective frames how patients view their outcomes, including success versus failure, decision satisfaction versus regret, and risks.

This chapter is intended to introduce the basic elements of SDM to clinicians who treat patients with claudication due to peripheral artery disease (PAD). We will review the definition of SDM and associated terminology, approaches to practicing and measuring SDM, and specific considerations related to claudication. An overview of evidence and evidence gaps related to SDM for claudication is also provided as a framework for considering the challenges that must be navigated for integration into both research and clinical practice.

Shared Decision-Making Definitions, Measurement, and Relevant Terminology

Shared decision-making has been defined as: "an approach where clinicians and patients share the best available evidence when faced with the task of making decisions, and where patients are supported to consider options to achieve informed preferences." [2, 3] Although SDM falls within the more general concept of *patient-centered care*, some have advocated approaching the patient as a person (rather than vice versa). The term *patient* denotes an individual within a specific medical context (e.g., a clinical encounter, prescription, or insurance plan), while a *person* more broadly considers social contexts that influence how options are prioritized and may determine whether outcomes are viewed as failure versus success [4]. Approaching SDM from the perspective of centering on the patient as a person (rather than the medical encounter) therefore considers a broader view of how treatment and illness are experienced by the patient, family, caregivers, and other decision partners [5].

Patient preferences and values are related concepts that are both integral to SDM. *Preferences* refer to which specific treatment options the patient prefers (or prefers to avoid) most among those presented for consideration [6]. *Values* instead refers to the underlying *attributes* (or factors) about a treatment option that are prioritized and motivate the preferences. For example, a patient may have a *preference* to avoid procedural interventions for claudication because they value risk avoidance as a treatment attribute. *Values clarification* refers to a structured process to help a patient understand their personal values, which some people may not be consciously aware of or able to describe. A variety of values clarification approaches have been described, including survey-based discrete choice experiments, ordinal scales, or best-worst order. Figure 18.1 shows an example of a choice card used to evaluate a patient's preference between two theoretical treatment options within a discrete choice survey; each option is displayed based on five different treatment-specific attributes. Qualitative approaches, including visualization of best case versus worst case scenarios, have also been described as approaches for values clarification related to surgical procedures [7, 8].

Mutual understanding between the patient and clinician is a prerequisite for SDM, and clinician-patient dialogue must therefore manage emotions and

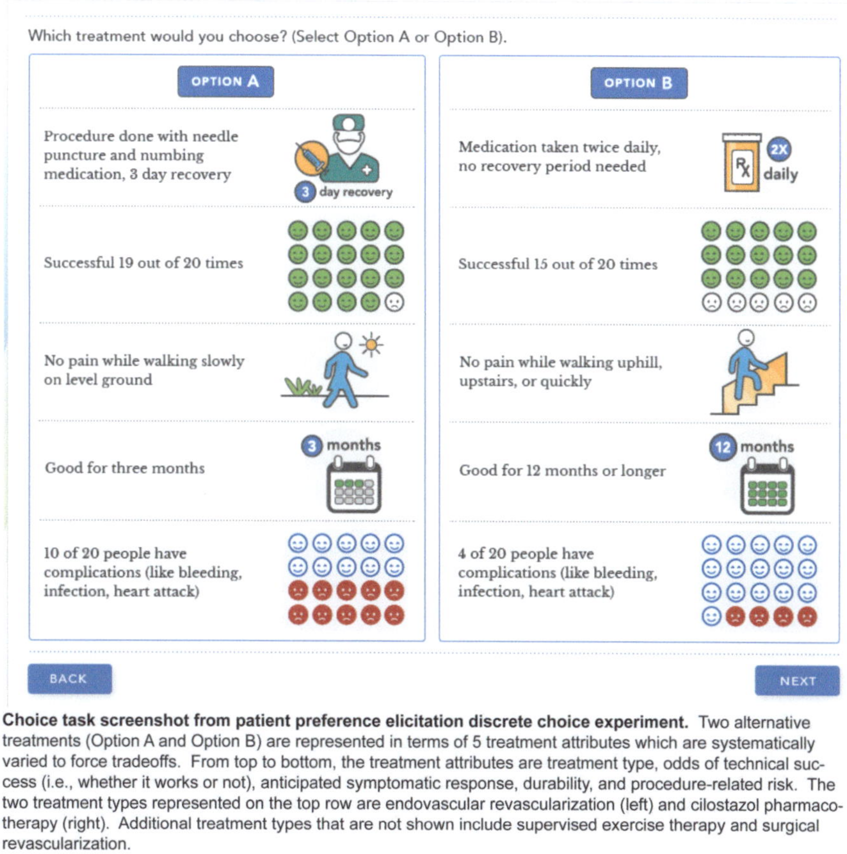

Fig. 18.1 Choice task screenshot from patient preference elicitation discrete choice experiment. Two alternative treatments (option A and option B) are represented in terms of five treatment attributes which are systematically varied to force tradeoffs. From top to bottom, the treatment attributes are treatment type, odds of technical success (i.e., whether it works or not), anticipated symptomatic response, durability, and procedure-related risk. The two treatment types represented on the top row are endovascular revascularization (left) and cilostazol pharmacotherapy (right). Additional treatment types that are not shown include supervised exercise therapy and surgical revascularization

psychological factors that arise during the process [2]. Tools used to assist patients and clinicians in SDM are referred to as *decision aids*. These tools are intended to support and catalyze patient contributions to SDM by making patient values and preferences clear [9]. The International Patient Decision Aids Standards (IPDAS) Collaboration has proposed decision aid criteria, reporting guidelines, instrument assessments, and checklists. [10, 11] Minimum IPDAS qualifying criteria for decision aids are summarized in Table 18.1 [12].

SDM instruments assess whether SDM took place related to a given decision or clinical encounter and may also quantify SDM. SDM instruments are often based on a survey administered after a clinical encounter or discussion with an

Table 18.1 Minimum International Patient Decision Aids Standards (IPDAS) Collaboration qualifying criteria for decision aids

Describes the condition (health or other) related to the decision
Describes the decision that needs to be considered (the index decision)
Identifies the target audience
Has information about the positive features of the options (e.g., benefits and advantages)
Has information about the negative features of the options (e.g., harms, side effects, and disadvantages)
Describes what it is like to experience the consequences of the options (e.g., physical, psychological, social)

opportunity for SDM has occurred. The *reporter*, sometimes alternatively referred to as the respondent, is the individual whose perspective on SDM is elicited through completion of the instrument. The reporter may be the patient, the clinician, or an observer present during the interaction. *Generic* SDM instruments are designed to be used in a variety of populations and contexts. *Disease-specific* instruments are intended to be used within circumstances defined by a diagnosis and/or treatment. Even generic instruments may nonetheless specify populations and/or reporters for intended use. For example, the Observer OPTION MCC instrument is designed for use for triadic decision-making between older patients with multiple chronic conditions, clinicians, and caregivers [13]. Table 18.2 summarizes generic SDM instruments referenced by the Agency for Healthcare Research and Quality [14].

SDM can and should be part of clinical practice, and it is important to emphasize that neither a decision aid nor an SDM instrument must be utilized for SDM to occur. Choice, option, and decision talk have been proposed as key steps for SDM within clinical practice by Elwyn et al. [2] *Choice talk* involves making sure that the patient is aware that more than one reasonable option is available. *Option talk* consists of sharing information and evidence about the options that are being considered. The final step, *decision talk*, refers to considering the options together with preferences and deciding which is the best [2].

Ethical and Practical Considerations Related to Shared Decision-Making

Since the concept of SDM emerged in the early 1980s, over 80 trials have demonstrated associated benefits that include increased patient knowledge and more active patient involvement [2]. According to the United States Preventative Services Task Force, patients have the right to be informed and participate in their healthcare decisions. The value for SDM therefore should not be assessed solely based on health outcomes, but also as an ethical right [9].

Caution has been advised against overreliance on decision aids and risk calculators for SDM [15]. Because these tools are often either clinician- or patient-facing, their use should not be assumed to establish partnership between both parties that is essential for SDM. Complete delegation of the decision to the patient is also inconsistent with SDM, and places the entire ownership burden to the patient. Dialogue

Table 18.2 Generic shared decision measures

Instrument	Full name	Reporter	Items (N)	Format	Notes
SDM-Q-9 [31, 32]	The 9-item shared decision-making questionnaire	Patient	9	Multiple choice, single response based on six-point ordinal scale	Complementary physician instrument available
SDM process 4 [33]	Shared decision-making process survey	Patient	4	Multiple choice, single response; variable response options between items	Includes separate instruments based on whether decisions involve 2 or >2 options
collaboRATE [34]	collaboRATE measure	Patient, parent, or patient representative	3	Multiple choice, single response based on ten-point ordinal scale	5-point scale alternative also available
SURE [35, 36]	SURE test version for clinical practice	Patient	4	Multiple choice, single response based on "yes" or "no" options	Developed based on the Ottawa decision support framework
SDM-Q-Doc [31, 32]	The 9-item shared decision-making questionnaire	Physician	9	Multiple choice, single response based on six-point ordinal scale	Complementary patient instrument available
OPTION(5) [37, 38]	The observer OPTION[5] measure	Observer of a clinic encounter	5	Multiple choice, single response based on 0–4 ordinal scale	Designed as a more efficient version of OPTION(12) instrument

(continued)

Table 18.2 (continued)

Instrument	Full name	Reporter	Items (N)	Format	Notes
OPTION(12) [38, 39]	OPTION observing patient involvement	Observer of a clinic encounter	12	Multiple choice, single response based on 0–4 ordinal scale	In addition to multiple choice items, form also includes patient and physician demographic information
OPTION MCC [13]	Observer OPTION^{MCC}	Observer of a clinic encounter	7	Multiple choice, single response based on 0–4 ordinal scale for clinicians and 0–2 ordinal scale for patients/ informal providers	Measures triadic decision-making and generates separate scores for clinicians, patients, and informal caregivers; developed for older patients with multiple chronic conditions

Items listed identified and available through the Agency for Healthcare Research and Quality [14]

between parties that includes discussion of options and preference elicitation before both parties choose together instead allows shared ownership of the decision while supporting the patient's autonomy [15].

As noted above, some have advocated for approaching the patient as a person (rather than vice versa). A *patient* denotes an individual within a specific medical context (e.g., a clinical encounter, prescription, or insurance plan), while a *person* more broadly considers social contexts that influence how options are prioritized and may determine whether outcomes are viewed as failure versus success [4]. Although clinicians might refer to a patient as a *claudicant* based on that diagnosis, describing them instead as *person with claudication* conveys more person-centered perspective. Approaching SDM from the perspective of centering on the person (rather than the medical encounter) therefore considers a broader view of how treatment and illness are experienced not only by the patient, but also their family, caregivers, and other decision partners [5].

Several factors influence the relative importance of SDM during a given encounter, including: the familiarity between the patient and the clinician, the severity and temporal stability of claudication symptoms, and response to current or previous treatments. For example, SDM is probably less important during a visit for stable, mild symptoms that are not lifestyle-limiting, especially if a plan of care is already established to avoid treatment escalation unless symptoms worsen. In contrast, SDM is critically important when: (1) there is uncertainty regarding the best treatment strategy; (2) when symptoms have worsened since the previous visit; or (3) when the visit is for a second opinion after the patient has already received recommendations from another clinician. This last scenario may indicate discordance between what the patient is seeking and what the previous clinician recommended, dissatisfaction with a previous recommendation or outcome, or uncertainty regarding the best strategy. Conversely, SDM may not be helpful if there is no equipoise (i.e., there is a clear best option), the patient's request conflicts with clinical evidence or clinician judgment, or the options are restricted by legal or institutional policies [16].

Potential for benefit of a given intervention has been proposed as a criterion for how an option is presented by the clinician, with recommendation by the clinician when an intervention with high or moderate certainty of benefit [9]. When certainty is lower or the net benefit is small, SDM that includes discussion of both positive and negative features of an intervention becomes critical to determine whether the option is worthwhile or not from the patient's perspective. When there is no clear benefit or negative features may outweigh the positive, it may be appropriate to bring up an option only if the patient asks [9].

Caution has been advised against overreliance on decision aids and risk calculators for SDM. These tools are often either clinician- or patient-facing, and cannot be assumed to establish the partnership between both parties that is essential for SDM. Complete delegation of the decision to the patient is also inconsistent with SDM, and places the entire ownership burden to the patient. Dialogue between parties that includes discussion of options and preference elicitation before they choose together allows both partners to instead share in ownership of the decision while still supporting the patient's autonomy.

Claudication-Specific Barriers and Facilitators to Shared Decision-Making

The simplest circumstances for SDM would be a choice between two treatment alternatives that must be made only once. Examples of such "either-or" choices include a decision related to a screening test or a vaccination where the alternatives are either to proceed or not. Claudication treatment selection, in contrast, involves significantly greater complexity from several perspectives. Because claudication is a chronic disease, treatment does not involve a curative scenario and instead requires lifelong post-diagnostic management. This premise is critical for the patient to understand, because it amplifies the importance of a decision to pursue revascularization or not. Figure 18.2 illustrates how symptom severity, quality of life, and treatment intensity can be used in combination to describe appropriate treatment intensity, undertreatment, and overtreatment.

Preoperative discussion of both durability and the implications of patency loss are therefore critical to SDM when revascularization is being considered. Patients with the misperception tjat post-revascularization symptomatic improvement is equivalent to cure of their peripheral artery disease, especially those who are smokers, may demand revascularization prematurely without medical optimization and/or before trying walking exercise therapy or cilostazol pharmacotherapy. Additionally, when smoking cessation is presented as a criterion for revascularization (without discussion of the long-term benefits), patients may be primed to

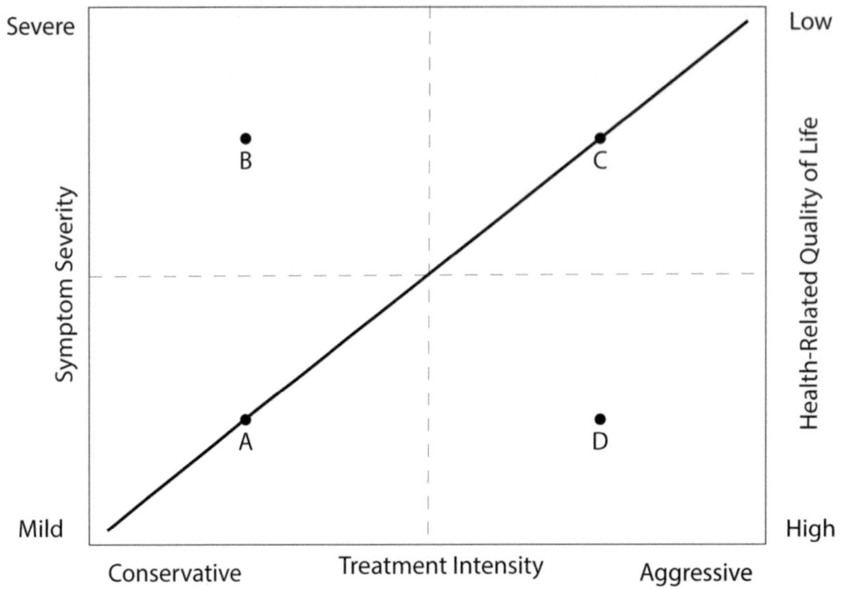

Anticipated correlation between PAD symptom severity, treatment intensity, and health-related quality of life (HRQoL). X-axis indicates treatment intensity. Y-axis indicates symptom severity on the right and health-related quality of life (HRQoL) on the left. Solid line represents ideal correlation between these factors. Each point represents a theoretical patient. Patients A and C received appropriate treatment intensity based on their symptoms and HRQoL. Patient B, who has severe symptoms and poor HRQoL, is under-treated. Patient D, who has mild symptoms and good HRQoL, received aggressive treatment and therefore was over-treated.

Fig. 18.2 Anticipated correlation between PAD symptom severity, treatment intensity, and health-related quality of life (HRQoL). X-axis indicates treatment intensity. Y-axis indicates symptom severity on the right, and HRQoL on the left. Solid line represents ideal correlation between these factors. Each point represents a theoretical patient. Patients A and C received appropriate treatment intensity based on their symptoms and HRQoL. Patient B, who has severe symptoms and poor HRQoL, is under-treated. Patient D, who has mild symptoms and good HRQoL, received aggressive treatment and therefore was over-treated

relapse postoperatively. Rather than returning to baseline claudication symptoms, many patients who experience loss of patency after revascularization instead progress to limb-threatening ischemia. Higher rates of amputation have been observed among patients with claudication treated with revascularization [17], underscoring the importance of medical optimization, exercise therapy, and cilostazol as due diligence prior to considering procedural interventions. These considerations have potential to influence not only the initial decision to perform revascularization or not, but also potentially support patient adherence to risk reduction pharmacotherapy and tobacco abstinence. It is also probable that these considerations would support adherence to exercise therapy and/or cilostazol pharmacotherapy among patients receiving one or both of these treatments prior to consideration of revascularization. SDM supports a conscientious mindset toward more aggressive treatment strategies, and supports mutual expectations between the clinician and patient regarding the appropriateness of the indications, risk tolerance, and implications of complications or patency loss.

As appropriate use criteria are increasingly proposed in response to scrutiny around overtreatment [18], SDM is a worthwhile investment to ensure mutual understanding and minimize decisional regret. Because claudication treatment decisions are revisited periodically during follow-up, clinicians have an opportunity to follow interval responses to treatment interventions that inform subsequent counseling and decisions. Longitudinal follow-up also provides an opportunity to develop trust with patients, confirming the priorities and treatment plan or making changes if needed.

Treatment selection for claudication is complex because of the multiple options that are available and may be implemented individually, sequentially, or simultaneously. For example, exercise therapy and cilostazol may be implemented in a staged fashion or in combination. Furthermore, these treatments can be continued post-revascularization (although there is little evidence regarding how often they are continued versus abandoned once revascularization has been performed).

Claudication treatment is also complex because patients are treated with interventions that may affect one or both legs depending upon the baseline symptom laterality and the intervention(s) performed. Exercise therapy and cilostazol are patient-level treatment interventions that affect both legs, while revascularization may be limited to one leg at a time. It is also common for patients with asymmetric leg symptoms to unmask symptoms in their contralateral leg following revascularization of the leg with the more severe symptoms at presentation as their walking increases from baseline. Preparing patients for this possibility helps them understand the anticipated course and need for periodic reassessment.

Multiple comorbid conditions are common among patients with claudication and may introduce potential uncertainty regarding the incremental benefit achievable through a given treatment intervention. For example, a patient with atypical leg symptoms who also suffers from peripheral neuropathy and balance problems may experience less walking improvement through treatment of their PAD if these other conditions are also contributing to leg pain and walking impairment at baseline. Similarly, a patient with pulmonary disease or congestive heart failure may have less potential for walking improvement through aggressive treatment of claudication if these other diagnoses impart a ceiling effect that limits their maximum walking speed, distance, or duration due to reasons other than leg pain. The implications of multiple chronic comorbid conditions among patients with claudication and potential implications for achievable walking improvement through treatment of claudication are summarized as a conceptual model in Fig. 18.3.

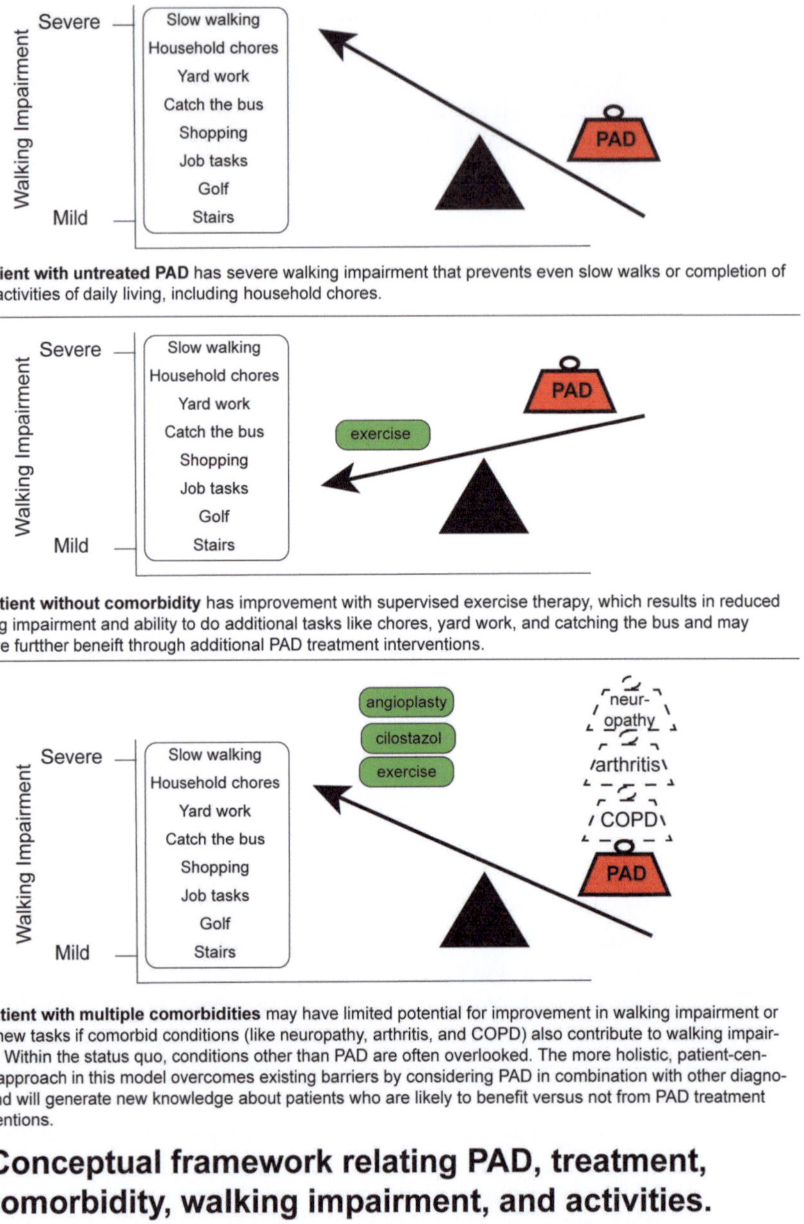

Fig. 18.3 Conceptual framework relating PAD, treatment, comorbidity, walking impairment, and activities

Lack of information, lack of access, and lack of trust have been proposed as potential barriers to guideline-based treatment and therefore contributors to clinical outcomes disparities among women and minority patients [9]. Accordingly, SDM also may have potential to mitigate these barriers and thereby improve patients' willingness to seek diagnosis and treatment of claudication, including implementation of guideline-based medical therapy.

Evidence and Evidence Gaps Related to Shared Decision-Making for Claudication

Preferences Related to Shared Decision-Making and Treatment Options

A growing number of studies support the importance of SDM for claudication based on qualitative, survey, and mixed methods designs. Key factors suggesting that greater SDM is needed for claudication include: heterogeneity in patient preferences, lack of patient awareness that multiple options exist, experiences suggesting that options are not presented to patients, and perceptions that treatment outcomes are unsuccessful.

In a survey exploring experienced versus desired roles in treatment choices among patients undergoing vascular procedures, 90% of participants indicated a preference for discussion of all options under consideration, while only 54% indicated that they were offered a choice. Among respondents with PAD in the same study, 35% indicated that none of their treatments received were successful [19].

A focus group study of patients with symptomatic PAD identified five treatment-specific attributes deemed relevant to values and SDM: the specific treatment interventions under consideration (i.e., some participants specifically either wanted or wanted to avoid one or more treatment options), the chance of technical success (i.e., would the treatment work or not work at all), the degree of symptomatic improvement anticipated with a technically successful treatment, durability of the treatment outcome, and treatment-related risk [20]. Within these attributes, it is important to acknowledge that treatment interventions may be technically unsuccessful even if they are not revascularization procedures. For example, a patient may be referred to supervised exercise therapy but unable to participate, or prescribed cilostazol but unable to tolerate the medication; these are technical failures. There was significant heterogeneity among patient experiences related to their treatment selection process in this study, with some participants describing clinicians ignoring their input and lack of trust in clinician recommendations. These attributes were subsequently used to identify distinct preference "phenotypes" among patients with symptomatic PAD that may be used to support SDM, including tailored management and communication strategies. [20]

Smolderen et al. evaluated patient knowledge and preferences for claudication treatments using a cross-sectional survey among patients with claudication [21]. Results indicated that only 54% of participants knew that there was more than one way to treat claudication, and only 47% indicated that they were offered more than one option. Consistent with other studies discussed above, the authors also observed significant variability in preferences between different treatment goals; "improving quality of life" (which might have a different definition from one patient to another) was identified as the most important treatment goal.

In a cross-sectional survey study among patients with claudication, Powell et al. identified significant heterogeneity in treatment goals [22]. Participants in this study were invited to indicate self-reported goals. Sixty-two percent of participants indicated that an increase in walking distance or duration without stopping was their primary treatment goal. Among this subgroup, most participants indicated walking distance and duration improvement cut points ≥0.5 miles (2640 feet) or 30 min without stopping, respectively, as minimum improvements needed for them to consider a given treatment intervention successful. These levels of improvement greatly exceed distances of 8–20 m considered as minimum important differences in the 6-min walk test, a measure increasingly used to assess claudication treatment outcomes [23]. This mismatch between significant improvement based on group-wise mean statistics versus individual patient perceptions underscores the importance of mutual understanding between patients and clinicians as a prerequisite for SDM. Otherwise, a patient who prefers aggressive management of claudication may end up disappointed by a treatment outcome that they consider unsuccessful even though the strategy chosen was consistent with their values. Clinicians therefore must consider what results are reasonably achievable and include this information when discussing treatment options. Moreover, 23% of respondents in the study by Powell et al. self-reported a treatment goal different from increased walking distance or duration [22]. Examples of self-reported goals included outdoor recreation, employment or home-related work tasks, climbing stairs, walking uphill, and shopping. These observations suggest that an open-ended question about an individual's goals is a valuable component of a clinic visit, especially for a new patient.

Reed et al. used a discrete choice experiment to quantify tradeoffs that patients would accept between reducing risk of clinically driven target vessel revascularization (i.e., repeat interventions due to loss of patency or restenosis) versus mortality risk [24]. This study was conducted within the context of use of a paclitaxel-associated device or not. Results demonstrated, perhaps surprisingly to many clinicians, that most patients would accept an incremental increase in 5-year mortality risk as tradeoff for lower risk of reintervention. Patient-level variability in this study was also significant, however, and a significant minority of patients (40%) chose the lower mortality treatment alternative >87% of the time.

Disease-Specific Decision Aids for Claudication and PAD

Two disease-specific decision aids for PAD are summarized in Table 18.3. Both are available only in English.

The *Peripheral Arterial Disease: Should I Have Surgery?* instrument is a decision aid for individuals deciding whether to have a surgical procedure (angioplasty

Table 18.3 Decision aids developed for patients with peripheral artery disease

Instrument	Format	Target population	Options presented (N)	Options (Description)	Compares probabilities	Limitations
Peripheral arterial disease: Should I have surgery? [25]	Web or paper	Individuals deciding whether to have a surgical procedure (angioplasty or bypass surgery) for peripheral arterial disease	2	Have angioplasty or surgery Try medicine or specialized exercise program to reduce leg pain	No	Not claudication-specific. Does not include option to do nothing. Does not distinguish between procedural interventions. Does not force tradeoffs between options.
Show me PAD [26, 27]	Web, video, paper, PDF	Patients with a new diagnosis of mild-severe claudication	4	Supervised exercise therapy Claudication medications Angioplasty/stents/ bypass surgery Doing nothing	Yes	Designed for newly diagnosed patients. Unclear applicability to follow up visits after failed interventions. Does not distinguish between procedural interventions. Does not force tradeoffs.

Items summarized based on instrument, format, target population, options, probabilities, and limitations or bypass surgery) for peripheral arterial disease. It is available in electronic format or paper format, and presents two options: Have angioplasty or surgery; or try medicine or specialized exercise program to reduce leg pain [25]. Advantages of this instrument include its simplicity due to two alternatives based on a context of considering procedural intervention or not. Disadvantages include absence of probabilities, lack of specificity for claudication, lack of an option to do nothing, and non-differentiation between surgical versus endovascular procedures as distinct options.

The *Show Me PAD* instrument is a decision aid for patients with a new diagnosis of mild to severe claudication and presents four treatment options: supervised exercise therapy, cilostazol pharmacotherapy, procedural intervention, or doing nothing [26, 27]. This decision aid has been evaluated in prototype format and is currently in beta testing. The patient serves as the instrument respondent. Strengths of this decision aid include comparison of outcome probabilities and inclusion of the option to do nothing (which is often an appropriate choice among patients with claudication). Disadvantages of *Show Me PAD* are that it has not been extensively tested beyond prototype phase, does not force tradeoffs (i.e., it is possible for the respondent to rate each option equally), and that it is only for newly diagnosed patients. This instrument therefore may not be as useful for patients that are not recently diagnosed or have had previous treatment interventions.

Ongoing Studies

Personalized outcomes forecasts are presently being evaluated as a means of supporting treatment of patients with claudication by physical therapists [28]. This interrupted time series study is being conducted in the Netherlands to evaluate whether personalized outcomes forecasts can support personalized care based on patient needs and priorities of individualized treatment outcomes. The study intervention includes a decision support system that includes visualization of exercise therapy outcomes based on similar patient "neighbors" within a large national database. SDM is one of the primary study outcomes that will be assessed based on the OPTION 5 instrument [13].

Summary

SDM has immense potential to contribute to person-centered claudication care, including avoidance of over- or under-treatment, and setting clear goals or expectations. Integration into clinical practice will require structured and efficient approaches to overcome barriers related to clinician time and preference heterogeneity between individual patients. Claudication-specific values clarification and decision aid tools have potential to support clinical practice and research implementation in the future, but will require more extensive validation to support widespread adoption [29]. Clinician training and policy-based incentives based on value to the patient also have potential to support SDM implementation in the future [30].

References

1. Gornik HL, Aronow HD, Goodney PP, Arya S, Brewster LP, Byrd L, et al. 2024 ACC/AHA/AACVPR/APMA/ABC/SCAI/SVM/SVN/SVS/SIR/VESS guideline for the Management of Lower Extremity Peripheral Artery Disease: a report of the American College of Cardiology/American Heart Association Joint Committee on Clinical Practice Guidelines. Circulation. 2024;149(24):e1313–410.
2. Elwyn G, Frosch D, Thomson R, Joseph-Williams N, Lloyd A, Kinnersley P, et al. Shared decision making: a model for clinical practice. J Gen Intern Med. 2012;27(10):1361–7.
3. Elwyn G, Laitner S, Coulter A, Walker E, Watson P, Thomson R. Implementing shared decision making in the NHS. BMJ. 2010;341:c5146.
4. Lynn J, McKethan A, Jha AK. Value-based payments require valuing what matters to patients. JAMA. 2015;314(14):1445–6.
5. Clayman ML, Gulbrandsen P, Morris MA. A patient in the clinic; a person in the world. Why shared decision making needs to center on the person rather than the medical encounter. Patient Educ Couns. 2017;100(3):600–4.
6. Witteman HO, Ndjaboue R, Vaisson G, Dansokho SC, Arnold B, Bridges JFP, et al. Clarifying values: an updated and expanded systematic review and meta-analysis. Med Decis Mak. 2021;41(7):801–20.
7. Baggett ND, Schulz K, Buffington A, Marka N, Hanlon BM, Zimmermann C, et al. Surgeon use of shared decision-making for older adults considering major surgery: a secondary analysis of a randomized clinical trial. JAMA Surg. 2022;157(5):406.
8. Kruser JM, Nabozny MJ, Steffens NM, Brasel KJ, Campbell TC, Gaines ME, et al. "Best case/worst case": qualitative evaluation of a novel communication tool for difficult in-the-moment surgical decisions. J Am Geriatr Soc. 2015;63(9):1805–11.
9. US Preventive Services Task Force, Davidson KW, Mangione CM, Barry MJ, Nicholson WK, Cabana MD, et al. Collaboration and shared decision-making between patients and clinicians in preventive health care decisions and US preventive services task force recommendations. JAMA. 2022;327(12):1171.
10. Holmes-Rovner M, Moumjid N, Llewellyn-Thomas H, O'Kane M, Thomson R, Stacey D, et al. IPDAS 2005: criteria for judging the quality of patient decision aids. International Patient Decision Aids Standards (IPDAS) Collaboration; 2005.
11. International Patient Decision Aids Standards (IPDAS) Collaboration [Internet]. [cited 2025 Jan 12]. Available from: https://decisionaid.ohri.ca/IPDAS/index.html
12. Joseph-Williams N, Newcombe R, Politi M, Durand MA, Sivell S, Stacey D, et al. Toward minimum standards for certifying patient decision aids: a modified Delphi consensus process. Med Decis Mak. 2014;34(6):699–710.
13. Pel-Littel RE, Buurman BM, van de Pol MH, Yilmaz NG, Tulner LR, Minkman MM, et al. Measuring triadic decision making in older patients with multiple chronic conditions: Observer^{MCC}. Patient Educ Couns. 2019;102(11):1969–76.
14. Measures, data, and funding for shared decision making research. Content last reviewed May 2023. Agency for Healthcare Research and Quality. Rockville, MD. [Internet]. [cited 2025 Jan 12]. Available from: https://www.ahrq.gov/sdm/measures-data-funding/index.html#sdm-measures
15. Kopecky KE, Urbach D, Schwarze ML. Risk calculators and decision aids are not enough for shared decision making. JAMA Surg. 2019;154(1):3–4.

16. van der Horst DEM, Garvelink MM, Bos WJW, Stiggelbout AM, Pieterse AH. For which decisions is shared decision making considered appropriate?—a systematic review. Patient Educ Couns. 2023;106:3–16.
17. Golledge J, Moxon JV, Rowbotham S, Pinchbeck J, Yip L, Velu R, et al. Risk of major amputation in patients with intermittent claudication undergoing early revascularization. Br J Surg. 2018;105(6):699–708.
18. Forsyth AM, Simons JP. An assessment of the Society for Vascular Surgery appropriate use criteria for the management of intermittent claudication: key findings and considerations for implementation. Ann Vasc Surg. 2024;107:13–6.
19. Corriere MA, Avise JA, Peterson LA, Stafford JM, Easterling D, Boone DS, et al. Exploring patient involvement in decision making for vascular procedures. J Vasc Surg. 2015;62(4):1032.
20. Corriere MA, Barnard R, Saldana S, Guzman RJ, Boone D, Easterling D, Burke G, Ip E: Characterizing Treatment Preference "Phenotypes" Among Patients With Symptomatic Peripheral Artery Disease to Support Identification of Concordant Treatment and Communication Strategies, Abstract, Oral Presentation, Vascular Annual Meeting 2020, Virtual, 2020, Journal of Vascular Surgery. 2020;72(1):e77–e77.
21. Smolderen KG, Romain G, Gosch K, Arham A, Provance JB, Spertus JA, et al. Patient knowledge and preferences for peripheral artery disease treatment. Vasc Med. 2023;28(5):397–403.
22. Powell CA, Kim GY, Edwards SN, Aalami O, Treat-Jacobson D, Byrnes ME, et al. Characterizing patient-reported claudication treatment goals to support patient-centered treatment selection and measurement strategies. J Vasc Surg. 2023;77(2):465.
23. McDermott MM, Tian L, Criqui MH, Ferrucci L, Conte MS, Zhao L, et al. Meaningful change in 6-minute walk in people with peripheral artery disease. J Vasc Surg. 2021;73(1):267–276.e1.
24. Reed SD, Sutphin J, Wallace MJ, Gonzalez JM, Yang JC, Reed Johnson F, et al. Quantifying patients' preferences on tradeoffs between mortality risk and reduced need for target vessel revascularization for claudication. Vasc Med. 2024;2024:1358863X241290233.
25. Peripheral arterial disease: should I have a procedure or surgery? [Internet]. [cited 2025 Jan 12]. Available from: https://www.healthwise.net/ohridecisionaid/Content/StdDocument.aspx?DOCHWID=ue4756
26. Show me PAD decision aid for peripheral artery disease [Internet]. ShowMe-PAD. [cited 2025 Jan 12]. Available from: https://showme-pad.org/
27. Smolderen KG, Pacheco C, Provance J, Stone N, Fuss C, Decker C, et al. Treatment decisions for patients with peripheral artery disease and symptoms of claudication: development process and alpha testing of the SHOW-ME PAD decision aid. Vasc Med. 2021;26(3):273–80.
28. Sinnige A, Kittelson A, Rutgers KM, Marcellis LHM, Van Der Wees PJ, Teijink JAW, et al. Nationwide implementation of personalized outcomes forecasts to support physical therapists in treating patients with intermittent claudication: protocol for an interrupted time series study. Zhou J, editor. PLoS One. 2023;18(7):e0288511.
29. Sepucha KR, Scholl I. Measuring shared decision making. Circ Cardiovasc Qual Outcomes. 2014;7(4):620–6.
30. Hess EP, Coylewright M, Frosch DL, Shah ND. Implementation of shared decision making in cardiovascular care. Circ Cardiovasc Qual Outcomes. 2014;7(5):797–803.
31. Kriston L, Scholl I, Hoelzel L, Simon D, Loh A, Haerter M. The 9-item shared decision making questionnaire (SDM-Q-9). Development and psychometric properties in a primary care sample. Patient Educ Couns. 2010;80(1):94–9.
32. Doherr H, Christalle E, Kriston L, Haerter M, Scholl I. Use of the 9-item shared decision making questionnaire (SDM-Q-9 and SDM-Q-doc) in intervention studies—a systematic review. PLoS One. 2017;12(3):e0173904.
33. Fowler FJ, Sepucha KR, Stringfellow V, Valentine KD. Validation of the SDM process scale to evaluate shared decision-making at clinical sites. J Patient Exp. 2021;8:23743735211060811.
34. Barr PJ, Thompson R, Walsh T, Grande SW, Ozanne EM, Elwyn G. The psychometric properties of CollaboRATE: a fast and frugal patient-reported measure of the shared decision-making process. J Med Internet Res. 2014;16(1):e2.

35. Legare F, Kearing S, Clay K, Gagnon S, D'Amours D, Rousseau M, et al. Are you SURE? Assessing patient decisional conflict with a 4-item screening test. Can Fam Phys. 2010;56(8):E308–14.
36. Ferron Parayre A, Labrecque M, Rousseau M, Turcotte S, Légaré F. Validation of SURE, a four-item clinical checklist for detecting decisional conflict in patients. Med Decis Mak. 2014;34(1):54–62.
37. Barr PJ, O'Malley AJ, Tsulukidze M, Gionfriddo MR, Montori V, Elwyn G. The psychometric properties of observer OPTION[5], an observer measure of shared decision making. Patient Educ Couns. 2015;98(8):970–6.
38. Stubenrouch FE, Pieterse AH, Falkenberg R, Santema TKB, Stiggelbout AM, van der Weijden T, et al. OPTION[5] versus OPTION[12] instruments to appreciate the extent to which healthcare providers involve patients in decision-making. Patient Educ Couns. 2016;99(6):1062–8.
39. Elwyn G, Hutchings H, Edwards A, Rapport F, Wensing M, Cheung WY, et al. The OPTION scale: measuring the extent that clinicians involve patients in decision-making tasks. Health Expect. 2005;8(1):34–42.

19 Non-traditional and Emerging Treatments for Intermittent Claudication

Dominique M. Dockery, Louis M. Messina, and Douglas W. Jones

Introduction

The need for more effective therapies for intermittent claudication has never been greater. Relative to coronary artery disease, peripheral artery disease (PAD) is an undertreated and under-investigated condition. Recent publications on patients undergoing revascularization for intermittent claudication have raised serious concerns about their long-term effectiveness [1–4]. After 5–8 years of follow-up, revascularization strategies for intermittent claudication lose their early benefits. Moreover, they do not result in any long-term improvement in patient-reported outcomes, including health-related quality of life [1–3]. Of greatest concern is that revascularization is associated with a 2.9-fold higher rate of progression to chronic limb-threatening ischemia and a 4.5-fold increased amputation rate compared to patients managed conservatively [4].

Current Management Guidelines

The 2024 ACC/AHA/AACVPR/APMA/ABC/SCAI/SVM/SVN/SVS/SIR/VESS Guidelines for the management of lower extremity PAD recommend that patients with intermittent claudication should be prescribed either single antiplatelet therapy with aspirin or clopidogrel versus low-dose aspirin and rivaroxaban 2.5 mg twice daily to prevent major adverse cardiovascular events and major adverse limb events [5]. The only recommended drug therapy for limb symptoms in intermittent claudication is cilostazol (100 mg twice daily 30 min before or 2 h after meals). A recently

D. M. Dockery · L. M. Messina · D. W. Jones (✉)
Division of Vascular and Endovascular Surgery, University of Massachusetts Chan Medical School, Worcester, MA, USA
e-mail: Dominique.Dockery@umassmemorial.org; Louis.Messina@umassmemorial.org; Douglas.Jones@umassmemorial.org

W. P. Robinson III, J. P. Simons (eds.), *The Patient-Centered Approach to Claudication*, https://doi.org/10.1007/978-3-032-02460-2_19

published study of a randomized, open-label, multicenter, 24-week clinical trial for patients with intermittent claudication showed the addition of 2.5 mg of rivaroxaban twice daily to aspirin 100 mg daily improved walking distance by 68 m during a 6-min walk test compared to aspirin alone, suggesting that low-dose anticoagulation may have a role in claudication symptom management as well [6]. Finally, all patients with claudication should undergo a structured exercise program, including supervised exercise therapy and community-based (including structured home-based) programs. Other recommendations include lipid-lowering (i.e., high-intensity statin) and antihypertensive therapy, management of diabetes, and smoking cessation.

In most cases, revascularization is reserved for patients who have failed the above interventions and experience severe, lifestyle-limiting claudication. Ideally, revascularization should only be performed after smoking cessation. Despite their poor long-term durability, bypass and endovascular treatments are still regularly performed.

Just as there is wide variation in treatment methods, claudication symptoms may vary considerably from patient to patient. Symptoms of PAD do not always correlate directly with a patient's ankle-brachial index (ABI), and a particular ABI value does not predict symptomatology. Although hemodynamic measures are important to monitor disease progression, classification of patient symptoms and disability is paramount. Given that long-term outcomes of revascularizations for intermittent claudication are suboptimal, the decision to proceed with intervention should be carefully considered, particularly regarding patient risk. Thus, there is a need to identify other non-revascularization-based treatments to serve patients better. This chapter will describe novel pharmacologic, non-invasive, and biologic therapies being implemented for claudication.

Pharmacologic

Established pharmacologic agents may increase pain-free walking distance in patients with claudication and slow the progression to lifestyle-limiting disease. Most practitioners are comfortable using antiplatelet agents and anticoagulation, but other non-traditional agents may offer some additional improvement through mechanisms that increase nitric oxide availability. These agents are readily available, non-invasive, and relatively inexpensive additions to the treatment paradigm for patients with claudication.

Nitric Oxide

One of the most compelling novel treatments for claudication targets increased nitric oxide bioavailability to restore endothelial function. Derived from endothelial nitric oxide synthase (eNOS), nitric oxide dilates smooth muscle, promotes angiogenesis, inhibits platelet aggregation, and reduces inflammation [7]. Endothelial nitric oxide synthase is a dimer composed of two monomers linked by tetrahydrobiopterin (BH4), commonly referred to as "coupled eNOS". Under conditions of oxidant stress induced by cardiovascular risk factors such as hypercholesterolemia, BH4 concentrations are reduced, and eNOS devolves into monomers: "uncoupled eNOS" (Fig. 19.1). Under these conditions, L-arginine, the substrate for eNOS, produces superoxide rather than nitric oxide, which amplifies the oxidant stress induced by the risk factor. The oxidant stress-induced endothelial dysfunction makes arteries more susceptible to plaque formation and creates a prothrombotic state, leading to PAD. Nitric oxide is also essential for dilating and elongating collateral arteries, a form of arteriogenesis that dilates pre-existing arteries. Thus, restoration of endothelial cell nitric oxide bioavailability can inhibit plaque formation and enlarge collateral arteries. For this reason, many clinical trials of L-arginine supplementation were initiated to reverse endothelial dysfunction. However, results were unexpectedly mixed, including those showing no clinical benefit or that L-arginine supplementation worsened the outcomes.

For decades, various studies have examined L-arginine supplementation and its effects. One of the first studies from 1998 utilized twice daily 8 g doses of intravenous L-arginine for 3 weeks and found that pain-free walking distance improved by 230 m and absolute walking distance by 155 m [8]. For oral supplementation, the results have been mixed. One of the largest randomized clinical trials on this topic was the Nitric Oxide in Peripheral Arterial Insufficiency (NO-PAIN) study, which compared 3 g of oral arginine a day versus placebo [9]. Although L-arginine levels were increased, flow-mediated vasodilation and urinary nitrogen levels were paradoxically higher in the placebo group. Moreover, pain-free walking distance was also higher in the placebo group than in the L-arginine group, suggesting possible harm from L-arginine administration. This concern was also suggested in a trial of L-arginine after acute myocardial infarction [10]. L-arginine did not increase ejection fraction nor vasodilation, but increased mortality causing early termination of

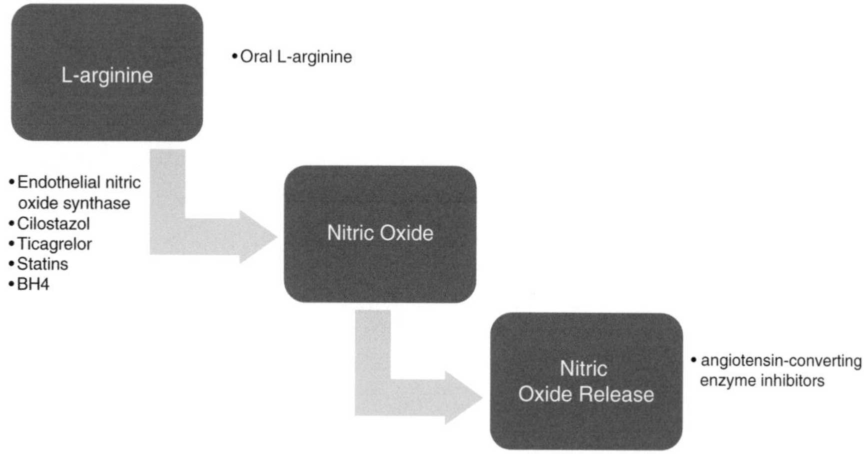

Fig. 19.1 Nitric oxide pathway and acting drugs

the study. However, other small studies have found success with oral administration. A Polish study analyzed walking distance in patients with claudication, with mild to severe symptoms, who received 12 g of L-arginine or a placebo daily for 28 days. They found that all patients in the L-arginine arm had improved pain-free walking distance from 80 to 428 m and total walking distance from 158 to 687 m [11]. Another study utilized food bars enriched with 3.3 g of L-arginine and found that patients who consumed two bars daily over 2 weeks had a 66% increase in pain-free walking distance and a 23% increase in total walking distance [12]. However, this effect was not demonstrated in patients who only consumed one bar per day, which was a similar dose to the NO-PAIN study. This might imply that oral supplementation of arginine may need to be greater than 3 g daily to impact walking distance.

In addition to administering L-arginine alone, its effect may be improved when L-arginine is paired with other constituents that regulate nitric oxide derived from eNOS activity.

In one animal model of hindlimb ischemia, supplementation of L-arginine with BH4 and L-ascorbate led to synergistic effects that decreased oxidant stress, and increased eNOS activity, muscle nitric oxide, collateral artery enlargement, and limb blood flow [13]. L-arginine or BH4 alone had no effect on these variables. The reduction of oxidant stress maintained endothelial nitric oxide synthase in a functional dimeric form, enhancing nitric oxide production. Based on this, isolated L-arginine administration in the presence of cardiovascular risk factor-induced oxidant stress may not be able to increase eNOS activity, potentially explaining the lack of clinical benefits seen in prior studies.

In addition to oral or intravenous supplementation, there has also been interest in the use of L-arginine during angiography. The LargPAD Trial included patients with claudication, rest pain, or minor tissue loss and infused 50 mg, 100 mg, or 500 mg of L-arginine intra-arterially during diagnostic angiography in diseased superficial femoral arteries [14]. Endothelium-dependent relaxation was measured using intravascular ultrasound and a Doppler FloWire (Volcano Corporation, Rancho Cordova, CA) and levels of nitric oxide/arginine were measured via chemiluminescence and mass spectrometry. Serum arginine and nitric oxide levels increased by 43.6% and 85%, respectively. The most effective dose response was seen at 100 mg, which caused the greatest increase in endothelial function.

Carnitine has also been studied as an over-the-counter supplement to increase pain-free walking distance in patients with intermittent claudication. The acyl derivative, propionyl-L-carnitine, plays a role in the metabolism of fatty acids by stimulating oxidative phosphorylation, which increases energy production and helps improve endothelial function. A systematic review of over 1400 randomized participants across 12 studies found that carnitine supplementation was associated with increased walking distances. However, all groups were compared to placebo and not standard treatment, which limits their applicability. In these studies, the dosing of propionyl-L-carnitine was 1–2 grams orally or intravenously per day. Maximal walking performance improved 50.86 m or 26% in the intervention group [15]. Pain-free walking distance also improved by 31%, and there was an improvement in ABI of 0.09. Overall, the risk profile was low and comparable to that seen in the placebo group, suggesting that L-carnitine is a safe, inexpensive, and non-invasive way to potentially increase pain-free walking distance in patients who have intermittent claudication.

Approved Therapies

Medications currently on the market to treat vascular risk factors, such as hyperlipidemia and hypertension, have also been proposed as therapies to treat intermittent claudication (Table 19.1). Many of these drugs, including cilostazol, ticagrelor, and statins, are thought to be beneficial due to a mechanism similar to that of L-arginine by acting on the endothelial nitric oxide synthase pathway to increase serum nitric oxide (Fig. 19.2). Angiotensin-converting enzyme (ACE) inhibitors increase nitric oxide production by multiple mechanisms, including inhibiting the generation of angiotensin II, which decreases nitric oxide production, and inhibiting the degradation of bradykinin, which stimulates nitric oxide release. Thus, drugs that act on nitric oxide synthase or increase nitric oxide release are targets for claudication therapies.

Although statins are routinely used in patients with claudication to lower low-density lipoprotein cholesterol levels and reduce cardiovascular risk, they have also been shown to reduce oxidative stress by multiple pathways. These include reducing the production of reactive oxygen species, increasing antioxidant pathways, and regulating oxidation pathways, including the endothelial nitric oxide synthase pathway. Independent of their effects on low-density lipoprotein cholesterol levels and after controlling for ABI severity, statin use improved results in the 6-min walk test in one clinical study [16]. Patients who were on statin therapy walked nearly 60 feet further with a faster walking velocity and higher summary performance score. However, one major limitation of this study was that statin type and dose were not recorded. Another study focused on using simvastatin, a low- to medium-intensity

Table 19.1 Common therapeutics with proposed benefit in PAD

Drug name	Drug class	Common indications	Proposed mechanism
Statins (atorvastatin, rosuvastatin, simvastatin, pravastatin, etc.)	HMG-CoA reductase inhibitors	Hyperlipidemia	Act on nitric oxide synthase to increase nitric oxide availability
Lisinopril, enalapril, ramipril, etc.	ACE-inhibitors	Hypertension	Increased nitric oxide release via decreased production of angiotensin II and inhibition of bradykinin degradation
Colchicine	Anti-gout	Gout, pericarditis	Anti-inflammatory properties
Canakinumab, anakinra, tolicizumab, ustekinumab	Pro-inflammatory interleukin inhibitors	Autoimmune diseases	Anti-inflammatory properties

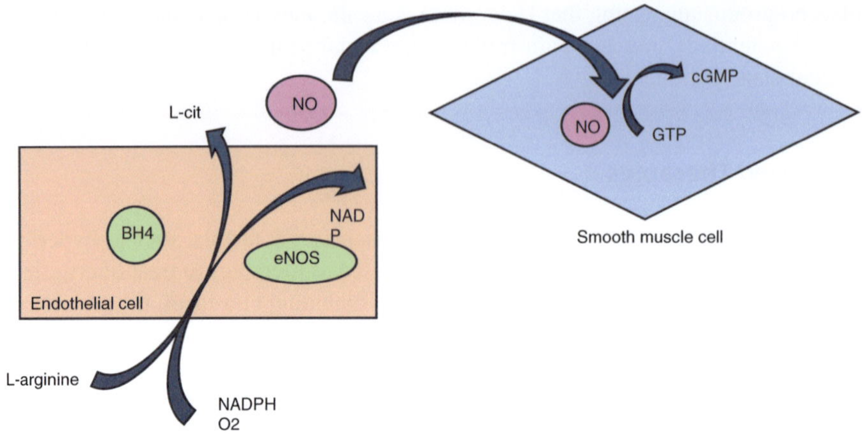

Fig. 19.2 Schematic of the role of tetrahydrobiopterin and the structure of endothelial nitric oxide synthase

statin at dosages of either 20 mg or 40 mg. In over 4000 patients, there was a reduced risk of new or worsening claudication by up to 38% [17]. Overall, statins are a relatively well-tolerated medication that many vascular surgery patients are already taking for hyperlipidemia. In those patients who have not initiated statin therapy but are reporting claudication and have evidence of atherosclerosis, it is advisable to start statins regardless of cholesterol levels.

ACE inhibitors such as lisinopril and enalapril also act on the nitric oxide pathway. Primarily, they work to increase nitric oxide release by preventing production of angiotensin II, which diminishes nitric oxide production [18]. They also inhibit degradation of bradykinin which in turn stimulates local release of nitric oxide. In one meta-analysis of four randomized studies, the use of ACE inhibitors was associated with an increase in maximal walking distance by 126 meters and an increase in ankle-brachial index (ABI) by 0.09 [19]. The authors also found increases in pain-free walking distance by 86 m. Another meta-analysis, including nine clinical trials, found that there were no significant benefits to ACE inhibitor therapy [20]. However, when analyzed separately, many of the included studies reported significant improvements in walking distance (over 130 m) with ramipril therapy. Just as is the case with statins and hyperlipidemia, many patients have hypertension as a comorbidity and may already be on ACE inhibitor therapy. Thus, the preferred use of ACE inhibitors may treat hypertension and have a beneficial effect on claudication symptoms. In patients without hypertension, adding this medication may also provide benefit if they have adequate blood pressure to withstand the addition of an ACE inhibitor. These effects can be considered as relevant when selecting anti-hypertensive therapies.

Chronic inflammation contributes to the development of atherosclerosis and plaque instability and efforts to reduce it may play a significant role in treating PAD and claudication. Recent studies have investigated the use of anti-inflammatory agents, such as colchicine and specific interleukin inhibitors, in managing claudication. These drugs target inflammatory pathways involved in vascular damage and could offer novel benefits in symptom management and disease progression. In a retrospective cohort study with nearly 70,000 patients, colchicine therapy was initiated for PAD and patients were followed for roughly 4.5 years. The risk of major adverse limb events, revascularization, and amputations was lower in patients taking colchicine with a hazard ratio of 0.75 [21]. These patients were also found to have a lower risk of cardiovascular death. Although any length of colchicine use was associated with decreased major adverse limb events, a dose-dependent effect was observed with decreased events if treatment time was extended. These effects were similar in all groups including those with the concomitant use of statins.

Interleukins, tumor necrosis factor-α, and P-selectin, which play a role in regulating the inflammatory response, have been studied for their potential role in the treatment of PAD [22]. Interleukins (ILs) play an important role in the development and progression of PAD. A recent comprehensive literature review showed that five pro-inflammatory interleukins (IL-1β, IL-2, IL-5, IL-6, and IL-8) and one pro-atherogenic interleukin (IL-12) were positively correlated with PAD diagnosis and progression [23]. In contrast, two anti-inflammatory interleukins (IL-4 and IL-10) were protective against PAD diagnosis and adverse limb events. IL-6 and IL-8 were the most strongly correlated with PAD.

Most of the current studies investigating drugs that act on these interleukins have examined cardiovascular outcomes, though they also offer promise for use in PAD. Some of the drugs being studied include: inclacumab (p-selectin inhibition), infliximab/etanercept (anti-TNFα), canakinumab (IL-1β inhibition), anakinra (IL-1 receptor antagonism), tolicizumab (IL-6 receptor inhibition), and ustekinumab (IL-12/23 inhibition) [24]. In one study, the investigators hypothesized that IL-1β signaling decreases plaque progression in lower extremity arteries and increases pain-free walking distance in patients with intermittent claudication [25]. Thirty-eight patients (mean age 65 years; 71% male) who had claudication confirmed by symptoms and ABI were randomized 1:1 to receive canakinumab (150 mg subcutaneously) or placebo monthly for up to 12 months. Markers of systemic inflammation, interleukin-6, and high-sensitivity C-reactive protein were reduced significantly as early as 1 month after initiation of treatment. MRI showed no evidence of plaque progression in the femoral artery in either placebo-treated or canakinumab-treated patients. However, placebo-adjusted maximum and pain-free walking distance (58 m) improved as early as 3 months after treatment with canakinumab. Further studies are needed to investigate these as targets for patients who have intermittent claudication.

Investigational Therapeutics

Managing claudication effectively is crucial for improving patients' mobility and quality of life. While conventional treatments include lifestyle modifications, medications, and revascularization-based strategies, emerging non-pharmacological approaches, such as intermittent pneumatic compression (IPC) and extracorporeal shockwave therapy are gaining attention. In theory, these therapies may offer a relatively easy and non-invasive method to treating claudication that can be used as an adjunct to medical and exercise therapy.

Intermittent Pneumatic Compression

IPC involves using a device that applies sequential pressure, up to/greater than 100 mmHg, to the lower limbs through inflatable cuffs. These cuffs are inflated and deflated in a pattern that mimics the natural muscle contractions that occur during walking which enhances venous return. The effectiveness of IPC is contingent upon regular and proper use. Patients typically need to use the IPC device several times a week for sessions lasting between 30 and 60 min, like that of exercise therapy. Therefore, this may act as an alternative for patients who are unable to adhere to walking programs. Ensuring patient adherence to the treatment regimen is important. Education on the correct use of IPC devices and addressing any potential discomfort or inconvenience associated with the treatment can help improve patient compliance.

The primary mechanism of IPC is to enhance venous return, thereby increasing the arteriovenous pressure gradient/flow [26]. One proposed mechanism is via attenuation of precapillary arteriolar vasoconstriction after the decrease in venous pressures. Lastly, it has been thought that this promotes the release of nitric oxide, leading to vasodilation [26].

Several studies have investigated the efficacy of IPC in treating claudication. Clinical trials have demonstrated that IPC can lead to significant improvements in walking distance and functional capacity. One meta-analysis including eight controlled trials with nearly 300 patients with claudication found that the average walking distance of patients receiving compression was 125 m further than their control counterparts [27]. The majority of those studies included IPC of the calf and foot, one utilized just the foot, and one trialed intermittent non-pneumatic mechanical compression, though treatment times varied. Although secondary outcomes varied in the meta-analysis, an improvement in ABI was found in five of seven individual studies, and popliteal artery flow was increased in one of four studies. Overall, these treatments led to improved quality of life in three of four studies.

Another study looked at three different groups (patients with claudication without prior revascularization, patients who had undergone infrainguinal autologous bypass, and controls) and the use of IPC in the thigh, calf, and both thighs/calves [28]. They found that popliteal inflow velocities increased in all groups with thigh/calf IPC having the highest hemodynamic benefits. The percentage increase of median mean velocity with the use of IPC increased by 51% in un-revascularized patients with claudication, 78% in bypass patients, and 95% in controls [28]. Therefore, even though the effect is not as strongly observed in patients with vascular disease, there was still an increase in native or autologous arterial velocity and flow via a non-invasive, at-home technique.

While IPC offers a non-invasive alternative, cost and accessibility can be barriers to widespread adoption. The initial investment in IPC devices and ongoing maintenance may be prohibitive for some patients or healthcare systems. However, as technology advances and becomes more affordable, IPC could become a more accessible option for a broader population though its effectiveness has not been convincingly proven.

Extracorporeal Shockwave Therapy

Extracorporeal shockwave therapy involves the application of acoustic waves to targeted tissues via a transmitter which penetrates the tissue and stimulates various biological processes (Fig. 19.3). One of the primary mechanisms by which this is believed to benefit patients with claudication is through the promotion of arteriogenesis by inducing mechanical stress in tissues, activating endothelial cells and growth factors; this was originally studied in the cardiology literature [29]. This angiogenic effect is theorized to improve blood supply to ischemic tissues, potentially alleviating symptoms by enhancing collateral circulation. Lastly, it is hypothesized that the shockwaves generated could have anti-inflammatory effects and promote the release of anti-inflammatory cytokines and reduce pro-inflammatory markers.

One randomized trial of patients with unilateral claudication randomized 15 patients to shockwave therapy to the calf for 3 months (three times per week, 20 min per session) and 15 to sham treatment [30]. Primary outcomes were pain-free and maximum walking distance with secondary outcomes including ABI change, treatment tolerability, and quality of life. They found that pain-free walking distance increased 276% and maximum walking distance by 167% at 12 weeks in the treatment arm compared to 35% and 11% in the sham arm [30]. Importantly, no adverse effects were observed in this study though the average pain score was higher in patients receiving therapy but decreased over time with sequential treatments. No

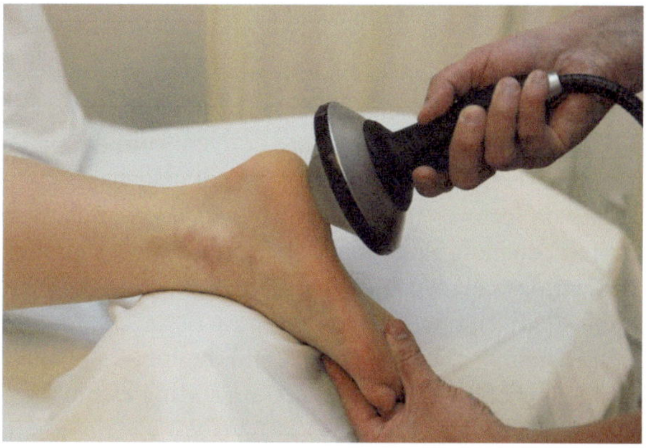

Fig. 19.3 Example of extracorpeal shockwave therapy on the foot. (Crevenna, R., Mickel, M., Schuhfried, O. et al. Focused Extracorporeal Shockwave Therapy in Physical Medicine and Rehabilitation. *Curr Phys Med Rehabil Rep* **9**, 1–10 (2021). https://doi.org/10.1007/s40141-020-00306-z)

differences were observed in ABI pre- and post-treatment. However, quality of life improved in the treatment group at both 4 and 12 weeks.

A large, randomized placebo-controlled study confirmed these effects in 138 patients over a 12-week period [31]. The study protocol included 100 impulses in the calf three times a week for 3 weeks. The primary outcome was changes in physical function with secondary outcomes of walking distances and ABI change. At 12 weeks, the shockwave group had higher physical function scores with a mean difference of 3.8, but this was not found to be a statistically significant difference [31]. However, patients also had longer pain-free (34.1 m) and maximum (51.4 m) walking distances. Overall, shockwave therapy was safe and well tolerated.

Extracorporeal shockwave therapy represents an innovative approach to managing claudication. By promoting angiogenesis, improving collateral circulation, and reducing inflammation and pain, this therapy may offer potential for symptomatic improvement. Like intermittent pneumatic compression, the upfront cost and implementation may be difficult at first. More studies are required to demonstrate effectiveness convincingly.

Biologics

Over the past few decades, there has been an emphasis on personalized medicine and the use of biologics. Countless research studies have examined stem cell therapies to regenerate tissues or restore normal function, particularly in oncologic therapy and fields such as orthopedic surgery. Biologics are emerging as a potential therapeutic option for the treatment of claudication. They leverage the body's immune system and biological processes, offering a novel approach to enhance vascular health by targeting the underlying inflammatory pathways and promoting angiogenesis. As research continues to evolve, understanding the role of biologics in PAD treatment may redefine management strategies and improve the prognosis for affected individuals.

Stem Cell Therapy

Several types of stem cells have shown promise in PAD and claudication: autologous hematopoietic stem cells, mesenchymal stem cells, and endothelial progenitor cells. Autologous stem cells are derived from the patient's own body and are commonly harvested from bone marrow, adipose tissue, or peripheral blood after the use of growth factors. These transfusions have no risk of immune rejection but may be limited depending on a patient's health. Mesenchymal stem cells can differentiate into various cell types giving them significant regenerative potential. They can be harvested from bone marrow, adipose tissues, and umbilical cords. Lastly, endothelial progenitor cells are involved in angiogenesis and are isolated from peripheral blood and bone marrow after certain sorting techniques. Overall, there are relatively few studies examining the use of stem cells for claudication and further research is needed to determine the feasibility and efficacy of these methods.

One of the largest autologous stem cell studies included 81 patients; 25 had severe claudication, and the remaining had chronic limb-threatening ischemia [32]. These patients were randomized to either intra-arterial bone marrow-derived stem cell injection at the site of occlusion or sham injection. Their primary endpoints were a significant increase in ABI, or the partial pressure of oxygen measured on the skin surface, as well as transcutaneous pressure of oxygen. Secondary endpoints for patients with claudication were >50% improvement in pain-free walking distance. There was 100% technical success in the study with no significant adverse events identified. Overall, patients who received stem cells were more likely to have an improvement in ABI >0.1 and transcutaneous pressure of oxygen improvement of >15% at the midfoot and lower foot [32]. For the patients with severe claudication, there was an improvement in transcutaneous pressure of oxygen but no significant improvement in ABI. Additionally, no statistically significant difference was noted in this study for improvement in pain-free walking distance. Although not all outcomes had significant improvement, this study demonstrated that for patients with advanced disease, intra-arterial stem cell injection may have some beneficial effects. Further studies are needed to determine efficacy and safety profiles.

Most studies on mesenchymal stem cells have involved either diabetic foot ulcers or CLTI-related tissue loss, mostly in animal models. Although not directly studied in patients with claudication, similar methods may be extrapolated to this population in the future. Vascular endothelial growth factor (VEGF) plasmids have been used in mouse models, where hind limb ischemia was induced by ligating the profunda and superficial femoral arteries. Treatment was associated with increased concentrations of VEGF by up to 2.5-fold compared to untransfected cells [33]. This was associated with improved perfusion by 26% in transfected mice within 3 weeks, and limb salvage increased by 3.5-fold. Although this study showed success in an animal model for CLTI, further human clinical trials are needed to understand the use of mesenchymal stromal cells in PAD fully.

Exercise therapy also increases circulating endothelial progenitor cells. A randomized trial of 60 patients with claudication analyzed the effects of a 12-week exercise therapy program on endothelial progenitor cell quantities after a treadmill test [34]. The program included five weekly sessions with 45 min of aerobic activity (walking on a flat surface or slight incline) and 15 min of circuit training (calisthenic exercises). Circulating endothelial progenitor cells increased significantly after 24 h with larger quantities after the 12-week program [34]. Additionally, patients had improvements in pain-free walking time and maximum walking time which was positively correlated with the change in endothelial progenitor cell concentration and was an independent determinant for pain-free walking time. Exercise may increase circulating progenitor cells and improve walking capacity, though a causal relationship has not been proven.

While these studies are promising, stem cell therapy for claudication remains an evolving field. Challenges such as optimizing cell delivery methods, ensuring long-term efficacy, and managing potential risks must be addressed. Further large-scale, long-term studies are needed to establish standardized protocols and confirm the safety and effectiveness of these therapies.

Nanotherapy

Nanotherapy, or nanomedicine, involves the use of nanotechnology for medical applications. Nanoparticles, particles with sizes ranging from 1 to 100 nm, offer unique advantages in drug delivery, imaging, and therapeutic interventions due to their small size and high surface area. In the context of claudication, nanotherapy can potentially enhance treatment efficacy through targeted drug delivery and promotion of vascular regeneration. One application that most vascular surgeons are familiar with is paclitaxel-coated angioplasty balloons, which utilize nanoparticles to encapsulate paclitaxel for improved drug delivery during angioplasty. However, other uses have been described in the treatment of claudication.

Nanoparticles can be engineered to improve the solubility and stability of preexisting oral therapeutic agents, ensuring more effective delivery to the targeted site. This has been studied using pentoxifylline, a hemorheologic agent commonly used to treat claudication. Pentoxifylline is metabolized by the liver with extensive first-pass metabolism and thus has a large reduction in therapeutic levels after a short duration of time, exhibiting a half-life of 1–2 h with an absolute bioavailability of 20–30%. A study in male rats utilized a self-nano-emulsifying drug delivery system consisting of oil, surfactant, and co-surfactant and found bioavailability increased 1.5-fold as compared to the pure drug [35]. A similar study utilized lipid nanocarrier-loaded gelatin capsules with the administration of cilostazol. Once the optimal dosing and solubility were reached, rabbits were given either the conventional tablet suspension, the enhanced capsule with cilostazol, or a control-enhanced capsule. They found increased cilostazol release due to a bioavailability 1.74 times higher than the commercial tablets [36]. The enhanced capsules also had a longer shelf life than did tablets alone at 526 days. Although bioavailability improved in both studies, there have been no human models to discuss the impact of increased bioavailability on claudication symptoms. More studies are once again necessary, but the use of nanoparticles to improve drug bioavailability could potentially lead to a positive dose-effect response.

Nanoparticles can also improve drug delivery for other therapeutics such as prostaglandin E1, which is currently limited in use as it necessitates daily intravenous infusions due to the low stability of lipid emulsions. Prostaglandins have been found to promote vasodilation and platelet inhibition while also modulating immune responses. A study in rats utilized femoral ligation to produce ischemia and then observed activity on a rodent treadmill [37]. Researchers mixed prostaglandin E1 with nanoparticles and used immunohistochemical analysis to determine angiogenesis and enzyme immunoassay to determine prostaglandin levels. Prostaglandin E1 had a better drug profile and was able to be detected at the lesion on the day after administration, whereas the lipid emulsion/standard drug was not [37]. This then led to improved angiogenesis at the site of ligation with improvement in walking speed in only the nano-enhanced formulations. Although no human studies have yet to be described, nanoparticles may make prostaglandin use more feasible for widespread use in patients with claudication, promoting angiogenesis and improving symptoms.

Nanotherapy represents a novel approach to treating claudication and peripheral artery disease. By leveraging the unique properties of nanoparticles for targeted drug delivery and vascular regeneration, nanotherapy offers the potential to significantly improve treatment outcomes. As research progresses, addressing current challenges and optimizing nanotherapy applications will be crucial for integrating these innovative technologies into standard clinical practice.

Summary

Novel therapies for claudication are rapidly evolving, with several innovative approaches currently under investigation in clinical trials. New pharmacologic approaches, non-invasive devices, stem cell therapy, and nanotherapy offer new avenues for addressing the limitations of traditional treatments. While early results from these studies are promising, further research is needed to confirm their efficacy, safety, and long-term benefits. The continued advancement of these novel therapies may significantly improve the management of claudication and enhance the quality of life for patients suffering from intermittent claudication due to PAD.

References

1. Djerf H, Millinger J, Falkenberg M, Jivegård L, Svensson M, Nordanstig J. Absence of long-term benefit of revascularization in patients with intermittent claudication: five-year results from the IRONIC randomized controlled trial. Circ Cardiovasc Interv. 2020;13(1):e008450. https://doi.org/10.1161/CIRCINTERVENTIONS.119.008450. Epub 2020 Jan 15. PMID: 31937137.
2. Holeman TA, Chester C, Hales JB, Zhang Y, Johnson CE, Brooke BS. Long-term patient-reported outcomes among patients undergoing revascularization vs medical therapy for intermittent claudication. J Vasc Surg. 2024;80(2):466–477.e4. https://doi.org/10.1016/j.jvs.2024.03.455. Epub 2024 Apr 10. PMID: 38608965; PMCID: PMC11260535.
3. Gunnarsson T, Gottsäter A, Bergman S, Troëng T, Lindgren H. Eight-year outcome after invasive treatment of infrainguinal intermittent claudication: a population-based analysis from the Swedish vascular register (Swedvasc). SAGE Open Med. 2020;8:2050312120926782. https://doi.org/10.1177/2050312120926782. PMID: 32547751; PMCID: PMC7249589.
4. Madabhushi V, Davenport D, Jones S, Khoudoud SA, Orr N, Minion D, Endean E, Tyagi S. Revascularization of intermittent claudicants leads to more chronic limb-threatening ischemia and higher amputation rates. J Vasc Surg. 2021;74(3):771–9. https://doi.org/10.1016/j.jvs.2021.02.045. Epub 2021 Mar 26. PMID: 33775749.
5. Gornik HL, Aronow HD, Goodney PP, Arya S, Brewster LP, Byrd L, Chandra V, Drachman DE, Eaves JM, Ehrman JK, Evans JN, Getchius TSD, Gutiérrez JA, Hawkins BM, Hess CN, Ho KJ, Jones WS, Kim ESH, Kinlay S, Kirksey L, Kohlman-Trigoboff D, Long CA, Pollak AW, Sabri SS, Sadwin LB, Secemsky EA, Serhal M, Shishehbor MH, Treat-Jacobson D, Wilkins LR. 2024 ACC/AHA/AACVPR/APMA/ABC/SCAI/SVM/SVN/SVS/SIR/VESS

guideline for the Management of Lower Extremity Peripheral Artery Disease: a report of the American College of Cardiology/American Heart Association Joint Committee on clinical practice guidelines. Circulation. 2024;149(24):e1313–410. https://doi.org/10.1161/CIR.0000000000001251. Epub 2024 May 14. PMID: 38743805.

6. Ramacciotti E, Volpiani GG, Britto KF, Agati LB, Ribeiro CM, Aguiar VCR, Paganotti A, Pereira FM, Caffaro RA, Krakauer R, Rached HRS, Fareed J, Wolosker N, Anand SS, Eikelboom JW, Chang C, Lopes RD. Rivaroxaban for patients with intermittent claudication. NEJM Evid. 2024;3(9):EVIDoa2400021. https://doi.org/10.1056/EVIDoa2400021. Epub 2024 Aug 26. PMID: 39185955.
7. Falconer D, Papageorgiou N, Salem K, Lim WY, Katsargyris A, Avgerinos E, Tousoulis D. Nitric oxide donors for peripheral artery disease. Curr Opin Pharmacol. 2018;39:77–85. https://doi.org/10.1016/j.coph.2018.02.009. Epub 2018 Mar 26. PMID: 29587164.
8. Böger RH, Bode-Böger SM, Thiele W, Creutzig A, Alexander K, Frölich JC. Restoring vascular nitric oxide formation by L-arginine improves the symptoms of intermittent claudication in patients with peripheral arterial occlusive disease. J Am Coll Cardiol. 1998;32(5):1336–44. https://doi.org/10.1016/s0735-1097(98)00375-1. PMID: 9809945.
9. Wilson AM, Harada R, Nair N, Balasubramanian N, Cooke JP. L-arginine supplementation in peripheral arterial disease: no benefit and possible harm. Circulation. 2007;116(2):188–95. https://doi.org/10.1161/CIRCULATIONAHA.106.683656. Epub 2007 Jun 25. PMID: 17592080.
10. Schulman SP, Becker LC, Kass DA, Champion HC, Terrin ML, Forman S, Ernst KV, Kelemen MD, Townsend SN, Capriotti A, Hare JM, Gerstenblith G. L-arginine therapy in acute myocardial infarction: the Vascular Interaction With Age in Myocardial Infarction (VINTAGE MI) randomized clinical trial. JAMA. 2006;295(1):58–64. https://doi.org/10.1001/jama.295.1.58. PMID: 16391217.
11. Micker M, Krauss H, Ast J, Chęciński P, Jabłecka A. The influence of oral supplementation of L-arginine on intermittent claudication in patients with peripheral arterial disease of the lower extremities. Acta Angiol. 2007;13:1–14.
12. Maxwell AJ, Anderson BE, Cooke JP. Nutritional therapy for peripheral arterial disease: a double-blind, placebo-controlled, randomized trial of HeartBar®. Vasc Med. 2000;5(1):11–9. https://doi.org/10.1177/1358836X0000500103.
13. Yan J, Tie G, Messina LM. Tetrahydrobiopterin, L-arginine and vitamin C act synergistically to decrease oxidant stress and increase nitric oxide that increases blood flow recovery after hindlimb ischemia in the rat. Mol Med. 2012;18(1):1221–30. https://doi.org/10.2119/molmed.2011.00103.revised. PMID: 23212846; PMCID: PMC3510301.
14. Kashyap VS, Lakin RO, Campos P, Allemang M, Kim A, Sarac TP, Hausladen A, Stamler JS. The LargPAD trial: phase IIA evaluation of l-arginine infusion in patients with peripheral arterial disease. J Vasc Surg. 2017;66(1):187–94. https://doi.org/10.1016/j.jvs.2016.12.127. Epub 2017 Mar 30. PMID: 28366306.
15. Kamoen V, Vander Stichele R, Campens L, De Bacquer D, Van Bortel L, de Backer TL. Propionyl-L-carnitine for intermittent claudication. Cochrane Database Syst Rev. 2021;12(12):CD010117. https://doi.org/10.1002/14651858.CD010117.pub2. PMID: 34954832; PMCID: PMC8710338.
16. McDermott MM, Guralnik JM, Greenland P, Pearce WH, Criqui MH, Liu K, Taylor L, Chan C, Sharma L, Schneider JR, Ridker PM, Green D, Quann M. Statin use and leg functioning in patients with and without lower-extremity peripheral arterial disease. Circulation. 2003;107(5):757–61. https://doi.org/10.1161/01.cir.0000050380.64025.07. PMID: 12578881.
17. Pedersen TR, Kjekshus J, Pyörälä K, Olsson AG, Cook TJ, Musliner TA, Tobert JA, Haghfelt T. Effect of simvastatin on ischemic signs and symptoms in the Scandinavian simvastatin survival study (4S). Am J Cardiol. 1998;81(3):333–5. https://doi.org/10.1016/s0002-9149(97)00904-1. PMID: 9468077.
18. Goyal A, Cusick AS, Thielemier B. ACE inhibitors. [Updated 2023 Jun 26]. In: StatPearls [Internet]. Treasure Island: StatPearls Publishing; 2024. Available from: https://www.ncbi.nlm.nih.gov/books/NBK430896/

19. Barrons RW, Woods JA. The roles of ACE inhibitors in lower extremity peripheral artery disease. Am J Ther. 2016;23(1):e7–15. https://doi.org/10.1097/MJT.0000000000000011. PMID: 24786850.
20. Hunter MR, Cahoon WD Jr, Lowe DK. Angiotensin-converting enzyme inhibitors for intermittent claudication associated with peripheral arterial disease. Ann Pharmacother. 2013;47(11):1552–7. https://doi.org/10.1177/1060028013501803. PMID: 24285767.
21. Lin DS, Huang KC, Lin TT, Lee JK, Lin LY. Effects of colchicine on major adverse limb and cardiovascular events in patients with peripheral artery disease. Mayo Clin Proc. 2024;S0025-6196(24):00249-0. https://doi.org/10.1016/j.mayocp.2024.05.004. Epub ahead of print. PMID: 39115507.
22. Saenz-Pipaon G, Martinez-Aguilar E, Orbe J, González Miqueo A, Fernandez-Alonso L, Paramo JA, Roncal C. The role of circulating biomarkers in peripheral arterial disease. Int J Mol Sci. 2021;22(7):3601. https://doi.org/10.3390/ijms22073601. PMID: 33808453; PMCID: PMC8036489.
23. Djahanpour N, Ahsan N, Li B, Khan H, Connelly K, Leong-Poi H, Qadura M. A systematic review of interleukins as diagnostic and prognostic biomarkers for peripheral artery disease. Biomolecules. 2023;13(11):1640.
24. Antonopoulos AS, Papanikolaou E, Vogiatzi G, Oikonomou E, Tousoulis D. Anti-inflammatory agents in peripheral arterial disease. Curr Opin Pharmacol. 2018;39:1–8. https://doi.org/10.1016/j.coph.2017.11.001. Epub 2017 Nov 21. PMID: 29169069.
25. Russell KS, Yates DP, Kramer CM, Feller A, Mahling P, Colin L, Clough T, Wang T, LaPerna L, Patel A, Lawall H, Shennak MM, Fulmer J, Nikol S, Smith WB, Müller OJ, Ratchford EV, Basson CT. A randomized, placebo-controlled trial of canakinumab in patients with peripheral artery disease. Vasc Med. 2019;24(5):414–21.
26. van Bemmelen PS, Mattos MA, Faught WE, Mansour MA, Barkmeier LD, Hodgson KJ, Ramsey DE, Sumner DS. Augmentation of blood flow in limbs with occlusive arterial disease by intermittent calf compression. J Vasc Surg. 1994;19(6):1052–8. https://doi.org/10.1016/s0741-5214(94)70217-9. PMID: 8201706.
27. Oresanya L, Mazzei M, Bashir R, Farooqui A, Athappan G, Roth S, Choi ET, van Bemmelen P. Systematic review and meta-analysis of high-pressure intermittent limb compression for the treatment of intermittent claudication. J Vasc Surg. 2018;67(2):620–628.e2. https://doi.org/10.1016/j.jvs.2017.11.044. PMID: 29389425.
28. Delis KT, Husmann MJ, Cheshire NJ, Nicolaides AN. Effects of intermittent pneumatic compression of the calf and thigh on arterial calf inflow: a study of normals, claudicants, and grafted arteriopaths. Surgery. 2001;129(2):188–95. https://doi.org/10.1067/msy.2001.110023. PMID: 11174701.
29. Cai HY, Li L, Guo T, Wang YU, Ma TK, Xiao JM, Zhao L, Fang Y, Yang P, Zhao HU. Cardiac shockwave therapy improves myocardial function in patients with refractory coronary artery disease by promoting VEGF and IL-8 secretion to mediate the proliferation of endothelial progenitor cells. Exp Ther Med. 2015;10(6):2410–6. https://doi.org/10.3892/etm.2015.2820. Epub 2015 Oct 20. PMID: 26668649; PMCID: PMC4665829.
30. Harwood AE, Green J, Cayton T, Raza A, Wallace T, Carradice D, Chetter IC, Smith GE. A feasibility double-blind randomized placebo-controlled trial of extracorporeal shockwave therapy as a novel treatment for intermittent claudication. J Vasc Surg. 2018;67(2):514–521.e2. https://doi.org/10.1016/j.jvs.2017.07.105. Epub 2017 Sep 22. PMID: 28943002.
31. Cai P, Pymer S, Ibeggazene S, Raza A, Hitchman L, Chetter I, Smith G. Extracorporeal shockwave for intermittent claudication and quality of life: a randomized clinical trial. JAMA Surg. 2024;159(6):625–32. https://doi.org/10.1001/jamasurg.2024.0625. PMID: 38598227; PMCID: PMC11007658.
32. Sharma S, Pandey NN, Sinha M, Kumar S, Jagia P, Gulati GS, Gond K, Mohanty S, Bhargava B. Randomized, double-blind, placebo-controlled trial to evaluate safety and therapeutic efficacy of angiogenesis induced by intraarterial autologous bone marrow-derived stem cells in patients with severe peripheral arterial disease. J Vasc Interv Radiol. 2021;32(2):157–63. https://doi.org/10.1016/j.jvir.2020.09.003. Epub 2020 Nov 25. PMID: 33248918.

33. Park JS, Bae SH, Jung S, Lee M, Choi D. Enrichment of vascular endothelial growth factor secreting mesenchymal stromal cells enhances therapeutic angiogenesis in a mouse model of hind limb ischemia. Cytotherapy. 2019;21(4):433–43. https://doi.org/10.1016/j.jcyt.2018.12.007. Epub 2019 Mar 15. PMID: 30879964.
34. Pasqualini L, Bagaglia F, Ministrini S, Frangione MR, Leli C, Siepi D, Lombardini R, Marini E, Naeimi Kararoudi M, Piratinskiy A, Pirro M. Effects of structured home-based exercise training on circulating endothelial progenitor cells and endothelial function in patients with intermittent claudication. Vasc Med. 2021;26(6):633–40. https://doi.org/10.1177/1358863X211020822. Epub 2021 Jun 21. PMID: 34151646.
35. Shailendrakumar AM, Ghate VM, Kinra M, Lewis SA. Improved oral pharmacokinetics of pentoxifylline with palm oil and capmul® MCM containing self-nano-emulsifying drug delivery system. AAPS PharmSciTech. 2020;21(4):118. https://doi.org/10.1208/s12249-020-01644-w. PMID: 32318890.
36. Sallam MA, Marín Boscá MT. Optimization, ex vivo permeation, and stability study of lipid nanocarrier loaded gelatin capsules for treatment of intermittent claudication. Int J Nanomedicine. 2015;10:4459–78. https://doi.org/10.2147/IJN.S83123. PMID: 26203244; PMCID: PMC4508069.
37. Ishihara T, Yamashita Y, Takasaki N, Yamamoto S, Hayashi E, Tahara K, Takenaga M, Yamakawa N, Ishihara T, Kasahara T, Mizushima T. Prostaglandin E1—containing nanoparticles improve walking activity in an experimental rat model of intermittent claudication. J Pharm Pharmacol. 2013;65(8):1187–94. https://doi.org/10.1111/jphp.12080. Epub 2013 May 21. PMID: 23837586.

Differences Between Published Guidelines and Consensus Statements on the Management of Claudication: Society for Vascular Surgery, American College of Cardiology/American Heart Association, and European Society for Vascular Surgery

20

Tian Zhang

Background

Peripheral arterial disease (PAD) is a complex disease process that has major implications on the health and quality of life of millions of patients in the United States as well as globally [10]. As its prevalence increases, with the increasing age of the American population and growing incidence of comorbid diseases, it accounts for a significant amount of healthcare resources in the United States. These healthcare costs can be attributed not only to the disease itself but also to the associated comorbid conditions, as seen in Fig. 20.1 [20].

Peripheral arterial disease may manifest in different forms: asymptomatic PAD, intermittent claudication, and chronic limb-threatening ischemia (CLTI). Although the guidelines from the aforementioned major Western societies have many similarities, there are differences noted in the management of these patients which will be discussed below.

Clinical Assessment for Claudication

History and Physical

The clinical assessment for PAD includes the history and physical examination, differential diagnoses, and diagnostic testing. Risk factors for PAD are also assessed,

T. Zhang (✉)
Division of Vascular Surgery, Southern Illinois University School of Medicine, Springfield, IL, USA
e-mail: tzhang@siumed.edu

W. P. Robinson III, J. P. Simons (eds.), *The Patient-Centered Approach to Claudication*, https://doi.org/10.1007/978-3-032-02460-2_20

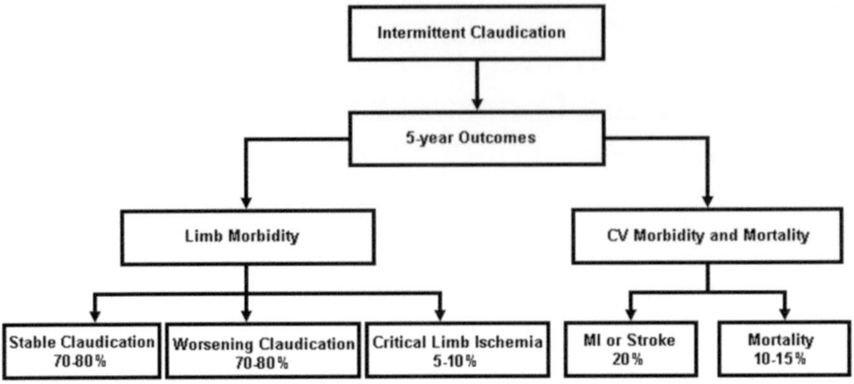

Fig. 20.1 The natural history of patients with claudication treated with noninvasive management. (Adapted from Society et al. [36])

including hypertension, diabetes, and tobacco use. According to the SVS, there are three subsets of PAD: asymptomatic PAD, intermittent claudication, or critical limb ischemia (CLI) [36]. Critical limb ischemia in more contemporary literature has been renamed as critical limb-threatening ischemia (CLTI). In general, all three guidelines refer to three clinical subsets of PAD: asymptomatic PAD, chronic symptomatic PAD or intermittent claudication, and CLTI. The inclusion of acute limb ischemia by the ACC/AHA as a subset of PAD does not correlate in the SVS or ESVS guidelines, and the discussion of the management of acute limb ischemia is excluded in the practice guidelines of the latter two societies.

Diagnostic Testing

If the history and physical examination identifies a patient with signs or symptoms of PAD, diagnostic testing to confirm the diagnosis is performed. The ankle brachial index (ABI), has been a longstanding cornerstone in diagnosis, although it is not without its limitations. Its benefits include its simplicity, noninvasive nature, minimal risks, and low cost. The three major societies agree in the utility of using the ABI as the primary method for establishing the diagnosis of PAD. They feel it is reasonable to use the ABI for asymptomatic patients who are at "elevated risk for PAD." The definition of this differs between societies. The SVS defines this population as individuals aged >70, smokers, diabetics, patients with an abnormal pulse examination, or those who have other established cardiovascular disease. The AHA/ACC defines this group as individuals ≥65; age 50–64 with risk factors for atherosclerosis (diabetes, history of smoking, dyslipidemia, hypertension), chronic kidney disease, or family history of PAD; age < 50 with diabetes and one additional risk factor for atherosclerosis; or any individual with known atherosclerotic disease in another vascular bed. The ESVS follows the WHO guidelines, which could include anyone ≥70 years; or those aged 45–69 with at least one risk factor for PAD. In addition, there is agreement that the appropriateness of using the ABI as a screening tool for both the general population as well as patients with cardiovascular risk factors but without symptoms, is unknown. It is important to consider and rule out other potential differential diagnoses that may mimic symptoms of PAD. The 2015 SVS guidelines and the 2024 ESVS guidelines pay particular attention to the consideration of neurogenic claudication, given its prevalence and symptom overlap with PAD.

Physiologic tests such as segmental pressure measurements, pulse volume recording, toe pressures/toe brachial index, and even exercise ABIs enhance the usefulness of noninvasive testing. Standardized criteria for its reporting allow it to be used broadly with excellent reproducibility. In patients for whom the ABI is unreliable or inconclusive, or for patients who need revascularization, additional imaging such as duplex ultrasound, magnetic resonance angiography (MRA), computed tomography angiography (CTA), or catheter-based angiography of the lower extremities is available to help guide management. These tests have variable but generally good sensitivity and specificity for lesions. Duplex ultrasound can be technologist-dependent but is noninvasive and without risk to the patient. CTA and MRA offer excellent spatial resolution but have limitations of their own: CTA requires use of iodinated contrast and radiation exposure, and MRA uses gadolinium, which is contraindicated in patients with severe renal dysfunction. Catheter-based angiography offers excellent anatomic information and is the gold standard according to the SVS practice guidelines, but is invasive and therefore has procedural risks, also requires iodinated contrast and radiation exposure, and is generally reserved for planned revascularization. For patients with claudication managed with guideline-directed medical therapy (GDMT) alone, risks of these advanced imaging studies outweigh any potential benefit.

Medical Therapy

Medical therapy is an important part of the management of patients with claudication to reduce the risk of major adverse cardiac events (MACE) and mortality. The SVS and ACC/AHA note that much of the data for risk factor modification for patients with PAD is extrapolated from patients studied for secondary prevention in coronary artery disease.

Antiplatelet and Antithrombotic Therapy

Antiplatelet and antithrombotic medications are key mainstays of medical therapy for patients with claudication, to reduce the risk of MI, stroke, and death given their burden of atherosclerosis [2]. Numerous studies have studied combinations of single antiplatelet therapy with various antiplatelet medications, dual antiplatelet therapies with multiple combinations of medications, as well as low-dose direct oral anticoagulation rivaroxaban in the management of patients with cardiovascular disease [11]. ESVS and SVS guidelines give a class of recommendation (COR) 1 and level of evidence (LOE) A recommending patients to have single antiplatelet therapy for secondary cardiovascular prevention. Dual antiplatelet therapy can be considered but with the large degree of heterogeneity in this patient population, specific situations are not addressed. In patients with symptomatic PAD, the AHA/ACC guidelines give the strongest COR 1 and LOE A to administering single antiplatelet therapy or low-dose rivaroxaban (2.5 mg twice daily) combined with low-dose aspirin. This is a marked difference in comparison to the ESVS guidelines, which gives a more measured recommendation of COR 2a and LOR B due to the lack of data comparing aspirin plus rivaroxaban to clopidogrel alone, mitigated by the higher risk of bleeding in the aspirin plus rivaroxaban group. The SVS guidelines predate the release of the VOYAGER and COMPASS trials and do not comment on the use of rivaroxaban in this patient population [8, 11].

In patients who have not undergone intervention for their claudication and without other atherosclerotic disease such as coronary artery disease, the value of dual antiplatelet therapy is unknown. In patients who have received revascularization, the AHA/ACC guidelines give the stronger COR 1 and LOE A to treating patients with low-dose rivaroxaban (2.5 mg twice daily) combined and low-dose aspirin. Adding low-dose rivaroxaban is shown to reduce ischemic events at the cost of a higher risk of major bleeding in both the COMPASS trial and the VOYAGER PAD trial, although the VOYAGER PAD trial specifically assessed patients who had undergone lower extremity revascularization [8, 11]. Due to this, the ESVS guidelines suggest patients who have undergone revascularization for claudication may be candidates for either dual antiplatelet therapy or dual pathway inhibition, such as single antiplatelet with rivaroxaban with a COR of 2a and LOE of B. ACC/AHA guidelines do stipulate that the use of dual antiplatelet therapy after endovascular therapy is extrapolated from coronary data. Again, the SVS guidelines do not comment on the addition of dual pathway inhibition due to the age of the guidelines preceding the release of the major trials studying this combination of pharmacotherapy.

The use of dual antiplatelet therapy combined with full oral anticoagulation has been studied, and data has shown an increased risk of major and minor bleeding complications [1, 21, 23]. Specific to the PAD patient population, this combination has not been effective in reducing major adverse limb events (MALE) or major adverse cardiac events (MACE) and the increase of major bleeding complications has rendered it to be inadvisable. Because of this, the use of full-intensity oral anticoagulation with dual antiplatelet therapy solely for the treatment of symptomatic PAD is not recommended by any of the guidelines.

Lipid-Lowering Therapy for PAD

Dyslipidemia is a common risk factor for patients with PAD, given its role in accelerating advanced atherosclerosis. Statin therapy has been shown to improve both cardiac (MACE) and limb (MALE) outcomes and should be prescribed for all patients with PAD, with historical goals to achieve a low-density lipoprotein cholesterol (LDL-C) level <70 mg/dL as per the ACC/AHA and <100 mg/dL or to <70 mg/dL in very high-risk individuals as per the SVS [7, 18]. ESVS has recommendations to decrease LDL levels to <55 mg/dL (<1.4 mmol/L) and decrease it by ≥50% if baseline values are within 55–110 mg/dL. Despite numerous trials demonstrating the benefit of statins, rates of its use in this patient population remain suboptimal. Currently, the AHA/ACC cholesterol guideline makes a COR 1, LOE A recommendation to prescribing high-intensity statin therapy with a goal to reduce LDL-C levels by ≥50% in patients who are ≤75 years old. The largest study comes from the US Department of Veterans Affairs health care system, and showed lower rates of amputation and death in patients who were treated with statins [4].

Studying the effects of the use of adjunctive or alternative agents to statin therapy is still ongoing, and for the PAD population, results are part of an overall study on patients with combined cardiovascular disease. Nonetheless, the ACC/AHA recommends the use of proprotein convertase subtilisin-kexin type 9 (PCSK9) inhibitors in patients with PAD who have not achieved an LDL-C of <70 [17]. ESVS recognizes the limitations of the data regarding PCKS9 inhibitors, given it was designed to treat patients with coronary artery disease, and therefore cannot give recommendations. Due to its novel formulation, the SVS guidelines precede the advent of PCSK9 inhibitors onto the market and do not comment on it. Similarly, the use of ezetimibe in this patient population is not well defined. A subgroup analysis of the IMPROVE-IT trial with extracoronary atherosclerotic disease showed a lower rate of MACE with the addition of ezetimibe, but there is no data to support its use to reduce the risk of MALE [7]. Nevertheless, the ACC/AHA cholesterol guideline recommendations do include the use of ezetimibe for patients who atherosclerotic cardiovascular disease who have not achieved an LDL target of <70, a recommendation echoed by SVS and ESVS.

Antihypertensive Therapy

Hypertension is a common cardiovascular risk factor and contributing cause of atherosclerosis. Treatment of hypertension in patients with PAD is necessary to reduce the risk of MACE. However, much of the data is extrapolated from patients with overall cardiovascular disease, and there is less guidance specific to PAD patients. The current ACC/AHA hypertension clinical practice guideline has a COR 1 recommendation for a goal blood pressure of <130/80 in patients with cardiovascular disease [40]. ESVS recommends goals of ≤120–129/80 mmHg in patients <70 years and to ≤130–139/80 mmHg in patients ≥80 years. In patients with PAD and hypertension, the selective use of angiotensin-converting enzyme (ACE) inhibitors or angiotensin-receptor blockers is recommended to reduce the risk of MACE [3]. However, there was no difference in MALE, including major amputation [3]. SVS guidelines do recommend the use of ACE inhibitors, but do not mention specific blood pressure goals to reduce adverse outcomes in these patients.

Smoking Cessation

Tobacco use, particularly in the form of cigarette smoking, is a well-known aggravating cause of accelerated atherosclerosis. Smoking cessation is important for reducing the severity of PAD as well as its deterioration from milder subsets into chronic limb-threatening ischemia, and cardiovascular mortality and is given a COR of 1 and LOE of A by all three guidelines. Patients who smoke should be continually encouraged to continue cessation efforts. Combining nonpharmacological and pharmacological approaches can increase the success rates of smoking cessation. In recent years, electronic nicotine delivery systems are increasingly used, but its efficacy in aiding in smoking cessation is unknown, and there is limited data studying the risk of its use with the development and/or progression of PAD. The ESVS practice guideline is the only one that recognizes a possible reduction in cardiovascular risk compared to traditional cigarette smoking, and therefore endorsed use of these alternatives to achieve complete nicotine abstinence. Second-hand smoke has been associated with an increased risk of death, stroke, and cardiovascular disease, as well as the development of PAD [24, 31]. However, its effects on limb-based outcomes in patients with claudication are unknown.

Diabetes Management

Diabetes is a key risk factor for the development of PAD, and its management is important for improving outcomes. Management of diabetes should include a multidisciplinary approach to address diet, exercise, weight management, glycemic control, and podiatric care. Multiple studies have shown a link between elevated hemoglobin A1c values and MALE. Recently, glucagon-like peptide-1 (GLP-1) agonists and sodium-glucose cotransporter-2 (SGLT-2) inhibitors have been shown to reduce MACE and lower extremity amputation in patients with type 2 diabetes and cardiovascular disease, which includes PAD, although the presence of PAD was found in the minority of patients studied [9, 19, 25]. The SVS does not comment on the effectiveness of GLP-1 agonists or SGLT-2 inhibitors in this patient population. Unlike the ACC/AHA cholesterol management guidelines, however, the guidelines for the management of diabetes do not include specific therapy goals such as a targeted hemoglobin A1c level by the ACC/AHA although the SVS and ESVS guidelines state a goal of achieving a hemoglobin A1c of <7.0%.

Medications for Symptoms

Cilostazol is a phosphodiesterase III inhibitor and acts to improve endothelial function by producing vasodilation as well as reducing platelet aggregation. It has been shown to improve walking distance and quality of life, although did not change ABI values [5]. There have been studies showing some benefit of cilostazol in improving primary patency of bare metal stents in the femoropopliteal segment and reducing restenosis at 1 year [37]. It has been given a COR of 1 and LOE of A by the ACC/AHA in the management of patients with claudication. ESVS and SVS guidelines note the improvement in walking distance but offer a more nuanced stance on its use in this population. However, it is contraindicated in patients with congestive heart failure of any severity. Pentoxifylline and chelation therapy have not been shown to improve maximal walking distance in patients with claudication and are not recommended.

Exercise Therapy

In all three guidelines, structured exercise therapy (SET) is noted to be an important part of treatment for claudication due to PAD. Mechanisms behind any improvement are not yet well understood, but hypotheses include improved efficiency of skeletal muscle fiber contractions at a cellular and macroscopic level, improved endothelial cell function, collateral artery enlargement, and reduced inflammatory response.

The definition of "structured exercise therapy" includes both supervised exercise therapy as well as structured community-based exercise programs. There are key differences noted in the setting difference, with supervised exercise therapy primarily used in a hospital or outpatient facility with direct supervision by qualified health care professional(s). Exercise duration, frequency, length as well as individual session instructions are given. In a structured community-based exercise program, the patient's therapy is self-directed in a home, community, or neighborhood setting, with physician counseling required beforehand on how to begin, maintain, and progress the therapy. Physician supervision may include use of in person or virtual coaching sessions to maintain continued understanding and compliance, as well as to assess for necessary changes.

Overall, all three guidelines have a strong recommendation for the use of structured exercise therapy for symptomatic peripheral arterial disease. The class of recommendation and quality of evidence are high, with most notable improvements seen in walking performance and quality of life [14, 28]. However, it is noted that specific functional measures for structured exercise therapy have differed. Trials showing long-term benefits of SET for patients with claudication have persisted from 18 months up to 7 years [12, 29]. However, a 6-min walk test used in a trial for SET did not show continued improvement of walking 6 months after cessation of therapy [27]. These discordant results underscore a lack of universally accepted criteria for assessing improvement in qualitative and functional outcomes for SET in patients with claudication.

It is noted that despite the health benefits associated with SET in this patient population, its strong class of recommendation, level of evidence supporting its use, and Medicare coverage, referral rates for its use are low at approximately 2% [35]. Access to hospital or outpatient facilities may be a barrier, and community-based exercise programs help with adherence. In addition, frequent assessments with patients undergoing SET may also promote retention.

Intervention

All three guidelines suggest a measured approach to intervention in patients with claudication. The importance of determining functionally limiting symptoms and their response to exercise therapy and guideline-directed medical therapy (GDMT) is the first step in management, which should precede assessing if a patient is a candidate for invasive intervention. Those who have an adequate response to exercise therapy and GDMT and who no longer have significant functional impairment should not undergo revascularization. This is a stance shared by all three guidelines. For patients who do not improve with exercise therapy and GDMT, consideration for invasive intervention can be given. Anatomic and quantitative evaluation is used to determine hemodynamically significant lesions, using noninvasive vascular lab studies to help corroborate lesion significance. The decision to pursue revascularization requires multifactorial consideration: patient symptoms, degree of functional limitation and its limitation on the patient's quality of life, response to medical therapy, short- and long-term outcomes of revascularization weighed against short- and long-term procedural risk and potential need for repeat intervention(s). The guidelines recommend a patient-centered approach and actively involving the patients in the decisions around their care.

Endovascular and surgical therapies are briefly discussed in the AHA/ACC guidelines, but are more extensively discussed in the SVS and ESVS guidelines. Endovascular therapies include using catheter-based techniques and any adjunctive procedures as based on lesion characteristics, operator experience, and available technologies with differences in different anatomic locations. These include percutaneous transluminal angioplasty, drug-coated balloon angioplasty, stent technologies, lithotripsy, and atherectomy. The AHA/ACC guidelines do not offer specific guidelines on the appropriateness of use of individual modalities of intervention, but the SVS and ESVS guidelines offer more recommendations based on anatomic complexity, which are discussed below (Fig. 20.2).

Aortoiliac Segment

Multiple trials have compared endovascular interventions with medical therapy for patients with aortoiliac and/or femoropopliteal disease who present with claudication [12, 26, 32]. Overall, these studies have shown that intervention can be very effective to improve functional outcomes such as walking performance and quality of life. As seen in the CLEVER (Claudication: Exercise versus Endoluminal Revascularization) trial, the addition of intervention with structured exercised therapy outperformed any single modality of treatment alone [30]. Similar results were seen in the endovascular revascularization and supervised exercise (ERAS) trial, with greater improvements seen in the combined endovascular revascularization plus SET group versus the SET group alone [13].

In the aortoiliac segment, both SVS and ESVS recommend endovascular therapy over open surgery for focal lesions causing claudication. However, for extensive

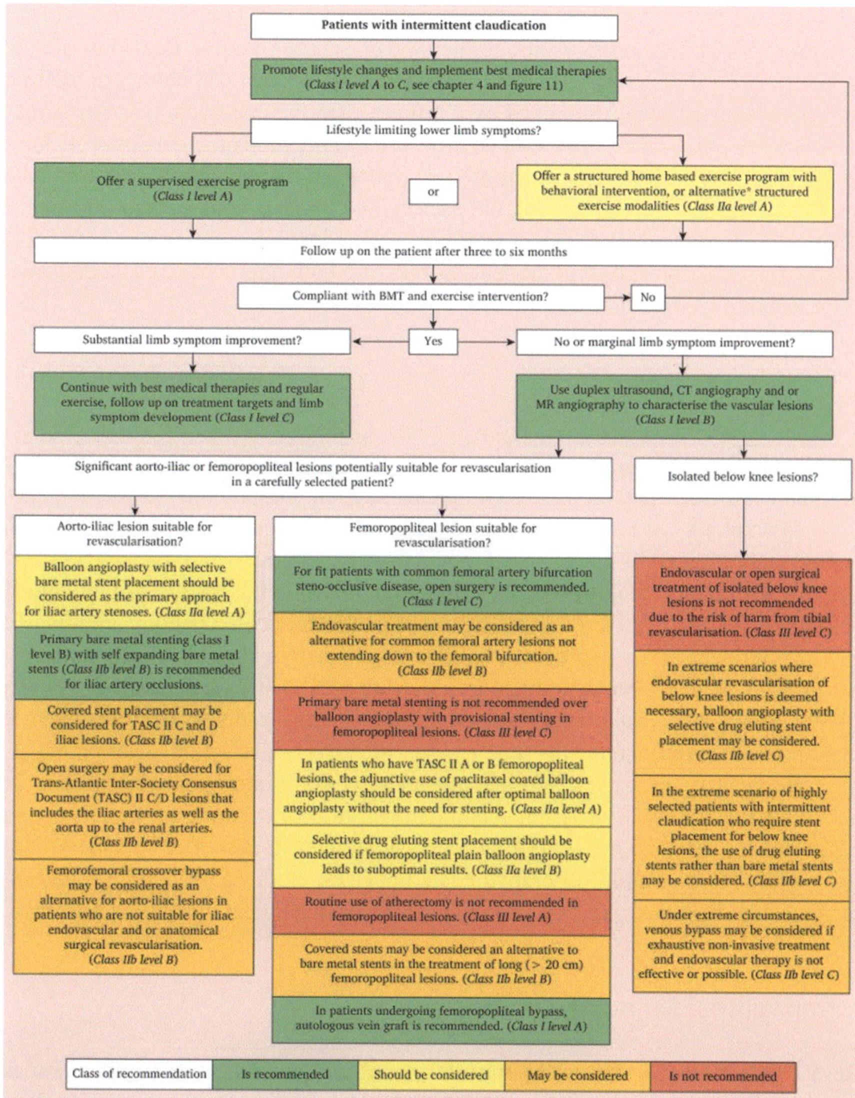

Fig. 20.2 Management strategy for patients with claudication. (Nordanstig et al. [33] (permission pending))

disease, open surgical techniques may be utilized. The ESVS guidelines do utilize the TASC II classification system for both aortoiliac and femoropopliteal lesions to guide management broadly into endovascular or open procedures, although they note that advanced endovascular techniques are available and may be suitable for even TASC II C/D lesions in both anatomic areas. The SVS guidelines recommend selective use of bare metal or covered stenting for iliac lesions, whereas the ESVS recommends primary bare metal stenting over primary balloon angioplasty due to the lower risk of distal embolization. The SVS does note however, that while simple angioplasty for iliac lesions has been a longstanding mainstay of endovascular therapy, it has largely been supplanted by a primary stenting approach. For more complex iliac lesions, such as the presence of severe calcification or aneurysmal changes as noted by the SVS, covered stents are recommended for use. ESVS does also note a role for covered stent placement, but uses TASC II C/D lesions as their criteria for necessitating covered stent placement. For lesions involving the common femoral artery, open surgery or hybrid procedures utilizing both open surgical and endovascular techniques should be employed.

Femoropopliteal Segment

The development of novel endovascular therapies has given physicians a wide array of tools with which to treat patients with claudication. Despite this, the heterogeneity and complexity of lesions remain a significant challenge for providers. Although endovascular therapy is widely used as an attractive alternative to open bypass surgery for femoropopliteal lesions, the optimal approach in this area is still undefined despite many comparative studies. The use of paclitaxel-coated balloon angioplasty can be considered after non-coated balloon angioplasty without the need for stenting in TASC II A/B femoropopliteal lesions with a COR of 2a and LOE of A by the ESVS. ESVS also recommends selective drug-eluting stents to be considered if there remain suboptimal results (i.e., residual stenosis or dissection) after plain balloon angioplasty. However, routine atherectomy for femoropopliteal lesions in patients with claudication is not recommended due to the lack of superiority in ESVS guidelines. The ACC/AHA and SVS guidelines do not offer specific guidelines with regard to antiproliferative coated devices. Both ESVS and SVS recommend using autologous saphenous vein grafts if open surgical bypass is performed.

Infrapopliteal Segment

Revascularization for the infrapopliteal vessels in patients with claudication is rarely performed, as isolated disease in this segment is an uncommon cause of claudication but is usually involved in patients with chronic limb-threatening ischemia. The ESVS cited two trials evaluating the endovascular treatment of intermittent claudication due to disease in the infrapopliteal segment: BIOLUX P-II and YUKON-BTK [34, 41]. Both trials offered small sample sizes and were not specific to patients with claudication only. Nevertheless, the YUKON-BTK trial randomized patients with focal infrapopliteal lesions to either sirolimus eluting stents or bare metal stents. One-year primary patency rates, amputation rates, and target vessel revascularization rates favored the sirolimus eluting stent group, and for this reason,

ESVS gave a measured recommendation of using drug eluting technology for isolated infrapopliteal lesions in the extreme scenario of highly selected patients with disabling claudication [34].

Follow-Up

Peripheral arterial disease is a chronic condition with correlation to overall cardiovascular health. Patients with PAD are at risk for major adverse cardiac events, such as MI, stroke, and death. Therefore, risk factor modification and longitudinal assessment is important in the care of these patients. Monitoring limb symptoms and functional status by using a history and physical examinations including pulse and foot examinations and noninvasive testing offers the ability to assess for the rare circumstance of progression to chronic limb-threatening ischemia. A multidisciplinary approach involving many care teams can facilitate cooperation and risk factor management to optimize outcomes for these patients [39, 42]. Adherence to tenets of exercise therapy and GDMT including antiplatelet and antithrombotic and statin therapies is an important pillar of care for these patients, as well as management of associated risk factors such as hypertension, diabetes, and ongoing tobacco use.

After revascularization, routine surveillance is recommended by all three guidelines to monitor for significant restenosis that may make prior interventions at risk for failure, with which prompt reintervention can improve outcomes and reduce major adverse limb events. The AHA/ACC guidelines reference the Society for Vascular Surgery guidelines in surveillance of bypass grafts and prior endovascular procedures, to perform ABI and arterial duplex ultrasound within the first 1–3 months post-procedure, at 6 months, 12 months, and then annually if the patient does not have new lower extremity signs or symptoms [42]. ESVS guidelines do recommend routine patient surveillance after interventions, but do not give timeline-based recommendations.

Conclusion

There are some notable differences in the practice guidelines established by the SVS, ACC/AHA, and ESVS, most of which revolve around the areas with still many unanswered questions. In addition, other differences may be attributed to the fact that the SVS guidelines were published in 2015 and a more recent update may resolve some of the minor conflicts. Given the burden of PAD on the microcosm of the individual patient as well as the macrocosm of the overall healthcare system, further research in claudication is needed to optimize patients' functionality, quality of life, and reduce strain on the greater healthcare system.

References

1. Anand S, Yusuf S, Xie C, et al. Oral anticoagulant and antiplatelet therapy and peripheral arterial disease. N Engl J Med. 2007;357:217–27.
2. Antithrombotic trialists collaboration. Collaborative meta-analysis of randomized trails of antiplatelet therapy for prevention of death, myocardial infarction, and stroke in high risk patients. BMJ. 2002;324:71–86.
3. Armstrong EJ, Chen DC, Singh GD, et al. Angiotensin-converting enzyme inhibitor or angiotensin receptor blocker use is associated with reduced major adverse cardiovascular events among patients with critical limb ischemia. Vasc Med. 2015;20:237–44.
4. Arya S, Khakharia A, Binney ZO, et al. Association of statin dose with amputation and survival in patients with peripheral artery disease. Circulation. 2018;137:1435–46.
5. Bedenis R, Stewart M, Cleanthis M, et al. Cilostazol for intermittent claudication. Cochrane Database Syst Rev. 2014;10:CD003748.
6. Bekken JA, Vroegindeweij D, Vos JA, et al. Two year results of the randomized DISCOVER trial comparing covered versus bare metal stents in the common iliac artery. Eur J Vasc Endovasc Surg. 2023;65:359–68.
7. Bonaca MP, Gutierrez JA, Cannon C, et al. Polyvascular disease, type 2 diabetes, and long-term vascular risk: a secondary analysis of the IMPROVE-IT trial. Lancet Diabetes Endocrinol. 2018;6:934–43.
8. Bonaca MP, Bauersachs RM, Anand SS, et al. Rivaroxaban in peripheral artery disease after revascularization. N Engl J Med. 2020;382:1994–2004.
9. Cosmi F, Laini R, Nicolucci A, et al. Semaglutide and cardiovascular outcomes in patients with type 2 diabetes. N Engl J Med. 2017;376:890.
10. Criqui MH, Langer RD, Fronek A, et al. Mortality over a period of 10 years in patients with peripheral arterial disease. N Engl J Med. 1992;326:381–6.
11. Eikelboom JW, Connolly SJ, Bosch J, et al. Rivaroxaban with or without aspirin in stable cardiovascular disease. N Engl J Med. 2017;377:1319–30.
12. Fakhry F, Rouwet EV, den Hoed PT, et al. Long-term clinical effectiveness of supervised exercise therapy versus endovascular revascularization for intermittent claudication from a randomized clinical trial. Br J Surg. 2013;100:1164–71.
13. Fakhry F, Spronk S, Van der Laan L, et al. Endovascular revascularization and supervised exercise for peripheral artery disease and intermittent claudication: a randomized clinical trial. JAMA. 2015;314:1936–44.
14. Golledge J, Singh TP, Alahakoon C, et al. Meta-analysis of clinical trials examining the benefit of structured home exercise in patients with peripheral artery disease. Br J Surg. 2019;106:319–31.
15. Gornik H, Aronow H, Goodney P, et al. ACC/AHA/AACVPR/APMA/ABC/SCAI/SVM/SVN/SVS/SIR/VESS Guideline for the management of lower extremity peripheral artery disease: a report of the American College of Cardiology/American Heart Association Joint Committee on clinical practice guidelines. Circulation. 2024;149(24):e1313–410.
16. Gouëffic Y, Torsello G, Zeller T, et al. Efficacy of a drug-eluting stent versus bare metal stents for symptomatic femoropopliteal peripheral artery disease: primary results of the EMINENT randomized trial. Circulation. 2022;146:1564–76.
17. Grundy SM, Stone NJ, Bailey AL, et al. AHA/ACC/AACVPR/AAPA/ABC/ACPM/ADA/AGS/APhA/ASPC/NMA/PCNA guideline on the management of blood cholesterol: a report of the American College of Cardiology/American Heart Association task force on clinical practice guidelines. Circulation. 2018;139:e1082–143.
18. Heart protection study collaborative group. Randomized trial of the effects of cholesterol-lowering with simvastatin on peripheral vascular and other major vascular outcomes in 20,536 people with peripheral arterial disease and other high-risk conditions. J Vasc Surg. 2007;45:645–54.

19. Heyward J, Mansour O, Olson L, et al. Association between sodium-glucose cotransporter 2 (SGLT2) inhibitors and lower extremity amputation: a systematic review and meta-analysis. PLoS One. 2020;15:e0234065.
20. Hirsch AT, Hartman L, Town RJ, et al. National health care costs of peripheral arterial disease in the Medicare population. Vasc Med. 2008;13:209–15.
21. Johnson W, Williford W, et al. Benefits, morbidity, and mortality associated with long-term administration of oral anticoagulant therapy to patients with peripheral arterial bypass procedures: a prospective randomized study. J Vasc Surg. 2001;35(3):13–21.
22. Koeckerling D, Raguindin PF, Kastrati L. Endovascular revascularization strategies for aortoiliac and femoropopliteal artery disease: a meta-analysis. Eur Heart J. 2023;44:935–50.
23. Efficacy of oral anticoagulants compared with aspirin after infrainguinal bypass surgery (the Dutch bypass oral anticoagulants or aspirin study): a randomised trial. Lancet. 2000;355:346–51.
24. Lu L, Mackay DF, Pell JP. Secondhand smoke exposure and risk of incident peripheral arterial disease and mortality: a Scotland-wide retrospective cohort study of 4045 non-smokers with cotinine measurement. BMC Public Health. 2018;18:348.
25. Marso SP, Daniels GH, Brown-Frandsen K, et al. Liraglutide and cardiovascular outcomes in type 2 diabetes. N Engl J Med. 2016;375:311–22.
26. Mazari FA, Gulati S, Rahman MN, et al. Early outcomes from a randomized, controlled trial of supervised exercise, angioplasty, and combined therapy in intermittent claudication. Ann Vasc Surg. 2010;24:69–79.
27. McDermott MM, Kibbe MR, Guralnik JM, et al. Durability of benefits from supervised treadmill exercise in people with peripheral artery disease. J Am Heart Assoc. 2019;8:e009380.
28. McDermott MM, Dayanidhi S, Kosmac K, et al. Effect of low-intensity vs high-intensity home-based walking exercise on walk distance in patients with peripheral artery disease: the LITE randomized clinical trial. JAMA. 2021;325:1266–76.
29. Murphy TP, Cutlip DE, Regensteiner JG, et al. Supervised exercise, stent revascularization, or medical therapy for claudication due to aortoiliac peripheral artery disease: the CLEVER study. J Am Coll Cardiol. 2015;65:999–1009.
30. Murphy TP, Cutlip DE, Regensteiner JG, et al. Supervised exercised, stent revascularization, or medical therapy for claudication due to aortoiliac peripheral artery disease: a randomized clinical trial. J Am Coll Cardiol. 2017;65:999–1009.
31. Ngu NL, McEvoy M. Environmental tobacco smoke and peripheral arterial disease: a review. Atherosclerosis. 2017;266:113–20.
32. Nordanstig J, Gelin J, Hensater M, et al. Walking performance and health-related quality of life after surgical or endovascular invasive versus non-invasive treatment for intermittent claudication—a prospective randomized trial. Eur J Vasc Endovasc Surg. 2011;42:220–7.
33. Nordanstig J, Behrendt CA, Baumgartner I, et al. European society for vascular surgery (ESVS) 2024 clinical practice guidelines on the management of asymptomatic lower limb peripheral arterial disease and intermittent claudication. Eur J Vasc Endovasc Surg. 2024;67(1):9–96.
34. Rastan A, Brechtel K, Krankenberg H, et al. Sirolimus-eluting stents for treatment of infrapopliteal arteries reduce clinical event rate compared to bare-metal stents: long-term results from a randomized trial. J Am Coll Cardiol. 2012;60:587–91.
35. Saxon JT, Safley DM, Men-Hurtado C, et al. Adherence to guideline-recommended therapy—including supervised exercise therapy referral—across peripheral artery disease specialty clinics: insights from the international PORTRAIT registry. J Am Heart Assoc. 2020;9:e012541.
36. Society for Vascular Surgery Lower Extremity Guidelines Writing Group, Conte M, Pomposelli F, Clair D, et al. Society for vascular surgery practice guidelines for atherosclerotic occlusive disease of the lower extremities: management of asymptomatic disease and claudication. J Vasc Surg. 2015;61(3):2S–41S.e1.
37. Soga Y, Hamasaki T, Edahiro R, et al. Sustained effectiveness of cilostazol after endovascular treatment of femoropopliteal lesions: midterm follow-up from the sufficient treatment of peripheral intervention by cilostazol (STOP-IC) study. J Endovasc Ther. 2018;25:306–12.

38. Twine C, Kakkos S, Aboyans V, et al. European society for vascular surgery (ESVS) 2023 clinical practice guidelines on antithrombotic therapy for vascular diseases. Eur J Vasc Endovasc Surg. 2023;65(5):626–89.
39. Venermo M, Sprynger M, Desormais I, et al. Editor's choice—follow-up of patients after revascularisation for peripheral arterial diseases: a consensus document from the European Society of Cardiology Working Group on aorta and peripheral vascular diseases and the European Society for Vascular Surgery. Eur J Vasc Endovasc Surg. 2019;58:641–53.
40. Whelton PK, Carey RM, Aronow WF, et al. 2017 ACC/AHA/AAPA/ABC/ACPM/AGS/APhA/ASPC/NMA/PCNA guideline for the prevention, detection, evaluation, and management of high blood pressure in adults: a report of the American College of Cardiology/American Heart Association Task Force on clinical practice guidelines. Hypertension. 2018;71:e13–e115.
41. Zeller T, Beschorner U, Pilge E, et al. Paclitaxel-coated balloon in infrapopliteal arteries: 12-month results from the BIOLUX P-II randomized trial (BIOTRONIK'S-First in man study of the Passeo-18 LUX drug releasing PTA balloon catheter vs the uncoated Passeo-18 PTA balloon catheter in subjects requiring revascularization of infrapopliteal arteries). JACC Cardiovasc Interv. 2015;8:1614–22.
42. Zierler RE, Jordan WD, Lal BK, et al. The Society for Vascular Surgery practice guidelines on follow-up after vascular surgery arterial procedures. J Vasc Surg. 2018;68:256–84.

Cost-Effectiveness of Claudication Treatment

21

Nader Zamani and Neal R. Barshes

Abbreviations

ICER	incremental cost-effectiveness ratio
PAD	peripheral artery disease
SET	supervised exercise therapy
QALY	quality-adjusted life-year

Introduction

The United States has more per capita health care spending than any other country in the world. In absolute monetary values, per capita spending in 2022 was 55% higher than Switzerland, the second highest-spending country and a country with a higher per capita gross domestic product. Health care spending in the United States comprises nearly 18% of the gross domestic product, a value also at least 50% more than the comparable figures in Canada, Australia, the United Kingdom, and European countries (which range from 10% to 13% of gross domestic product) [1–4].

Despite this, health outcomes in the United States—as measured by maternal mortality, life expectancy, or access to care—are not the best. Within the United States, this begs the question: is what we are getting what we are paying for? In other words, are our health care programs and interventions worth their additional costs? In the end, the resources of *all* health care systems are ultimately finite, so

N. Zamani · N. R. Barshes (✉)
Division of Vascular Surgery and Endovascular Therapy, Michael E. DeBakey Department of Surgery, Baylor College of Medicine/Michael E. DeBakey Veterans Affairs Medical Center, Houston, TX, USA
e-mail: zamani@bcm.edu; nbarshes@bcm.edu

W. P. Robinson III, J. P. Simons (eds.), *The Patient-Centered Approach to Claudication*, https://doi.org/10.1007/978-3-032-02460-2_21

while this question might seem most relevant to the United States, it is a question that should be asked in all health care systems throughout the world.

This question should be fundamental to vascular specialists treating patients with intermittent claudication, specifically when high technology and procedural costs offer relatively marginal improvements in function and no impact on patient survival. Intermittent claudication is a manifestation of peripheral artery disease that remains clinically stable for the majority of patients. With an annual amputation rate of 1%, treatment of claudication is centered on improving quality of life and walking performance. Guidelines by the ACC/AHA [5], the United Kingdom's National Institute for Health and Clinical Excellence (NICE) [6], and the Society for Vascular Surgery [7] support supervised exercise therapy and optimal medical management for the treatment of claudication. The decision to pursue revascularization, therefore, is based on a number of factors, among which include a patient's baseline functional status, severity of symptoms, life expectancy, and overall surgical risk.

The invasive treatment of claudication, especially using atherectomy, has been critiqued within our field of vascular surgery and in the general press. Alleged overtreatment of lower extremity PAD has resulted in Federal False Claims Act and Anti-Kickback Statute violation allegations and is the focus of a report in progress by the United States Department of Health and Human Services, expected to be published in 2025. So questioning the "value" or cost-effectiveness of interventions for claudication is very timely [8–11].

In this chapter, we will assess the cost-effectiveness of various health care interventions used in the management of intermittent claudication. We will explain the methodology of cost-effectiveness studies—the predominant means by which policy makers and health care providers answer the question of whether a particular intervention is worth its cost. We will review published cost-effectiveness estimates for claudication treatment, and we will discuss factors that might help vascular specialists generalize these findings to the care of individual patients within specific health care systems.

Defining Value and Cost-Effectiveness

Cost-Utility Analyses

Many types of economic analyses of health care programs exist, but the most commonly utilized—and the type we will focus on here—is a cost-effectiveness, or "cost-utility" analysis. In basic terms, cost-utility analyses compare the relative costs and outcomes of at least two health care interventions or programs used to treat a particular condition: most often the "standard" or conventional therapy compared to one or more alternatives. In doing so, cost-utility analyses produce estimates of the additional ("incremental") outcomes yielded by paying the additional ("incremental") costs associated with one treatment option compared to another.

Measuring Costs The costs that are captured and included in a cost-utility analysis depend on the perspective of the study itself. If performed from the health care perspective, the costs that are directly related to the intervention are captured. For example, this can include the cost of a particular operation, the postoperative pharmacotherapy that is required, the inpatient hospital stay, the outpatient office visits, etc. If a study is performed from a societal perspective, however, not only are these costs considered, but also other costs that may not be directly related to the health care sector. Examples might include patient- and caregiver-time costs, travel/transportation, and lost productivity [12].

The relevant costs for the management of intermittent claudication, in turn, are primarily those related to the health care perspective. These costs are incurred primarily due to the intervention/procedure offered to the patient. Though the time and cost of maintaining scheduled follow-up can be considered from a patient's or caregiver's perspective, the overall downstream costs of claudication therapy are not as significant as those incurred by the upfront intervention. The caveat to consider, however, is that if a patient improves symptomatically and is able to return to the workforce, this would certainly have a positive impact from a societal perspective that should not be discounted.

Measuring Effectiveness Effectiveness is any measurement of health benefit as defined by the particular study. Contemporary analyses largely use quality-adjusted life-years (QALYs) as a single measure that incorporates the product of both survival and health utility, a parameter similar to quality of life that is measured using various commonly-used questionnaires [13]. Specifically, cost-utility studies are a subtype of cost-effectiveness analyses that use QALYs as the measure of effectiveness. That QALYs can be estimated for all health care conditions is a feature that allows payers and policy makers to assess the relative impact of any health care intervention or program to be compared to any other, across disease processes (e.g., the addition of fluoride to drinking water for the prevention of dental caries versus high-risk percutaneous coronary interventions for patients with advanced heart failure). This feature has led to cost-utility studies using QALYs to be the most commonly-performed subtype of economic analysis within health care and the type preferred by many payers (including the National Health Service in the United Kingdom).

Interventions for claudication have focused on function, and thereby only would be expected to affect the health utility component of effectiveness as measured in QALYs. There have been no data analyses to suggest interventions for intermittent claudication impact survival.

Since cost-utility studies, by definition, are always comparisons, the single-most important result parameter is the incremental cost-effectiveness ratio, or ICER. The ICER is calculated as the ratio of the difference in incremental costs to the difference in incremental effectiveness between the intervention and its comparator [12, 13]. In this way, the ICER determines if the intervention's effectiveness justifies its cost. In other words, the ICER is used to directly determine if a particular intervention is cost-effective.

$$\text{ICER} = \left(\text{Cost}_{\text{intervention}} - \text{Cost}_{\text{comparator}}\right) / \left(\text{Effectiveness}_{\text{intervention}} - \text{Effectiveness}_{\text{comparator}}\right)$$

$$\text{ICER} = \left(\text{Cost}_{\text{intervention}} - \text{Cost}_{\text{comparator}}\right) / \left(\text{QALY}_{\text{intervention}} - \text{QALY}_{\text{comparator}}\right)$$

After researchers gather these estimates of costs and utilities, computerized simulation models—especially probabilistic Markov models—are often used to generate the total costs and QALYs based on a number of different parameters and health states that simulate a patient's progression after the intervention. Results of a study are then presented as the total costs, the QALYs gained or lost, as well as the incremental cost-effectiveness ratio. Using a model allows for researchers to incorporate varying sources of uncertainty into the evaluation and also improves generalizability of the findings of the analysis.

Interpreting ICERs After the ICER of the intervention has been calculated relative to the comparator, it is plotted on a cost-effectiveness plane (an example is provided in Fig. 21.1). This is a plot of the incremental costs on the vertical axis to incremental effectiveness (i.e., QALYs) on the horizontal axis. The baseline/comparator group is represented by the intersection of the two axes. If an ICER for an intervention falls in the upper-left quadrant, the intervention is more costly and less effective than the comparator (in other words: the intervention has worse outcomes/is not as beneficial). Therefore, it would not make sense for a society to adopt this intervention. In this scenario, the intervention is "*dominated*" (using cost-utility analysis terminology) by the baseline comparator. Conversely, if an ICER for an intervention falls in the lower-right quadrant, it is more effective and less expensive than the comparator. This describes a scenario for potential cost-savings. Here, the intervention is certainly cost-effective, and the intervention *dominates* the comparator.

If an ICER falls in the upper-right quadrant of the cost-effectiveness plane, however, greater interpretation is required. This quadrant represents an intervention that is more effective than the comparator, but achieves these outcomes at a greater cost. With unlimited resources, this intervention would be adopted regardless of its expense. However, in a system with finite resources, one must determine if that particular intervention's additional effectiveness justifies its cost. To do this, the ICER is compared to the willingness-to-pay threshold. An intervention in this quadrant is considered cost-effective if its ICER falls below the willingness-to-pay threshold.

Simply put, the willingness-to-pay threshold is the amount that a society is willing to pay to produce a health outcome [14]. These thresholds naturally vary between different societies, and though there is usually no explicit threshold, there

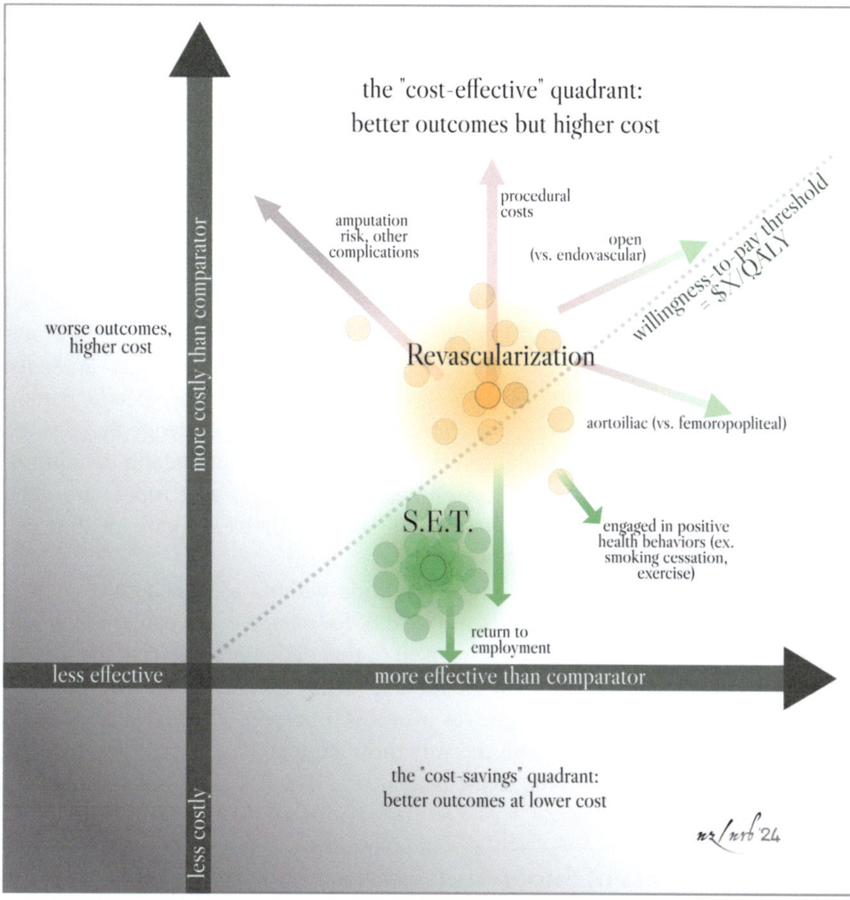

Fig. 21.1 Cost-effectiveness plane for intermittent claudication. Theoretical plot of incremental cost-effectiveness ratios (ICERs) for supervised exercise therapy (SET) and revascularization, each compared to a baseline treatment strategy of medical management alone. Arrows depict possible ways that point estimates may be influenced by different variables. If a treatment strategy is more effective than medical management and has an ICER that falls below the willingness-to-pay threshold, the strategy is considered cost-effective

are usually general ranges available in the literature. To illustrate, in the United States, an ICER below $50,000–$100,000 is generally considered cost-effective [15]. In other words, the United States is willing to pay up to $100,000 for an additional one QALY. The United Kingdom's National Institute for Health and Clinical Excellence (NICE) uses a threshold of £20,000–£30,000 (approximately $25,000–$38,000, exchange rates as of December 2024) [16]. In the Netherlands, the threshold is between €20,000 and €80,000 ($21,000–$84,000) and interestingly varies based on underlying disease severity [17]. Finally, in Scandinavia, the Swedish National Board of Health has indicated that an ICER below €50,000 ($53,000) is cost-effective [18, 19].

"Value" in Health Care

A term related to cost-effectiveness is "value". Since the publication of health care commentaries by Michael Porter, a well-known economist in the fields of economic theory and competitive strategy, "value" in health care has been largely defined as a patient's health outcomes achieved relative to the total cost required to achieve those outcomes over the complete cycle of care for that condition [20–22]:

Value = Outcomes / Total Cost

This has obvious similarities to the equation calculating ICERs in that outcomes are divided by costs. Different from cost-utilities analyses, however, is that outcomes and costs are not strictly quantified in QALYs and monetary amounts, respectively. Instead, Porter and colleagues refrain from advocating specific parameters that might quantify outcomes and costs and instead acknowledge that desired outcomes and definitions of "value" vary between patients and health conditions. Indeed, outcomes that have no direct clinical impact (e.g., wait times) are valid parameters in a Porterian "value" analysis due to the relative importance they can have with patients.

When considering a chronic medical condition without a defined cure, such as lower extremity peripheral artery disease (PAD), for example, the care cycle would involve everything related to the management of that patient's PAD from the time of diagnosis to the patient's death. This would involve any number of specific interventions or services that the patient receives over this timespan. Therefore, an inherent characteristic of value comes from the way those collective services for a medical problem, like PAD, are *delivered* to the patient.

Cost-Effectiveness of Supervised Exercise Therapy

Several economic analyses have been performed comparing supervised exercise therapy (SET) for claudication to medical management. These studies have been listed and described in the Table 21.1. In this context, "medical management" generally involves risk factor modification, antiplatelet and statin therapy, managing relevant comorbidities, smoking cessation, and advice on adopting an unsupervised/community-based walking regimen.

Authors in the United Kingdom, the Netherlands, and the United States have attempted to establish the costs and benefits of SET. Lee et al. performed a prospective cohort study of 70 patients (37 receiving medical management; 33 SET) [23]. At the time of publication in 2007, a 3-month SET regimen in the United Kingdom was reported to cost approximately £48 for a single patient, with an incremental cost-effectiveness ratio (ICER) of £1800 per QALY gained for the first year after the initiation of the exercise regimen. This is similar to the data presented by Bermingham et al. who performed an analysis using a review of previously published randomized controlled trials [24]. Assuming that patient compliance was equivalent between supervised and unsupervised walking therapy, their model generated an ICER of

Table 21.1 Key cost-effectiveness analyses for the treatment of intermittent claudication

Study characteristics			Cost-effectiveness analysis parameters					Results		
Author (year)	Location[a]	Diseased arterial segment	Data source	Treatment strategies[b]	Evaluation perspective[c]	Instrument for measuring health utility	Time horizon	Costs	QALYs gained	ICER
de Vries (2002) [29]	n/a	Not described	Boston registry; Groningen and Rotterdam databases	(1) SET (2) Endo (3) Open	Societal	EuroQol	5 yr	Not provided	Any revasc: 0.09–0.17	Endo vs. SET: $38,000
Treesak (2004) [33]	n/a	Aortoiliac	Pooled RCTs	(1) SET (2) Endo (angioplasty)	Societal	n/a (used pain-free walking distance)	6 mo	SET: $5000 Endo: $9300	SET: 123 per meter Endo: 54 per meter	SET dominates Endo
Lee (2007) [23]	United Kingdom	Not described	Prospective cohort (n = 70)	(1) Medical (2) SET	Health care	SF-36	1 yr	SET: £48	SET: +0.03	SET vs. Medical: £1800
Spronk (2008) [30]	The Netherlands	Aortoiliac, fempop	RCT (n = 151)	(1) Endo (angioplasty ± stenting) (2) SET	Societal	EuroQol SF-36	1 yr	Endo: €7000 SET: €2800	Endo: 0.01	Endo vs. SET: €230,000
van Asselt (2011) [25]	The Netherlands	Not described	RCT (n = 304)	(1) Medical (2) SET	Societal	EuroQol	1 yr	Medical: €2300 SET: €3400	Medical: 0.67 SET: 0.71	SET vs. Medical: €29,000

(continued)

Table 21.1 (continued)

Study characteristics			Cost-effectiveness analysis parameters					Results		
Author (year)	Location[a]	Diseased arterial segment	Data source	Treatment strategies[b]	Evaluation perspective[c]	Instrument for measuring health utility	Time horizon	Costs	QALYs gained	ICER
Bermingham (2013) [24]	n/a	Not described	Hypothetical cohort based on RCTs	(1) Medical (2) SET	Health care	EuroQol SF-36	2 yr	Medical: £2500 SET: £2700	Medical: 5.1 SET: 5.2–5.3	SET vs. Medical: £710–1600
Mazari (2013) [31]	United Kingdom	Fempop	RCT ($n = 178$)	(1) Endo (angioplasty) (2) SET (3) Endo + SET (Combination)	Societal	SF-36, VascuQol	1 yr	Endo: €7300 SET: €3900 Combo: €6900	Endo: 0.62 SET: 0.63 Combo: 0.65	Endo vs. SET: €380,000 Combo vs. SET: €150,000 Combo vs. Endo: €13,000
Reynolds (2014) [27]	USA	Aortoiliac	RCT ($n = 111$)	(1) Medical (2) SET (3) Endo (stenting)	Societal	EuroQol	10 yr	Medical: $29,000 SET: $33,000 Endo: $38,000	Medical: 5.71 SET: 6.01 Endo: 6.08	SET vs. Medical: $15,000 Endo vs. Medical: $25,000 Endo vs. SET: $69,000
van den Houten (2016) [34]	n/a	Not described	Hypothetical cohort based on RCTs	(1) SET (2) Endo (angioplasty ± stent)	Health care	EuroQol	5 yr	SET: €10,000 Endo: €17,000	SET: 2.8 Endo: 2.9	Endo vs. SET: €92,000

Djerf (2018) [18]	Sweden	Aortoiliac, fempop	RCT ($n = 158$)	(1) Medical (2) Revasc (72% endo; 28% open)	Health care	EuroQol	2 yr	Medical: €1900 Revasc: €8300	Medical: 1.25 Revasc: 1.41	Revasc vs. Medical: €43,000
Djerf (2021) [19]	Sweden	Fempop (SFA)	RCT ($n = 100$)	(1) Medical[a] (2) Endo (SFA stenting)	Health care	EuroQol, SF-36	2 yr	Medical: €4800 Endo: €11,000	Medical: 0.95 Endo:1.35	Endo vs. Medical: €24,000
Fakhry (2021) [37]	The Netherlands	Aortoiliac, fempop	RCT ($n = 212$)	(1) SET (2) Endo + SET (combination)	Societal (Health care perspective analyzed separately)	EuroQol	1 yr	SET: €6000 (€3000) Combo: €6100 (€4500)	SET: 0.051 Combo: 0.093	Combo vs. SET: €3800 (€35,000)
van Reijen (2022) [32]	The Netherlands	Aortoiliac	RCT ($n = 240$)	(1) SET (2) Endo	Societal	EuroQol	1 yr	SET: €2200 Endo: €4000	SET: 0.73 Endo: 0.82	Endo vs. SET: €21,000

Abbreviations: *ICER* incremental cost-effectiveness ratio (currency/QALYs gained), *mo* month, *RCT* randomized controlled trial, *SET* supervised exercise therapy, *QALY* quality-adjusted life year, *yr* year

[a]Location—applicable if the study is based on data from an RCT or cohort study

[b]"Endo" refers to endovascular revascularization (including angioplasty with or without stenting); "Open" refers to surgical revascularization (including bypass operations). Medical management includes recommendations for unsupervised exercise regimens

[c]Societal perspective—studies are categorized as adopting a societal perspective if there was any mention of accounting for any informal health care sector or non-health care sector costs (i.e., costs that are not directly related to the procedure itself)

£1600. As this falls below the generally accepted threshold of £20,000–£30,000 used by the UK's National Institute for Health and Clinical Excellence [16], this ICER for SET is interpreted as cost-effective. Notably, SET became even more cost-effective as patient compliance with the regimen increased, with an ICER as low as £710.

Other studies based on empiric data have also been consistent in the cost-effectiveness of SET but have provided slightly more expensive estimates. For example, van Asselt et al. provided an analysis of the EXITPAD study in which 304 patients with claudication were randomized to either walking advice (medical management) or SET. In this case, SET was specifically performed by a physical therapist with varying weekly frequency over the 12-month study [25, 26]. In this scenario, the ICER for SET was also favorable (about €29,000 per QALY gained).

Reynolds et al. analyzed 18-month data from the CLEVER trial which specifically studied patients with claudication due to disease in the aortoiliac segment [27]. SET included an average of 56 exercise sessions and 11 telephone encounters for maintenance thereafter. Over a 10-year time horizon, the projected total cost of SET was $33,000, versus $28,000 for medical management. Given a mean difference of 0.3 QALYs, the ICER for SET was $15,000 per QALY gained, not only consistent with prior analyses, but also adding to the body of evidence considering supervised exercise therapy economically attractive by conventional standards.

In summary, the estimates provided argue that SET is a cost-effective intervention for intermittent claudication. Consistent with this body of literature, the Centers for Medicare and Medicaid Services (CMS) issued a National Coverage Determination in 2017 announcing its coverage of supervised exercise therapy for patients with intermittent claudication [28]. Beneficiaries became eligible for up to 36 sessions of therapy over a 12-week period. There was also the possibility of an additional 36 sessions over a more extended timeframe following review by Medicare administrative contractors. For Medicare purposes, SET was defined as sessions that last 30–60 min, are delivered by "qualified auxiliary personnel [...] who are trained in exercise therapy for PAD," and take place in either a hospital outpatient setting or at a physician's office.

Of note, when interpreting these studies, their fixed time horizons should also be considered since the treatment of claudication may extend beyond those time constraints. For example, since implementing a SET regimen may also positively influence general cardiovascular health, SET could potentially have an impact beyond the time horizon studied. This would actually serve to underestimate the strategy's cost-effectiveness in the short term.

Cost-Effectiveness of Revascularization

A series of analyses have aimed to determine if the quality of life gained by revascularization justifies its additional cost. These studies have collectively used data from patient registries, primary randomized controlled trials, pooled data from literature reviews, and hypothetical patient cohorts [27, 29–35]. Not surprisingly, this data has produced mixed results, with incremental cost-effectiveness ratios for revascularization ranging anywhere from €21,000 [32] to €380,000 per QALY gained [31].

In general, the increased cost of revascularization is due to not only the higher initial cost of the intervention, but also the required follow-up, possible complications, and potential for subsequent procedures [30]. To illustrate, among those who undergo revascularization for claudication (be it endovascular or open), upwards of 35% require reintervention within a 2-year period [36]. Conversely, an analysis of a national Dutch insurance database indicated that within 2 years of diagnosis, revascularization was only required in 6.4% of patients treated with SET [36].

The following pairwise comparisons presented in this section aim to synthesize the available literature and relative cost estimates for endovascular and open revascularization in relationship to either medical management alone or SET.

Endovascular Revascularization Versus Medical Management

Despite the upfront costs, there are important observations that can impact interpretation of the costs and the effectiveness of endovascular therapy. Two studies have used empirically derived estimates to compare endovascular intervention to medical management alone [19, 27]. Reynolds et al. used data from 111 patients with claudication due to aortoiliac disease in the CLEVER trial to determine that endovascular intervention was associated with 1.20 QALYs gained over the 18-month study (which was 0.16 QALYs more than medical management). Over an 18-month period, the cost estimates for medical management, SET, and endovascular therapy were: $5000, $9000, and $14,000, respectively. This all ultimately translated to a favorable ICER of $41,000 compared to medical management [27]. Over a longer time horizon of 10 years, the ICER was even more acceptable (more cost-effective) at $25,000 per QALY gained.

Similarly, Djerf et al. performed a randomized controlled trial of 100 patients with claudication due to femoropopliteal disease. At 2 years, endovascular intervention on these lesions accounted for an increase in 0.12 QALYs over that of medical management, resulting in an ICER of €24,000 per QALY gained [19]. Therefore, endovascular intervention may be reasonable from a cost-effectiveness perspective when compared to medical management alone.

Endovascular Revascularization Versus SET

When compared directly to SET, however, the cost-effectiveness of endovascular therapy is not as clear-cut. Of the seven studies included in Table 21.1 that provide direct comparisons between endovascular intervention and SET, four have presented ICERs that are beyond the generally accepted willingness-to-pay thresholds [30, 31, 33, 34]. At face value, this would indicate that endovascular therapy is likely not cost-effective compared to SET (in other words: endovascular intervention is more expensive without providing substantial improvements in quality of life). It has even been speculated that SET would remain cost-effective even if up to 80% of patients ultimately require revascularization [35].

Even so, sensitivity analyses among a subset of patients with severe symptoms of lifestyle-limiting claudication reveal a 70% probability that endovascular intervention is cost-effective compared to SET at conventional willingness-to-pay thresholds [34]. Therefore, even though an endovascular-first approach for everyone with intermittent claudication is too expensive relative to its potential benefit, revascularization may be cost-effective among those with lower baseline quality-of-life scores and severe symptoms despite a trial of SET.

Along these lines, the combination of endovascular therapy plus SET may be more cost-effective than revascularization alone. Fakhry et al. used data from the ERASE trial, which randomized 212 patients with claudication to either SET alone, or the combination of endovascular intervention followed by SET [37]. From this Dutch study, the revascularization option was actually found to be cost-effective, associated with only €1500 more per patient over the 12-month study period, and accounting for an additional 0.04 QALYs (for an ICER of €35,000 per QALY gained). Though there was less adherence to exercise therapy, the authors hypothesize that the combination of revascularization and SET may work together to promote durability of the index revascularization. This is consistent with observations from Mazari et al. who noted that the reintervention rate among their cohort undergoing combination therapy (endovascular plus SET) was zero within the 12-month study period [31]. This combination was cost-effective when compared to those who underwent revascularization without supervised exercise.

Open Revascularization Versus SET

There is very little data dedicated to the cost-effectiveness of open revascularization for the treatment of intermittent claudication. An early assessment by de Vries et al. first suggested that the gain in effectiveness provided by open revascularization was not justified by its associated costs [29].

Others have approached the issue of cost-effectiveness from the perspective of grouping endovascular and open interventions together. However, these collective revascularization cohorts presented by Fokkenrood et al. and Djerf et al. both heavily favor endovascular interventions in their composition (77% and 72% endovascular, respectively) [18, 36]. Revascularization, as defined here, costs 4–5 times as much as either medical management or SET. However, considering that endovascular therapy forms the vast majority of cases in these aggregate studies, it is not possible to specifically evaluate the cost-effectiveness of open operations.

Keeping Interventions for Intermittent Claudication Within the Willingness-to-Pay Threshold

The ideal patient for the cost-effective treatment of intermittent claudication would be a relatively younger patient with lifestyle-limiting symptoms that prevent him or her from being employed (or at least to full capacity), has aortoiliac disease amenable to durable endovascular intervention or open surgical reconstruction (e.g. aortofemoral bypass), and will be enrolled in a supervised exercise therapy program after the intervention. Some of these factors are illustrated in Fig. 21.1.

From a societal perspective, employment is an additional factor that can alter the cost-effectiveness estimates. The possibility that an intervention can improve a patient's pain-free walking distance and quality of life to the point where they may return to employment would have a positive economic impact. This would drive the estimates for either SET or revascularization lower down on the cost-effectiveness plane and further away from the willingness-to-pay threshold, making either one more economically favorable.

In contrast, certain other factors would likely increase an ICER (thereby decreasing its cost-effectiveness). The above-described ICER estimates for endovascular intervention are largely based on plain balloon angioplasty with the use of stenting as indicated. Therefore, anything that increases procedural/technological costs without significantly adding utility would increase the ICER and reduce the probability of an intervention being below a willingness-to-pay threshold. As of 2010, the cost of angioplasty alone, atherectomy, and stenting have been reported as: $12,002, $14,972, and $16,234, respectively [35]. Undoubtedly, the costs of other endovascular technologies such as drug-coated balloons, drug-eluting stents, intravascular ultrasound, and lithotripsy must all be considered.

Some common sources of increased costs for endovascular interventions might be femoropopliteal disease. To illustrate, O'Brien-Irr et al. indicated that the costs of endovascular intervention for claudication significantly differed based on the pattern of disease and arterial segments involved [35]. Two-year costs for complex, long-segment stenoses/occlusions, for example, were estimated to be approximately $14,380 per patient, compared to $11,715 for short-segment proximal lesions ($p = 0.017$). The total cost of treating femoropopliteal lesions was also more expensive: $14,904 per patient, compared to $9311 for aortoiliac disease ($p < 0.001$) [35]. Further, among studies that analyzed only patients with aortoiliac disease, ICERs were favorable and ranged from €21,000 [32] to $69,000 [27]. On the other hand, patients with claudication due to femoropopliteal-level disease generated prohibitively high ICER estimates upwards of €380,000 per QALY gained, arguing against revascularization as a cost-effective strategy for this disease pattern [31].

Postoperative complications are also important considerations. Notably, revascularization for claudication has also been significantly associated with: (1) progression to chronic limb threatening ischemia (hazard ratio 2.9, 95% confidence interval of 2.0–4.2), and (2) a future lower extremity amputation (hazard ratio 4.5, 95%

confidence interval 2.2–9.5) [38]. Both of these scenarios drastically increase cost and decrease the effectiveness of revascularization. These are situations in which revascularization would clearly be dominated by SET.

In other words, femoropopliteal interventions on unemployed, older patients without significant disability are unlikely to be cost-effective, especially when technology expenses go beyond angioplasty alone. [NOTE: guidelines recommend against tibial interventions and bypasses to tibial targets because of a lack of clear clinical benefit (i.e., effectiveness). In cost-effectiveness analysis terminology, these interventions would be considered dominated (that is, worse clinical outcomes and higher costs) and should generally not be offered.]

Finally, unlike the field of traditional economics which assumes that individuals make decisions solely based on reason and self-interest, behavioral economics takes into account psychology when examining the mechanisms behind decision-making. This acknowledges that human behavior is often influenced by a number of intangible factors, such as societal pressures, cognitive biases, and erroneous information. Behavioral economics has been applied to the treatment of claudication to seek out common characteristics of those who adhere to community-based exercise regimens. Interestingly, individuals who have implemented at least one other beneficial health behavior (such as smoking cessation), those that are future-oriented, and those that regularly save money have a significantly higher predilection to adhere with unsupervised exercise regimens [39, 40].

Of note, these generalizations are based on cost-utility analyses that inherently have used different assumptions regarding disease progression, escalation of treatment strategies, background mortality rates, and health care utilization across countries that have starkly different health care delivery models. Though this international, heterogeneous body of literature has produced variable point estimates, these very characteristics help improve the generalizability of the cost-effectiveness data available for the treatment of intermittent claudication.

Conclusion

Compared to medical management alone, all interventions for intermittent claudication increase both cost and effectiveness. The available data is consistent in that supervised exercise therapy is the single-most cost-effective treatment strategy for claudication. From an economic perspective, SET is a first-line treatment strategy for claudication.

With respect to revascularization strategies, the data is more variable, but also supports a SET-first approach. The value of revascularization may be influenced by a host of different factors, including: procedural/technological costs, type of revascularization, complexity/anatomy of the arterial disease burden, reintervention rates, postoperative complications, the non-zero risk of limb loss, the degree to which quality of life may be improved, and behavioral tendencies. From an economic perspective, those that may benefit the most from revascularization include those with severely diminished baseline quality of life, those with symptoms due to aortoiliac disease, those who may return to the workforce, and those who have successfully stopped smoking. Furthermore, for patients who undergo revascularization, the addition of a dedicated supervised exercise regimen actually offers a more cost-effective treatment strategy over revascularization alone, despite its increased upfront costs.

The economic evaluations reviewed here provide important information that can help inform difficult decisions that surgeons make on a daily basis. The goal of treatment for claudication, as with any other vascular pathology, is to provide high-quality care in a way that is both efficient and limits costs to the overall health care system. By being economically and financially conscientious, vascular surgeons should continue to be at the forefront of promoting safe, cost-effective health care.

References

1. Wager E, McGough M, Rakshit S, Amin K, Cox C. How does health spending in the U.S. compare to other countries? https://www.healthsystemtracker.org/chart-collection/health-spending-u-s-compare-countries/ (2024). Accessed 13 Dec 2024.
2. OECD. Health spending. https://www.oecd.org/en/data/indicators/health-spending.html. Accessed 13 Dec 2024.
3. Gunja MZ, Gumas ED, Williams II RD. U.S. health care from a global perspective, 2022: accelerating spending, worsening outcomes. (2023, January, Commonwealth Fund). https://doi.org/10.26099/8ejy-yc74. Accessed 13 Dec 2024.
4. Rakshit S, Wager E, Hughes-Cromwick P, Cox C, Amin K. How does medical inflation compare to inflation in the rest of the economy? https://www.healthsystemtracker.org/brief/how-does-medical-inflation-compare-to-inflation-in-the-rest-of-the-economy (2024, Aug). Accessed 13 Dec 2024.
5. Hirsch AT, Haskal ZJ, Hertzer NR, Bakal CW, Creager MA, Halperin JL, et al. ACC/AHA 2005 Practice Guidelines for the management of patients with peripheral arterial disease (lower extremity, renal, mesenteric, and abdominal aortic): a collaborative report from the American Association for Vascular Surgery/Society for Vascular Surgery, Society for Cardiovascular Angiography and Interventions, Society for Vascular Medicine and Biology, Society of Interventional Radiology, and the ACC/AHA Task Force on Practice Guidelines (Writing Committee to Develop Guidelines for the Management of Patients With Peripheral Arterial Disease): endorsed by the American Association of Cardiovascular and Pulmonary Rehabilitation; National Heart, Lung, and Blood Institute; Society for Vascular Nursing; TransAtlantic Inter-Society Consensus; and Vascular Disease Foundation. Circulation. 2006;113(11):e463–654. https://doi.org/10.1161/CIRCULATIONAHA.106.174526.
6. Layden J, Michaels J, Bermingham S, Higgins B, Guideline Development G. Diagnosis and management of lower limb peripheral arterial disease: summary of NICE guidance. BMJ. 2012;345:e4947. https://doi.org/10.1136/bmj.e4947.
7. Society for Vascular Surgery Lower Extremity Guidelines Writing G, Conte MS, Pomposelli FB, Clair DG, Geraghty PJ, McKinsey JF, et al. Society for Vascular Surgery practice guidelines for atherosclerotic occlusive disease of the lower extremities: management of asymptomatic disease and claudication. J Vasc Surg. 2015;61(3 Suppl):2S–41S. https://doi.org/10.1016/j.jvs.2014.12.009.
8. Meltzer AJ. How to succeed in vascular surgery: a guide for the aspiring outlier. Vascular Specialist. https://vascularspecialistonline.com/how-to-succeed-in-vascular-surgery-a-guide-for-the-aspiring-outlier/ (2021, March 2). Accessed 13 Dec 2024.
9. Waldman A. Thousands of patients may be undergoing vascular procedures too soon or unnecessarily. ProPublica. https://www.propublica.org/

article/thousands-of-patients-may-be-undergoing-vascular-procedure-unnecessarily (2023, December 12). Accessed 13 Dec 2024.
10. DOJ. NIRP and founder to pay nearly $9M to resolve alleged kickback referral violations. United States Attorney's Office, Southern District of Texas. https://www.justice.gov/usao-sdtx/pr/nirp-and-founder-pay-nearly-9m-resolve-alleged-kickback-referral-violations (2024, August 20). Accessed 13 Dec 2024.
11. HHS. Utilization of peripheral vascular procedures and CMS's related program integrity efforts. U.S. Department of Health and Human Services, Office of Inspector General. https://oig.hhs.gov/reports-and-publications/workplan/summary/wp-summary-0000852.asp. Accessed 13 Dec 2024.
12. Sanders GD, Neumann PJ, Basu A, Brock DW, Feeny D, Krahn M, et al. Recommendations for conduct, methodological practices, and reporting of cost-effectiveness analyses: second panel on cost-effectiveness in health and medicine. JAMA. 2016;316(10):1093–103. https://doi.org/10.1001/jama.2016.12195.
13. Barshes NR, Chambers JD, Cantor SB, Cohen J, Belkin M. A primer on cost-effectiveness analyses for vascular surgeons. J Vasc Surg. 2012;55(6):1794–800. https://doi.org/10.1016/j.jvs.2012.02.026.
14. Shiroiwa T, Sung YK, Fukuda T, Lang HC, Bae SC, Tsutani K. International survey on willingness-to-pay (WTP) for one additional QALY gained: what is the threshold of cost effectiveness? Health Econ. 2010;19(4):422–37. https://doi.org/10.1002/hec.1481.
15. Menzel P. How should willingness-to-pay values of quality-adjusted life-years be updated and according to whom? AMA J Ethics. 2021;23(8):E601–6.
16. Gandjour A. Willingness to pay for new medicines: a step towards narrowing the gap between NICE and IQWiG. BMC Health Serv Res. 2020;20(343):1–7.
17. Schurer M, Matthijsse SM, Vossen CY, van Keep M, Horscroft J, Chapman AM, et al. Varying willingness to pay based on severity of illness: impact on health technology assessment outcomes of inpatient and outpatient drug therapies in the Netherlands. Value Health. 2022;25(1):91–103. https://doi.org/10.1016/j.jval.2021.08.003.
18. Djerf H, Falkenberg M, Jivegard L, Lindgren H, Svensson M, Nordanstig J. Cost-effectiveness of revascularization in patients with intermittent claudication. Br J Surg. 2018;105(13):1742–8. https://doi.org/10.1002/bjs.10992.
19. Djerf H, Svensson M, Nordanstig J, Gottsater A, Falkenberg M, Lindgren H. Editor's choice—cost effectiveness of primary stenting in the superficial femoral artery for intermittent claudication: two year results of a randomised multicentre trial. Eur J Vasc Endovasc Surg. 2021;62(4):576–82. https://doi.org/10.1016/j.ejvs.2021.07.009.
20. Porter ME. Value-based health care delivery. Ann Surg. 2008;248(4):503–9. https://doi.org/10.1097/SLA.0b013e31818a43af.
21. Porter ME. What is value in health care? N Engl J Med. 2010;363(26):2477–81. https://doi.org/10.1056/NEJMp1011024.
22. Porter ME, Lee TH. From volume to value in health care: the work begins. JAMA. 2016;316(10):1047–8. https://doi.org/10.1001/jama.2016.11698.
23. Lee HL, Mehta T, Ray B, Heng MS, McCollum PT, Chetter IC. A non-randomised controlled trial of the clinical and cost effectiveness of a supervised exercise programme for claudication. Eur J Vasc Endovasc Surg. 2007;33(2):202–7. https://doi.org/10.1016/j.ejvs.2006.08.005.
24. Bermingham SL, Sparrow K, Mullis R, Fox M, Shearman C, Bradbury A, et al. The cost-effectiveness of supervised exercise for the treatment of intermittent claudication. Eur J Vasc Endovasc Surg. 2013;46(6):707–14. https://doi.org/10.1016/j.ejvs.2013.09.005.
25. van Asselt AD, Nicolai SP, Joore MA, Prins MH, Teijink JA, Exercise Therapy in Peripheral Arterial Disease Study G. Cost-effectiveness of exercise therapy in patients with intermittent claudication: supervised exercise therapy versus a 'go home and walk' advice. Eur J Vasc Endovasc Surg. 2011;41(1):97–103. https://doi.org/10.1016/j.ejvs.2010.06.024.
26. Nicolai SP, Teijink JA, Prins MH, Exercise Therapy in Peripheral Arterial Disease Study G. Multicenter randomized clinical trial of supervised exercise therapy with or without

feedback versus walking advice for intermittent claudication. J Vasc Surg. 2010;52(2):348–55. https://doi.org/10.1016/j.jvs.2010.02.022.
27. Reynolds MR, Apruzzese P, Galper BZ, Murphy TP, Hirsch AT, Cutlip DE, et al. Cost-effectiveness of supervised exercise, stenting, and optimal medical care for claudication: results from the Claudication: Exercise Versus Endoluminal Revascularization (CLEVER) trial. J Am Heart Assoc. 2014;3(6):e001233. https://doi.org/10.1161/JAHA.114.001233.
28. Jensen JS, Ashby L, Schafer J, Dolan D. National coverage determination for supervised exercise therapy (SET) for symptomatic peripheral artery disease (PAD). https://www.cms.gov/medicare-coverage-database/view/ncacal-decision-memo.aspx?proposed=N&NCAId=287 (2017). Accessed 2024.
29. de Vries SO, Visser K, de Vries JA, Wong JB, Donaldson MC, Hunink MG. Intermittent claudication: cost-effectiveness of revascularization versus exercise therapy. Radiology. 2002;222(1):25–36. https://doi.org/10.1148/radiol.2221001743.
30. Spronk S, Bosch JL, den Hoed PT, Veen HF, Pattynama PM, Hunink MG. Cost-effectiveness of endovascular revascularization compared to supervised hospital-based exercise training in patients with intermittent claudication: a randomized controlled trial. J Vasc Surg. 2008;48(6):1472–80. https://doi.org/10.1016/j.jvs.2008.06.016.
31. Mazari FA, Khan JA, Carradice D, Samuel N, Gohil R, McCollum PT, et al. Economic analysis of a randomized trial of percutaneous angioplasty, supervised exercise or combined treatment for intermittent claudication due to femoropopliteal arterial disease. Br J Surg. 2013;100(9):1172–9. https://doi.org/10.1002/bjs.9200.
32. van Reijen NS, van Dieren S, Frans FA, Reekers JA, Metz R, Buscher H, et al. Cost effectiveness of endovascular revascularisation vs. exercise therapy for intermittent claudication due to iliac artery obstruction. Eur J Vasc Endovasc Surg. 2022;63(3):430–7. https://doi.org/10.1016/j.ejvs.2021.10.048.
33. Treesak C, Kasemsup V, Treat-Jacobson D, Nyman JA, Hirsch AT. Cost-effectiveness of exercise training to improve claudication symptoms in patients with peripheral arterial disease. Vasc Med. 2004;9(4):279–85. https://doi.org/10.1191/1358863x04vm570oa.
34. van den Houten MM, Lauret GJ, Fakhry F, Fokkenrood HJ, van Asselt AD, Hunink MG, et al. Cost-effectiveness of supervised exercise therapy compared with endovascular revascularization for intermittent claudication. Br J Surg. 2016;103(12):1616–25. https://doi.org/10.1002/bjs.10247.
35. O'Brien-Irr MS, Harris LM, Dosluoglu HH, Dryjski ML. Endovascular intervention for treatment of claudication: is it cost-effective? Ann Vasc Surg. 2010;24(6):833–40. https://doi.org/10.1016/j.avsg.2010.03.025.
36. Fokkenrood HJ, Scheltinga MR, Koelemay MJ, Breek JC, Hasaart F, Vahl AC, et al. Significant savings with a stepped care model for treatment of patients with intermittent claudication. Eur J Vasc Endovasc Surg. 2014;48(4):423–9. https://doi.org/10.1016/j.ejvs.2014.04.020.
37. Fakhry F, Rouwet EV, Spillenaar Bilgen R, van der Laan L, Wever JJ, Teijink JAW, et al. Endovascular revascularization plus supervised exercise versus supervised exercise only for intermittent claudication: a cost-effectiveness analysis. Circ Cardiovasc Interv. 2021;14(7):e010703. https://doi.org/10.1161/CIRCINTERVENTIONS.121.010703.
38. Madabhushi V, Davenport D, Jones S, Khoudoud SA, Orr N, Minion D, et al. Revascularization of intermittent claudicants leads to more chronic limb-threatening ischemia and higher amputation rates. J Vasc Surg. 2021;74(3):771–9. https://doi.org/10.1016/j.jvs.2021.02.045.
39. Sharath SE, Lee M, Kougias P, Taylor WC, Zamani N, Barshes NR. Delayed gratification and adherence to exercise among patients with claudication. Vasc Med. 2019;24(6):519–27. https://doi.org/10.1177/1358863X19865610.
40. Sharath SE, Lee M, Kougias P, Taylor WC, Zamani N, Barshes NR. Successful smoking cessation associated with walking behavior in patients with claudication. Ann Vasc Surg. 2019;56:287–93. https://doi.org/10.1016/j.avsg.2018.09.017.

Unmet Needs and New Horizons in Treating Patients with Claudication

22

Alejandra P. Rodriguez and Shirling Tsai

Intermittent Claudication and Its Treatments

Intermittent claudication (IC), a non-limb-threatening manifestation of peripheral artery disease (PAD), can produce significant impairment in mobility and quality of life (QOL) and can cause overall functional decline. Treatment of IC generally starts with risk factor modification and medical management. Exercise therapy has also been shown to improve walking distance, strength, and endurance in patients with PAD. Supervised exercise therapy (SET) involves a structured exercise program and has the most evidence for improvement of IC. Revascularization can also be done for patients with IC either in the form of endovascular or open techniques, however guidelines emphasize conservative management first for these patients. This chapter will address the challenges of medical management, particularly exercise therapy (ET) alone and in conjunction with revascularization, as well as some innovations under development to overcome these challenges.

General Challenges to the Treatment of Intermittent Claudication

Treatment of IC, both medical management and ET, is dependent on the patient's participation, access to ET programs, and provider knowledge of such treatment options. There are countless factors on a patient level that affect the success of ET. Some of these factors include baseline walking capacity, comorbid conditions, age, and health literacy. Also, the patient's motivation to exercise and partake in risk factor modification is arguably one of the most important factors to consider. It is

A. P. Rodriguez · S. Tsai (✉)
Division of Vascular and Endovascular Surgery, Department of Surgery, UT Southwestern Medical Center, Dallas, TX, USA
e-mail: alejandra.rodriguez@phhs.org; shirling.tsai@utsouthwestern.edu

W. P. Robinson III, J. P. Simons (eds.), *The Patient-Centered Approach to Claudication*, https://doi.org/10.1007/978-3-032-02460-2_22

also important to consider the accessibility of ET programs for patients. Transportation, distance to the nearest ET program, time constraints, and access to technology for virtual options should be considered when advising patients. Provider knowledge of SET for patient referrals, encouragement, and instruction has also been a challenge nationwide with only 50% of vascular surgeons offering SET to their patients with PAD [1]. When accounting for ambulatory providers treating PAD, it was found that in only 22% of office visits out of nearly 2000 had patients receiving exercise counseling [2]. Despite what seems like countless factors against the success of SET, there have been studies that aimed to address some of these barriers.

Supervised Exercise Therapy and Its Challenges

SET involves a structured exercise program focused on walking exercises for a minimum of 30–45 min per 60-min session for at least 3 times per week for a minimum of 12 weeks [3]. SET improves pain-free walking and maximum walking distance although it does not improve ankle brachial index (ABI), amputation, or mortality [4]. Long-term follow-up of patients after SET showed persistent benefits up to 18 months [5]. However, data on the durability of the benefits of SET are scarce and sometimes contradictory. When comparing supervised treadmill exercise, supervised resistance training, and attention control for 1 year, supervised therapy, particularly treadmill therapy, improved 6-min walk distance at 6 months but did not have persistent benefit at 1 year [6]. When looking out to 4 years after SET, there were few patients that continued exercising and these patients had a more notable decline in their walking ability [7]. This highlights the patient-specific factors that contribute to the durability of the benefits from SET and the diminishing adherence to exercise after completion of SET programs. Long-term sustainability of the benefits seen with SET programs is what many practices strive for and is often difficult to predict. Importantly, these programs require active participation and buy in from patients for successful completion, however the suggested parameters, intensity, modality, and frequency can be individualized [8].

New Horizons

While the advances in surgical and endovascular treatments for PAD have seen great advancements and adoption in recent years, exercise therapy programs for IC have not seen as great adoption into everyday practice. However, some solutions and novel approaches are emerging. Recent advances have ranged from techniques to promote engagement and reduce attrition, to building community ET programs in areas without dedicated SET facilities and incorporating new technologies to personalize treatment.

Maintaining Engagement

Patient's motivation is integral in the success and adherence to ET. Roughly only 40–50% of patients complete SET emphasizing the underutilization of and poor adherence to current programs [9]. Like any exercise program, results are not immediate and involve encouraging patients until the onset of moderate to severe ischemic pain. Patients with more severe symptoms often have high fear-avoidance and have been found to be more likely to avoid behaviors or actions that cause pain, such as exercising [10]. Managing expectations is important when embarking on ET. The use of personalized outcomes forecasts can be used by therapists and patients to contextualize treatment expectations and provide patient-centered treatment plans [11]. These outcome forecasts are derived from previous data of similar patients to forecast response to therapy. This gives the patient a potentially attainable goal and motivation to achieve that goal. Other strategies to motivate patient participation include the use of patient-defined treatment goals. However, this could have both positive and negative effects. When patients were able to choose their treatment goal of either increased walking distance, ability to perform specific tasks such as shopping without having to rest in a large store, or increased walking speed, it was noted that some patients chose potentially unattainable goals [12]. This emphasizes the importance of providers setting realistic expectations with their patients. These patient-defined goals show that patients' priorities can differ from what guidelines define as treatment success, which may contribute to the decline in participation.

A very important barrier to the long-term sustainability of SET is the availability and use of SET programs [1]. Despite the Centers for Medicare & Medicaid Services and most commercial insurance providers covering 12 weeks of SET there is still low utilization of available programs. One method to address this is to offer home-based ET with the involvement of primary care providers. Approximately 20% of patients with PAD are treated with medical management by their primary care providers which provides another important avenue for the implementation of ET [13]. Some home-based programs involve coaching from primary care-based counselors at regular intervals [14]. Alternative exercise programs have also been studied to address the lack of availability of SET programs, including community-based exercise therapy. There have been some studies that found that SET in community-based settings can be equally effective for IC in improving walking distance as a clinic-based SET program [15]. However, while these home-based programs offer convenient alternatives for patients, conventional SET remains the most effective in improving walking distance and quality of life when compared to programs with intermittent coaching or walking advice alone [16]. Even though the long-term durability of community-based SET and home-based programs remains an area for further research, it is still important for providers to be aware of these options so that they can make individualized referrals for their patients for programs that best meet their patients' needs.

Some studies aimed to increase adherence to SET through promoting behavioral changes. For example, patients with a future-directed mindset versus those who seek immediate results were more likely to engage in exercise [17]. Bolt et al. found that increasing the participant's knowledge, promoting a positive attitude and self-efficacy could contribute to patient adherence to SET and improved long-term outcomes [18]. The GOALS trial, a randomized control trial examining home-based ET found that the group with behavior interventions such as teaching self-regulatory skills, had better walking performance than those that did not receive these behavior strategies and this improvement was maintained at 12 months [19]. Similarly, virtual coaching with motivational interviewing techniques increased walking capacity and improved illness perception in patients with IC at 6 months after home-based ET [20].

Another proposed solution to the underutilization of SET is its automatic incorporation to the PAD treatment algorithm. The success of such programs is seen in the implementation of cardiac rehabilitation programs. Cardiac rehab is an interdisciplinary program that is customized to patients with cardiovascular disease and has a goal of secondary prevention. It is offered to all patients who undergo cardiac intervention and begins in the hospital setting and continues after discharge. It includes risk factor and lifestyle modification interventions such as weight management, nutrition counseling, smoking cessation, and exercise training [21]. Unlike the well-integrated cardiac rehabilitation programs that are built into many hospital treatment algorithms, PAD rehabilitation is not as well defined. The implementation of a PAD rehabilitation with similar core components as cardiac rehabilitation that could be offered to patients undergoing vascular interventions would potentially streamline optimal medical management.

While the first-line therapy for IC is medical management with SET there are patients who continue to have lifestyle-limiting symptoms. These patients are often offered either surgical or endovascular revascularization. When comparing percutaneous transluminal angioplasty (PTA), versus SET and in combination, it was found that the combination of SET with PTA was more effective in improving clinical outcome than either treatment alone in the femoral popliteal segment [22]. There were similar improvements in QOL measures when comparing SET versus PTA alone. Thus, implementation of an automatic referral to a rehabilitation program after vascular intervention may provide patients with streamlined care that would optimize medical management and perhaps improve walking performance for the longer term.

Technology and Intermittent Claudication

Since studies have demonstrated that successful exercise programs require structure and supervision, two of the main barriers to adherence to exercise programs have been geographical location and time constraints. Patients in rural areas may not have access to facilities for supervised exercise. Even patients who live in urban or suburban areas may incur significant commutes to a rehab facility for supervised exercise therapy, which can quickly become overwhelming when SET requires visits three times a week. Both barriers could potentially be overcome by virtual platforms, which have fewer geographical constraints and offer flexibility to be scheduled around work and family care.

Virtual Therapy

Even before the widespread adoption of smart devices, fitness monitors and step counters were employed to enhance home-based or remote exercise therapy. Whereas totally unsupervised, unstructured exercise therapy has no benefit [3], studies have demonstrated that a fitness monitor or step counter may function in part as a surrogate for supervision in a home-based exercise program.

In an effort to improve accessibility, recent studies have demonstrated that supervised home walking programs with step monitors [23] may offer similar benefits to traditional in-person SET and may outperform SET in terms of improving the ability to perform activities of daily living [24]. One of the earliest studies of home-based exercise with a step-counter reported the compliance and adherence to exercise therapy was over 80% in both the SET and home-based group, which is much higher than in other studies of SET, and certainly higher than what one would see in practice.

Digital health technologies, such as blood pressure cuffs, capture patient data that can be transmitted to and used by care teams to monitor chronic health problems (e.g., hypertension). Wearable digital health technologies, such as smart watches or skin-surface patches, allow for continuous data capture, often without requiring initiation by the wearer of the device [25]. The wSTEP trial was a small randomized controlled trial of patients with IC enrolled in either traditional SET vs. a feedback-enabled wrist-worn activity monitor in addition to SET [26]. Compared to previous trials using step counters, this trial used the latest technology, with a user-friendly interface and real-time feedback. Patients in the wrist-worn activity monitor group set daily activity targets, which were reviewed at study visits, and adjusted based on percentage of time the daily activity targets were met. Patients in the wrist-worn activity monitor group demonstrated significant improvement in maximum walking distance (MWD) at 3 and 6 months, sustained out to 12 months, whereas the SET only group did not show improvement in any of the above outcome measures. The ease with which new technologies can be used may further facilitate the development of virtual reality platforms that will extend the reach of traditional SET.

Conclusion

SET in addition to medical management remains the mainstay of treatment for IC. Many barriers to the implementation of SET programs have been described. It is the onus of the providers who treat patients with PAD to explore these challenges and work alongside their patients to implement these best practices. SET can be available to patients with PAD through clinic-based programs, community-based programs, or through integrating new technologies to reach patients otherwise unable to participate. Engaging in exercise therapy is ultimately a behavioral change, which may enhance or prolong the benefits of surgical interventions for IC and may need to be considered as part of post-operative care for patients undergoing interventions for IC.

References

1. Dua A, et al. National assessment of availability, awareness, and utilization of supervised exercise therapy for peripheral artery disease patients with intermittent claudication. J Vasc Surg. 2020;71(5):1702–7.
2. Berger JS, Ladapo JA. Underuse of prevention and lifestyle counseling in patients with peripheral artery disease. J Am Coll Cardiol. 2017;69(18):2293–300.
3. Gornik HL, et al. 2024 ACC/AHA/AACVPR/APMA/ABC/SCAI/SVM/SVN/SVS/SIR/VESS guideline for the Management of Lower Extremity Peripheral Artery Disease: a report of the American College of Cardiology/American Heart Association Joint Committee on Clinical Practice Guidelines. Circulation. 2024;149(24):e1313–410.
4. Lane R, et al. Exercise for intermittent claudication. Cochrane Database Syst Rev. 2017;12(12):Cd000990.
5. Murphy TP, et al. Supervised exercise, stent revascularization, or medical therapy for claudication due to aortoiliac peripheral artery disease: the CLEVER study. J Am Coll Cardiol. 2015;65(10):999–1009.
6. McDermott MM, et al. Durability of benefits from supervised treadmill exercise in people with peripheral artery disease. J Am Heart Assoc. 2019;8(1):e009380.
7. Menard JR, et al. Long-term results of peripheral arterial disease rehabilitation. J Vasc Surg. 2004;39(6):1186–92.
8. Treat-Jacobson D, et al. Optimal exercise programs for patients with peripheral artery disease: a scientific statement from the American Heart Association. Circulation. 2019;139(4):e10–33.
9. Donohue JK, et al. Socioeconomic factors predict successful supervised exercise therapy completion. J Vasc Surg. 2024;79(4):904–10.
10. Sharath SE, Kougias P, Barshes NR. The influence of pain-related beliefs on physical activity and health attitudes in patients with claudication: a pilot study. Vasc Med. 2017;22(5):378–84.
11. Sinnige A, et al. Impact of personalized outcomes forecasts on clinical reasoning of physical therapists in intermittent claudication: a vignette study. Phys Ther. 2022;102(7):pzac051.
12. Powell CA, et al. Characterizing patient-reported claudication treatment goals to support patient-centered treatment selection and measurement strategies. J Vasc Surg. 2023;77(2):465–473.e5.
13. Weissler EH, et al. Clinician specialty, access to care, and outcomes among patients with peripheral artery disease. Am J Med. 2022;135(2):219–27.
14. Wullink M, Stoffers HE, Kuipers H. A primary care walking exercise program for patients with intermittent claudication. Med Sci Sports Exerc. 2001;33(10):1629–34.
15. Bendermacher BL, et al. Supervised exercise therapy for intermittent claudication in a community-based setting is as effective as clinic-based. J Vasc Surg. 2007;45(6):1192–6.
16. Hageman D, et al. Supervised exercise therapy versus home-based exercise therapy versus walking advice for intermittent claudication. Cochrane Database Syst Rev. 2018;4(4):Cd005263.
17. Sharath SE, et al. Delayed gratification and adherence to exercise among patients with claudication. Vasc Med. 2019;24(6):519–27.
18. Bolt LJJ, et al. Assessment of behavioral determinants influencing success of supervised exercise therapy in patients with intermittent claudication: a cross sectional survey. Physiol Behav. 2020;215:112732.
19. McDermott MM, et al. Home-based walking exercise intervention in peripheral artery disease: a randomized clinical trial. JAMA. 2013;310(1):57–65.

20. Bearne LM, et al. Effect of a home-based, walking exercise behavior change intervention vs usual care on walking in adults with peripheral artery disease: the MOSAIC randomized clinical trial. JAMA. 2022;327(14):1344–55.
21. Mehra VM, et al. Systematic review of cardiac rehabilitation guidelines: quality and scope. Eur J Prev Cardiol. 2020;27(9):912–28.
22. Mazari FA, et al. Early outcomes from a randomized, controlled trial of supervised exercise, angioplasty, and combined therapy in intermittent claudication. Ann Vasc Surg. 2010;24(1):69–79.
23. Gardner AW, et al. Efficacy of quantified home-based exercise and supervised exercise in patients with intermittent claudication: a randomized controlled trial. Circulation. 2011;123(5):491–8.
24. Gardner AW, et al. Step-monitored home exercise improves ambulation, vascular function, and inflammation in symptomatic patients with peripheral artery disease: a randomized controlled trial. J Am Heart Assoc. 2014;3(5):e001107.
25. Spatz ES, et al. Wearable digital health technologies for monitoring in cardiovascular medicine. N Engl J Med. 2024;390(4):346–56.
26. Normahani P, et al. Wearable sensor technology efficacy in peripheral vascular disease (wSTEP): a randomized controlled trial. Ann Surg. 2018;268(6):1113–8.

Appendix

GET MOTIVATED!

HOW TO SUCCEED WITH A WALKING PROGRAM

MAKE A NEW HABIT
Set aside 60 minutes, 5 days a week, as your time to walk. Think about where you might do this – a track, a mall, a gym.

"BUT I CAN'T WALK"
The idea is to walk at a moderate pace, as far as you can until the pain stops you. *Then rest until it goes away.* Then do the same thing again. You will do cycles of this for the 60 minutes.

SET GOALS, MONITOR PROGRESS
By 12 weeks of exercise therapy, you should be able to recognize your progress – you will be able to walk significantly farther before you have to stop. It won't be perfect, but many patients find that they have improved enough to avoid discussion of surgery!

HEALTHY LIFESTYLE CHANGES, SMOKING CESSATION, MEDICATIONS, NO SURGERY REQUIRED

CLAUDICATION

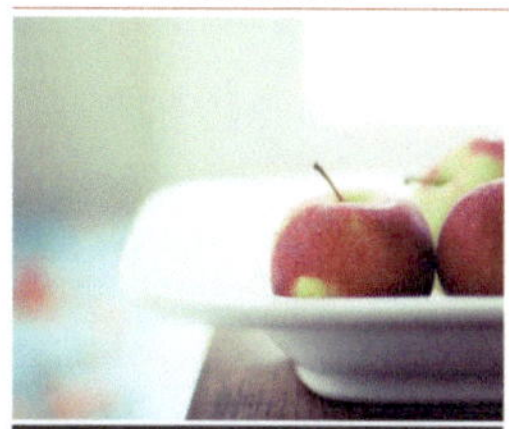

HEALTHY LIFESTYLE CHANGES

Resources

There are countless websites and videos about PAD. Be sure to find ones that differentiate claudication from more severe types of PAD, and then focus on the information about claudication. Remember! Claudication is not the same as gangrene and almost never leads to amputation.

Society for Vascular Surgery:
https://vascular.org/your-vascular-health

PERIPHERAL ARTERY DISEASE

Leg Claudication

A GUIDE FOR PATIENTS

GET HEALTHY NOW!

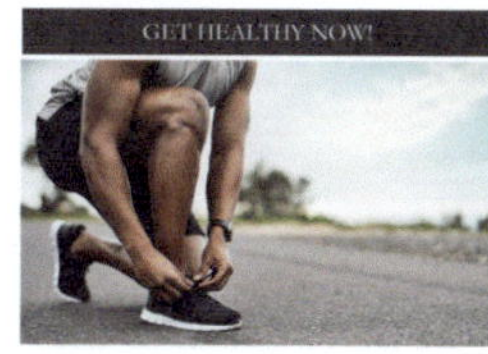

W. P. Robinson III, J. P. Simons (eds.), *The Patient-Centered Approach to Claudication*, https://doi.org/10.1007/978-3-032-02460-2

WHAT IS CLAUDICATION?

SYMPTOMS

If you experience pain, weakness, or fatigue of your calf, thigh, or buttock muscles when you walk, your healthcare provider may diagnose you with *intermittent claudication* due to peripheral artery disease (PAD). It is important to understand what this condition means for your overall health.

CLAUDICATION IS A TYPE OF PERIPHERAL ARTERY DIEASE

PAD is a condition where blockages build up in the arteries supplying blood to the legs. There are many reasons why these blockages can occur: smoking, diabetes, high cholesterol, high blood pressure, or a combination of these. This is the same process (called *atherosclerosis*) that causes the blockages of heart disease; people are often just less familiar with it in the legs.

Claudication is a mild form of PAD; it is different from gangrene. **It is very uncommon for claudication to lead to amputation. Surgery is not required to save your leg.**

CLAUDICATION AFFECTS YOUR LIFESTYLE

FOCUS ON HEART HEALTH

ARTERIES: HEART AND LEGS

PAD is associated with coronary artery disease (heart disease due to atherosclerosis). If you are diagnosed with claudication due to PAD, we don't want to ignore your leg symptoms, but we need to prioritize your heart.

MEDICATIONS FOR HEART HEALTH

Your healthcare provider will discuss medicines for heart health, such as aspirin and a statin medicine. Medications for blood pressure and diabetes are also important.

SMOKING CESSATION

If you are smoking, it is time to get serious about quitting. *This is perhaps the most important thing you can do for your health at this time!* Your healthcare provider can work with you to find ways to quit.

GET MOVING!

Your healthcare provider will evaluate you to ensure it is safe to start an exercise program. There are countless benefits to being physically active, including heart and mental health.

CLAUDICATION RARELY LEADS TO LIMB LOSS

HOW TO FEEL BETTER WITHOUT SURGERY

WHY WALKING HURTS

Claudication happens because there is a mismatch of supply-and-demand. That is, when you work your muscles by walking, they need more blood. But that blood can't get there because of the blockages. The pain you feel is just your muscles wanting more blood; this is *not* a sign of danger or serious damage!

NOT WHAT YOU MIGHT EXPECT

Claudication can be treated with walking therapy! Your muscles can learn to work more effectively with the blood they are getting by training them. Much like any physical activity or sport, we get better at it as we practice and train. In fact, a regular walking program has been shown to enlarge some of the small arteries that provide a natural detour around the blockages.

WHAT ABOUT SURGERY?

Some people do end up needing surgery. But surgery, even "minimally invasive" surgery, carries risk, including complications that lead to amputation … which is worse than if we did nothing to treat the claudication symptoms!

YOU CAN WALK FARTHER BY WALKING MORE!

Peripheral Artery Disease

What is PAD?

Peripheral artery disease (PAD) is a form of plaque build-up, or *atherosclerosis*, inside the blood vessels that bring oxygen-rich blood to the legs. One of the challenges to diagnosing PAD is that it can result in a wide range of different symptoms, including causing few or no symptoms at all. *The risks with each type of PAD are very different so it is important to know what type you have.*

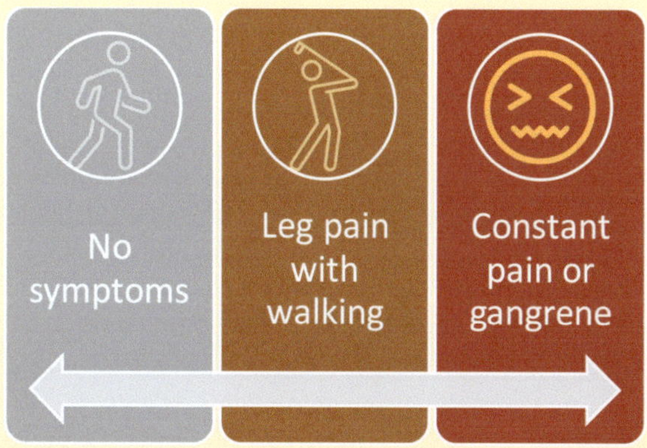

What is this type of PAD called?

Asymptomatic PAD	Intermittent Claudication	Chronic Limb Threatening Ischemia

What is the risk of losing my leg in the next few years?

Very low	Very low	High - Up to 50%

What should I do next to treat this condition?

Focus on heart health and reducing risks of atherosclerosis	1. Focus on heart health and reducing risks of atherosclerosis 2. Talk to your healthcare provider about a walking therapy program 3. It is often *not necessary* to do a procedure to improve the circulation	Seek timely consultation with a vascular specialist who can discuss options for improving the circulation

Index

W. P. Robinson III, J. P. Simons (eds.), *The Patient-Centered Approach to Claudication*, https://doi.org/10.1007/978-3-032-02460-2

T

MIX
Papier aus verantwortungsvollen Quellen
Paper from responsible sources
FSC® C105338

If you have any concerns about our products,
you can contact us on
ProductSafety@springernature.com

In case Publisher is established outside the EU,
the EU authorized representative is:
Springer Nature Customer Service Center GmbH
Europaplatz 3, 69115 Heidelberg, Germany

Printed by Libri Plureos GmbH
in Hamburg, Germany